माधव निदान

ENGLISH TRANSLATION OF MADHAVA NIDANA

डा. जनार्धन वि हेब्बार

Made with ♥ on the Notion Press Platform
www.notionpress.com

|| Jai Guruji ||

I, Dr. Janardhana V. Hebbar, dedicate this book at the holy feet of Sri Guruji – Swami Vivekananda and my spiritual Guru, Dr. A. Chandrashekhara Udupa MBBS, FAGE, Managing Director, Divine Park Trust (R), Saligrama, Udupi. (www.divinepark.org)

He guides, He energizes, He shows the path,
He holds my hand and makes me walk!

क्रम-सूची

क्रम-सूची

क्रम-सूची

Chief Editor

Dr Raghuram YS BAMS, MD(Ayu)

भूमिका

Madhava Nidana is written by Acharya Madhavakara. Madhavakara was the author of 'Rugvinishchaya'. The work Rugvinishchaya later came to be known as and become popular in the name 'Madhava Nidana'

Madhava nidana is mainly a compilation from the earlier works of Ayurveda such as Charaka Samhita, Sushruta Samhita, Ashtanga Samgraha, Ashtanga Hridaya and Ravigupta's Shuddhasara.

In spite of Madhava Nidana being a compilation of various previous works, Madhava Nidana enjoys an independent and respected status of being an important treatise. Verses on 'Nidana' available in various sections of Charaka Samhita, Sushruta Samhita and Ashtanga Sangraha etc. are compiled and quoted in Madhava Nidana. The verses are arranged in systematic manner.

Speciality – The major contribution and speciality of Madhavakara in his work Madhava Nidana is the order of arranging the names of diseases in his own style.

It is the first and one of the rare books or treatise which has been compiled in a systematic way, subject wise and covering the topics related to causes, premonitory symptoms, symptoms, pathogenesis, complications and prognosis of diseases.

Specialities of Madhava Nidana –

In his treatise Madhava Nidana, Madhavakara has composed the pathological aspects of a number of diseases pertaining to various branches of Ayurveda. The compilation is in below said order -

Chapter 1 – deals with basics of Nidana Panchaka (5 tools of examining a disease

Chapters 2-19, 22-37 and 49-54 – deals with topics related to Kaya Chikitsa (General systemic diseases like Jwara i.e. fever, Atisara i.e. diarrhoea etc)

Chapters 20-21 – deals with Graha or Bhuta vidya (toxicology, worm infestations)

Chapters 38 and 55 – deals with Shalya Chikitsa or surgical aspects

Chapters 56-60 – deals with Shalakya chikitsa (diseases pertaining to eye, ear, nose, throat, head, tongue, teeth etc)

Chapters 61-68 – deals with Kaumarabhritya (paediatrics, diseases

occurring in children)
Chapter 69 – deals with Agadatantra (toxicology)
In total, 79 diseases have been described in Madhavanidana

Systematic compilation – In Madhava Nidana the Nidana (causative factors), Purva Rupas (premonitory symptoms), Rupa (signs and symptoms), Samprapti (pathogenesis), Upadrava (complications) and Sadhya-Asadhyata (prognosis of the disease) are described in a systematic manner
Shula and Visphota – Madhava, for the first time recognized Shula (colic) and Visphota (vesicles and blisters) as independent entities, initially they were considered as symptoms of diseases
Names of new diseases – like Amavata, Parinamashoola, Annadrava shula, Medoroga, Shitapitta, Amlapitta, Masurika, Pakshmashata and Yonikanda were mentioned and described for the first time in Madhava Nidana
Madhava Chikitsa and Ratnamala – These two are the books probably written by 'Madhavakara' in which treatment of the diseases explained in Madhava Nidana have been explained and discussed
The new alignment of the diseases, which were arranged in the work of Madhavakara was followed by his successors like Vrinda Madhava, Chakrapanidatta, Govindadas in their treatises

Commentaries

Teeka or Commentaries on Madhava Nidana –

1. Madhukosha – written by Vijayarakshita and Srikanthadatta
2. Atankadarpana – written by Vachaspati

पावती (स्वीकृति)

Special thanks to **Dr Raghuram YS** for painstakingly editing the entire book.
Special thanks to my family members who have been supporting me unconditionally throughout this journey of Easy Ayurveda. Thank you for tolerating all the pains.
Smt. Padmakshamma (mother), Karthyayini (wife and staff), Smt. Vanamala (mother-in-law).
Daughters – Sadhvi & Chinmayi

Sister Sharada, brother-in-law Mr ShashiKumar, Tushar, Ms Sharada.
All my staff who make **Easy Ayurveda** possible, everyday.
Dr Sudarshan CH, Dr Shilpa Ramdas, Dr Renita D'Souza.
Mr Sachidananda Bhat, Smt. Nayana, Mr Nikhil and Smt. Sumangala.
My mentors - Dr MB Gururaja, Dr MS Krishnamurthy and Dr Prashanth BK

1

Madhava Nidana Chapter 1 Pancha Nidana Lakshana

Introduction

Madhava Nidana forms a part of 'Laghu Trayi' or lesser triad of Ayurvedic treatises, the other 2 being Sharangadhara Samhita and Bhavaprakasha. Madhava Nidana is a compilation of verses and references related to Nidana Panchaka of a disease (with exception of Upashaya and Anupashaya). Madhava Nidana excludes the treatment aspect and gives us a compilation of Nidanas for easy understanding of diseases. Here in this article we are learning about Madhava nidaana 1st chapter "Pancha Nidaana Lakshana".

Origin of 'Roga Vinischaya'

I have composed this 'Roga Vinischaya' treatise after offering my salutations and worship (prayers) to the holy feet of Lord Siva who is the chief cause for the creation, maintenance and destruction of the entire universe, one who bestows heaven and salvation and the protector of all the three worlds. I have composed this treatise based on the advice and motivation given to me by the revered physicians. The treatise also comprises the sayings of various sages on the complications, prognosis, causes, signs and symptoms of the diseases in brief.

प्रणम्य जगदुत्पत्तिस्थितिसंहारकारणम् |

स्वर्गापवर्गयोद्र्वारं त्रैलोक्यशरणं शिवम् ||१||
नानामुनीनां वचनैरिदानीं समासतः सद्भिषजां नियोगात् |
सोपद्रवारिष्टनिदानलिङ्गो निबध्यते रोगविनिश्चयोऽयम् ||२||
नानातन्त्रविहीनानां भिषजामल्पमेधसाम् |
सुखं विज्ञातुमातङ्कमयमेव भविष्यति ||३||

This will help the physicians having low intellect, not having precise knowledge of various shastras – treatises (and hence unable to study and understand them). This treatise named 'roga viniscaya' has been composed with an idea of helping such physicians to gain the knowledge of various diseases and also to understand them. (1-3)

Note – Here the author of this treatise claims and announces the objectives with which he has composed this treatise and the purpose and kinds of physicians it would serve.

Nidana Panchaka - Five means of understanding the diseases

निदानं पूर्वरूपाणि रूपाण्युपशयस्तथा |
सम्प्राप्तिश्चेति विज्ञानं रोगाणां पञ्चधा स्मृतम् ||४|| (वा. नि. अ. १)

The five means or tools of understanding the diseases are –

1. Nidana - causes, aetiology, aetiological factors of the disease,
2. Poorvaroopa - premonitory symptoms, prodromata of the disease
3. Roopa - signs and symptoms; clinical features, symptomatology of the disease,
4. Upasaya – diagnostic tests, pacification and aggravating factors which can be used for diagnosing the diseases through trial and error methods and also to differentiate one disease and the other through differential diagnosis and also to determine the prognosis of the diseases and
5. Sampraapti – pathogenesis of a disease, the process and pathway of formation of the disease (story of development of a disease, step by step)

These five means of understanding the diseases are called as Nidana Panchaka. (4)

Synonyms of Nidana

निमित्तहेत्वायतनप्रत्ययोत्थानकारणैः |
निदानमाहुःपर्यायैः... |५| (वा. नि. अ. १) |

The synonyms of Nidaana (causative factors or etiological factors of the disease) are –

Nimitta
Hetu

Ayatana
Pratyaya
Utthaana and
Kaaraṇa (5)

Purvarupa – Premonitory symptoms of the disease
...प्राग्रूपं येन लक्ष्यते ||५||
उत्पित्सुरामयो दोषविशेषेणानधिष्ठितः |
लिङ्गमव्यक्तमल्पत्वाद्व्याधीनां तद्यथायथम् ||६|| (वा. नि. अ. १) |
Poorvaroopa means 'premonitory symptoms' of the diseases. These are those signs and symptoms which appear earlier to the actual disease i.e., the purvarupas appear before the manifestation of the actual disease. These purvarupas are not specifically assignable to the doshas as they are mild in nature (not clearly recognizable) and few in numbers. (6)

Rupa – signs and symptoms of the disease
तदेव व्यक्ततां यातं रूपमित्यभिधीयते |
संस्थानं व्यञ्जनं लिङ्गं लक्षणं चिह्नमाकृतिः ||७|| (वा. नि. अ. १) |
The same premonitory signs and symptoms manifesting clearly in the later time are known as rupa i.e. 'signs and symptoms proper' or specific features of the disease. They synonyms of rupa are - vyanjana, linga, laksana, cinha and akriti. (7)

Upashaya
हेतुव्याधिविपर्यस्तविपर्यस्तार्थकारिणाम् |
औषधान्नविहाराणामुपयोगं सुखावहम् ||८||
विद्यादुपशयं व्याधेः स हि सात्म्यमिति स्मृतः |
विपरीतोऽनुपशयो व्याध्यसात्म्याभिसञ्ज्ञितः ||९|| (वा. नि. अ. १) |
Upashaya – factors (medicine, food, activity) subsiding the disease and thereby helping in diagnosing (or differentially diagnosing) a disease
Upashaya is the administration of medicine, food or activity which bring about sukha (comfort, relief of symptoms) to the patient; (thereby helping in diagnosis).They are of the following kinds viz:
1. Vipareeta (opposite) of hetu (cause), vyaadhi (disease) or both,
2. Vipareetha arthakaari (producing the opposite effect though not actually opposite) to either the hetu (cause), vyaadhi (disease) of both.
This (upasaya) is also known as saatmya (compatible). The opposite of

upashaya is anupasaya (increasing the discomfort) or asaatmya (incompatible) to the disease. (8-9)

Samprapti – pathogenesis of the disease

यथादुष्टेन दोषेण यथा चानुविर्सपता |
निर्वृत्तिरामयस्यासौ सम्प्राप्तिर्जातिरागतिः ||१०|| (वा. नि. अ. १) |

The process of manifestation of the disease, by the morbid doshas which are circulating all over the body is known as sampraapti. Jaati or aagati are the synonyms of samprapti. (10)

Types of Samprapti

सङ्ख्याविकल्पप्राधान्यबलकालविशेषतः |
सा भिद्यते यथाऽत्रैव वक्ष्यन्तेऽष्टौ ज्वरा इति ||११||
दोषाणां समवेतानां विकल्पोंऽशांशकल्पना |
स्वातन्त्र्यपारतन्त्र्याभ्यां व्याधेः प्राधान्यमादिशेत् ||१२||
हेत्वादिकात्स्न्यावयवैर्बलाबलविशेषणम् |
नक्तन्दिनर्तुभुक्तांशैर्व्याधिकालो यथामलम् ||१३|| (वा. नि. अ. १) |
इति प्रोक्तो निदानार्थः स व्यासेनोपदेक्ष्यते |१४| (वा. नि. अ. १) |

Sankhyaa, Vikalpa, Praadhaanya, Bala and Kaala are the five types of samprapti.

Name of the Samprapti Example

Sankhyaa Sampraapti → Counting jwaras (fevers) as eight in number etc. (types and subtypes of diseases)

Vikalpa Sampraapti → To point out a symptom or a disease as arising from a specific property of a particular dosha (fractional understanding)

Praadhaanya Sampraapti → To signify a disease as primary (or secondary)

Bala Sampraapti → To qualify a disease as severe or mild depending upon the cause etc. (to determine the strength and severity of a disease)

Kaala Sampraapti → To signify that a disease is severe during a particular period of time such as night, day, season, time of digestion of food, etc.

सर्वेषामेव रोगाणां निदानं कुपिता मलाः ||१४||
तत्प्रकोपस्य तु प्रोक्तं विविधाहितसेवनम् |१५|
(वा. नि. अ. १) |

The morbid (increased) doshas are considered to be the cause for all kinds of diseases. On the other hand, indulgence in different kinds of unhealthy foods or activities is considered to be the cause for morbid (abnormal) increase of the doshas. (14)

निदानार्थकरो रोगो रोगस्याप्युपजायते ||१५||
तद्यथा ज्वरसन्तापाद्रक्तपित्तमुदीर्यते |

Nidanarthakara Roga - Sometimes one disease might become a cause for another disease. Examples include-
Increased temperature of jwara (fever) may result in Raktapitta (bleeding disorders, purpura).

रक्तपित्ताज्ज्वरस्ताभ्यां शोषस्याप्युपजायते ||१६||
प्लीहाभिवृद्ध्या जठरं जठराच्छोथ एव च |
अर्शोभ्यो जाठरं दुःखं गुल्मश्चाप्युपजायते ||१७||

Raktapitta may cause manifestation of fever
Both jvara and raktapitta together may cause sosa (consumption, tuberculosis)
Pliha vrddhi (enlargement of spleen) may cause jathara roga (enlargement of abdomen)
Jathara (abdominal enlargement) may cause Sotha (oedema)
Arsas (piles) may become the cause for troublesome jathara dukha (abdominal pain) and also gulma (abdominal tumor)

(दिवास्वापादिदोषैश्च प्रतिश्यायश्च जायते) |
प्रतिश्यायादथो कासः कासात् सञ्जायते क्षयः |
क्षयो रोगस्य हेतुत्वे शोषस्याप्युपजायते ||१८||
(चि. नि. अ. ८) |

Divasvapna etc. doshas i.e., Sleeping at day time etc. (causative factors) might result into Pratisyaya (common cold)
Pratisyaya may lead to kasa i.e., cough
Kasa would lead to ksaya (emaciation) and
Ksaya might cause sosa roga (tuberculosis, consumption)

ते पूर्वं केवला रोगाः पश्चाद्धेत्वर्थकारिणः |१९|
(च. नि. अ. ८) |
कश्चिद्धि रोगो रोगस्य हेतुर्भूत्वा प्रशाम्यति ||१९||
न प्रशाम्यति चाप्यन्यो हेतुत्वं कुरुतेऽपि च |

एवं कृच्छ्रतमा नृणां दृश्यन्ते व्याधिसङ्कराः ||२०||
(च. नि. अ. ८) |

At the beginning the causative disease is just a mild symptom complex. In due course of time, it might become a major disease. Some of them may disappear when the second disease manifests. On the other hand, some others continue to persist even as the second disease exists (during the course of the second disease).
This would lead to a condition called vyadhi sankara i.e., coexistence of two or more diseases (like a syndrome) which is very troublesome. (15-20)

तस्माद्यत्नेन सद्वैद्यैरिच्छद्भिः सिद्धिमुद्धताम् |
ज्ञातव्यो वक्ष्यते योऽयं ज्वरादीनां विनिश्चयः ||२१||

So, the physician who desires to become successful should strive hard to understand the diagnosis of diseases like jwara etc. which will be described further on. (21)

इति श्रीमाधवकरविरचिते माधवनिदाने पञ्चनिदानलक्षणं समाप्तम् ||१||

Thus ends the chapter called 'Panchanidana Lakshana' in the book Madhava Nidana, written by Acharya Madhavakara.

2

Madhava Nidana Chapter 2 Jwara Nidanam

Origin / History of Jwara

दक्षापमानसङ्क्रुद्धरुद्रनिःश्वाससम्भवः ।
ज्वरोऽष्टधा पृथग्द्वन्द्वसङ्घातागन्तुजः स्मृतः ॥१॥

Long ago, Jwara was born from the wrath of Lord Rudra who had been insulted by Daksha. It is of eight types.

3 - One from each dosha (vataja, pittaja and kaphaja),

3 - One each from the combination of two dosas (vata pittaja,vata kaphaja, pitta kaphaja),

1 - One from the combination of all the three doshas (sannipātaja, tridosaja) and

1 - One from āgantu (external causes). (1)

The eight kinds of fever are as listed below –

Category of Jwara Names of Jwara

Eka doshaja → 1. Vataja 2. Pittaja 3. Kaphaja

Dwi dosaja / Dwandwa / Samsargaja → 4. Vata-pittaja 5. Vata-Kaphaja 6. Pitta-Kaphaja

Tridosaja / Sannipataja → 7. Vata-Pitta-Kaphaja

Agantuja (Caused by external causes) → 8. Agantuja

Jwara Samprapti – pathogenesis of fever

मिथ्याहारविहाराभ्यां दोषा ह्यामाशयाश्रयाः |
बहिर्निरस्य कोष्ठाग्निं ज्वरदाः स्यू रसानुगाः ||२||

Due to improper foods and activities, the Doshas (vāta, pitta and kapha) undergo an increase (individually or in combination). These vitiated doshas reach the āmāśaya (stomach and intestines) and expel the kosthāgni (digestion fire) to the exterior (skin and other tissues) and circulating along with rasa (dhātu) produces jwara. (2)

The events leading to manifestation of jwara (fever) – pathogenesis of jwara
Indulgence in improper foods and activities
Doshas undergo abnormal increase / aggravation either individually or in combination
The increased doshas reach the stomach / intestines
Causes expulsion of the gastric fire to the exterior
The same doshas circulate along with the blood plasma
Produce jwara – fever

Definition of Jwara

स्वेदावरोधः सन्तापः सर्वाङ्गग्रहणं तथा |
युगपद्यत्र रोगे च स ज्वरो व्यपदिश्यते ||३|| (सु.उ.तं.अ. ३९)

Jwara is defined as the disease in which there is obstruction to perspiration, increase of body temperature and pain all over the body. All these symptoms occur and exist together. (3)

Jwara Purvarupa – Premonitory symptoms

श्रमोऽरतिर्विवर्णत्वं वैरस्यं नयनप्लवः |
इच्छाद्वेषौ मुहुश्चापि शीतवातातपादिषु ||४||
जृम्भाऽङ्गमर्दो गुरुता रोमहर्षोऽरुचिस्तमः |
अप्रहर्षश्च शीतं च भवत्युत्पत्स्यति ज्वरे ||५||
(सामान्यतो विशेषात्तु जृम्भाऽत्यर्थं समीरणात् |
पित्तान्नयनयोर्दाहः कफादन्नारुचिर्भवेत् ||६||
रूपैरन्यतराभ्यां तु संसृष्टैर्द्वन्द्वजं विदुः |
सर्वलिङ्गसमवायः सर्वदोषप्रकोपजे) ||७||

Purvarupa Shrama - Fatigue,
Vivarnatva - discoloration of the skin,

Vairasya - bad taste in the mouth,
Nayana Plava - eyes full of tears,
Iccha Dvesho Muhushcapi Sheeta Vata Atapadishu - alternate like and dislike for cold wind and warm sunlight, etc.,
Jrumbha - yawning,
Angamarda - body ache,
Guruta - feeling of heaviness of the body,
Romaharsha - horripilation (body hairs standing on ends),
Aruchi - lack of appetite,
Tama - stupor,
Apraharsha - lack of interest in anything and
Sheeta - feeling of cold are the symptoms generally appearing earlier to the actual onset of fever (premonitory symptoms).
Even among these (premonitory symptoms),
Yawning will be more, if vātaja jwara were to manifest later,
Burning sensation will be found if pittaja jwara were to manifest later and
Lack of appetite will be found if kaphaja jwara were to manifest in future.
Similarly, the symptoms of two or three došhas will appear in fevers caused due to a combination of two or three doshas respectively. (4-7)

Symptoms of Vataja Jwara

वेपथुर्विषमो वेगः कण्ठौष्ठपरिशोषणम् |
निद्रानाशः क्षवस्तम्भो गात्राणां रौक्ष्यमेव च ||८||
शिरोहृद्गात्ररुग्वक्त्रवैरस्यं गाढविट्कता |
शूलाध्माने जृम्भणं च भवन्त्यनिलजे ज्वरे ||९||
(सु. उ. तं. अ. ३९) |

The symptoms of Vātaja jwara (fever due to the increase of vāta doṣa) are - shivering (chill, rigours), non-corresponding time of onset and exacerbation, severe dryness of the throat and lips, loss of sleep, absence of sneezing, roughness of the skin (or decrease of moisture in the body) pain in head, chest and body, bad taste in the mouth, hard and dry faeces, pain in the abdomen, distension of abdomen and too many yawning. (8-9)

Symptoms of Pittaja Jwara

वेगस्तीक्ष्णोऽतिसारश्च निद्राल्पत्वं तथा वमिः |
कण्ठौष्ठमुखनासानां पाकः स्वेदश्च जायते ||१०||
प्रलापो वक्त्रकटुता मूर्छा दाहो मदस्तृषा |

पीतविण्मूत्रनेत्रत्वं पैत्तिके भ्रम एव च ||११||
(सु. उ. तं. अ. ३९) |

The symptoms of Pittaja Jwara (fever due to the increase of pitta doṣa) are - very high temperature, diarrhoea, very little sleep, vomiting, ulcers in the throat, lips, mouth and nose, perspiration, delirium, bitter taste in the mouth, fainting, feeling of burning sensation all over the body, intoxication, thirst, yellow colouration of faeces, urine & eyes, etc., and giddiness. (10-11)

Symptoms of Kaphaja Jwara

स्तैमित्यं स्तिमितो वेग आलस्यं मधुरास्यता |
शुक्लमूत्रपुरीषत्वं स्तम्भस्तृप्तिरथापि च ||१२||
गौरवं शीतमुत्क्लेदो रोमहर्षोऽतिनिद्रता |
(स्रोतोरोधो रुगल्पत्वं प्रसेको लवणास्यता |
नात्युष्णगात्रता, च्छर्दिर्लालास्रावोऽविपाकता) |
प्रतिश्यायोऽरुचिः कासः कफजेऽक्ष्णोश्च शुक्लता ||१३||
(सु. उ. तं. अ. ३९) |

The symptoms of Kaphaja Jwara (due to increase of kapha doṣa) are - feeling of stiffness / cold all over the body, mild increase of temperature, lack of enthusiasm, sweet taste in the mouth, whitish urine and faeces, stiffness of extremities, abnormal feeling of contentment, feeling of heaviness, cold, nausea, horripilation, excessive sleep; obstruction to the channels, mild pains, excessive salivation, salty taste in the mouth, temperature is not very high, vomiting, saliva flowing out, indigestion of food, running nose, lack of appetite, cough and whitish eyes. (12-13)

Symptoms of Vatapitta Jwara

तृष्णा मूर्छा भ्रमो दाहः स्वप्ननाशः शिरोरुजा |
कण्ठास्यशोषो वमथू रोमहर्षोऽरुचिस्तमः ||१४||
पर्वभेदश्च जृम्भा च वातपित्तज्वराकृतिः |१५|
(सु. उ. तं. अ. ३९) |

The symptoms of Vata-pittaja jwara are - thirst, fainting, giddiness, burning sensation, loss of sleep, headache, dryness of throat and mouth, vomiting, horripilation, loss of taste (tastelessness), feeling of darkness before the eyes, pain in the small joints of hands and feet and yawning. - (14-15)

Symptoms of Vatakapha Jwara

स्तैमित्यं पर्वणां भेदो निद्रा गौरवमेव च ||१५||
शिरोग्रहः प्रतिश्यायः कासः स्वेदाप्रवर्तनम् |
सन्तापो मध्यवेगश्च वातश्लेष्मज्वराकृतिः ||१६||
(सु. उ. तं. अ. ३९) |

The symptoms of Vata-kaphaja jwara (fever caused by combination of increased vata and kapha doshas) are - feeling of stiffness / cold in the body, pain in the small joints of hands and feet, too much of sleep, feeling of heaviness of the body, headache common cold / running nose, cough, lack of perspiration (sweating) and moderate increase of body temperature. (15-16)

Symptoms of Kapha-pitta Jwara

लिप्ततिक्तास्यता तन्द्रा मोहः कासोऽरुचिस्तृषा |
मुहुर्दाहो मुहुः शीतं श्लेष्मपित्तज्वराकृतिः ||१७||
(सु. उ. तं. अ. ३९) |

The symptoms of Kapha-pittaja jwara are - coating of the tongue, manifestation of bitter taste in the mouth, drowsiness, delusion, cough, loss of taste, thirst, alternate feeling of heat and cold. (17)

Symptoms of Sannipata Jwara

क्षणे दाहः क्षणे शीतमस्थिसन्धिशिरोरुजा |
सास्रावे कलुषे रक्ते निर्भुग्ने चापि लोचने ||१८||
सस्वनौ सरुजौ कर्णौ कण्ठः शूकैरिवावृतः |
तन्द्रा मोहः प्रलापश्च कासः श्वासोऽरुचिर्भ्रमः ||१९||
परिदग्धा खरस्पर्शा जिह्वा स्रस्ताङ्गता परम् |
ष्ठीवनं रक्तपित्तस्य कफेनोन्मिश्रितस्य च ||२०||
शिरसो लोठनं तृष्णा निद्रानाशो हृदि व्यथा |
स्वेदमूत्रपुरीषाणां चिराद्दर्शनमल्पशः ||२१||
कृशत्वं नातिगात्राणां प्रततं कण्ठकूजनम् |
कोठानां श्यावरक्तानां मण्डलानां च दर्शनम् ||२२||
मूकत्वं स्रोतसां पाको गुरुत्वमुदरस्य च |
चिरात्पाकश्च दोषाणां सन्निपातज्वराकृतिः ||२३||
(च. चि. अ. ३) |

The symptoms of Sannipatajwara (caused by combination of all the three doshas) are - feeling of heat and cold alternately, pain in the bones and joints, headache, eyes full of tears, dirty, reddish and bulging out; ringing and pain in the ears, feeling of thorns pricking inside the throat, drowsiness, delusion, delirium, cough, difficulty in breathing (dyspnoea), loss of taste, giddiness, tongue angry red at its edges and rough, weakness of the limbs, excessive expectoration of sputum mixed with blood and bile, rolling of the head on the pillow, thirst, loss of sleep, pain in the heart (or region of the heart), elimination of small quantities of sweat, urine and faeces at long intervals, not much of wasting of the body, continuous moaning (feeble sound in the throat), appearance of dark red spots and patches on the skin, dumbness (unable to speak), ulceration of the orifices of the body, feeling of heaviness of the abdomen, doshas undergoing paka (return to normalcy) very slowly. (1-23)

Prognosis of Sannipata Jwara

दोषे विबद्धे नष्टेऽग्नौ सर्वसम्पूर्णलक्षणः ।
सन्निपातज्वरोऽसाध्यः, कृच्छ्रसाध्यस्ततोऽन्यथा ॥२४॥
(च. चि. अ. ३) ।

Sannipata jwara becomes incurable if the dosas are stagnated (profound and deep seated), if the digestive capacity of the patient is completely diminished and if all the symptoms are simultaneously manifested. Otherwise it is curable with difficulty. (24)

सन्निपातज्वरस्यान्ते कर्णमूले सुदारुणः ।
शोथः सञ्जायते तेन कश्चिदेव प्रमुच्यते ॥२५॥
(च. चि. अ. ३) ।

Sometimes there appears a profound swelling at the root of the ear at the end of the course of sannipata jwara and hardly anybody can get rid of it (it almost causes death). (25)

Agantuja Jwara

अभिघाताभिचाराभ्यामभिशापाभिषङ्गतः ।
आगन्तुर्जायते दोषैर्यथास्वं तं विभावयेत् ॥२६॥

Agantu Jwara is caused by - abhighata (assault by weapons), abhichara (sorcery and witchcraft), abhishapa (curse by godly men) and abhyanga (possession by evil spirits, infection by microorganisms). Even in such fevers the symptoms of doshas have to be recognised. (26)

Symptoms of different types of Agantuja Jwara

श्यावास्यता विषकृते तथाऽतीसार एव च |
भक्तारुचिः पिपासा च तोदश्च सह मूर्छया ||२७||
ओषधिगन्धजे मूर्छा शिरोरुग्वमथुः क्षवः |
कामजे चित्तविभ्रंशस्तन्द्राऽऽलस्यमभोजनम् ||२८||
(हृदये वेदना चास्य गात्रं च परिशुष्यति) |
भयात्प्रलापः शोकाच्च भवेत् कोपाच्च वेपथुः |
अभिचाराभिशापाभ्यां मोहस्तृष्णा च जायते ||२९||
भूताभिषङ्गादुद्वेगो हास्यरोदनकम्पनम् |३०|
(सु. उ. तं. अ. ३९) |

In agantu jwara caused by poison - bluish discolouration of the mouth, diarrhoea, loss of appetite, thirst, pain and fainting are seen.

In fever caused by smell of plants (pollen of flowers, etc.) - fainting, headache, vomiting and sneezing are seen.

In fever caused due to love or passion - mental aberration, stupor, inactivity or laziness and lack of interest in food, pain in the heart and emaciation of the body are the symptoms.

In fever caused due to fear and grief - the patient will be having delirium.

In fever caused due to anger - he will have tremors.

In fever caused due to sorcery and curse - the patient will be having delusion and thirst.

In fever caused due to possession by evil spirits - the patient will be highly emotional (irritable) and indulges in excess of laughing, weeping and shivering. (27-29)

Vata gets increased by lust, grief and fear. Pitta gets increased by anger. All the three doshas get increased from possession by evil spirits (or bacterial infection) and show their specific features. (30)

Vishama Jwara – meaning and pathogenesis

कामशोकभयाद्वायुः, क्रोधात् पित्तं, त्रयो मलाः ||३०||
भूताभिषङ्गात्कुप्यन्ति भूतसामान्यलक्षणाः |३१|

Doṣhas which have undergone slight / mild increase right from the beginning or the small quantities of doshas which have remained after the fever has gone away get aggravated once again due to consumption of unsuitable foods and activities, get lodged in one or the other dhātus (tissues) and produce Visama jwara (irregular or intermittent fevers). (31).

Types

सन्ततं रसरक्तस्थः, सोऽन्येद्युः पिशिताश्रितः ||३२||
मेदोगतस्तृतीयेऽह्नि त्वस्थिमज्जगतः पुनः |
कुर्याच्चतुर्थकं घोरमन्तकं रोगसङ्करम् ||३३||
(सु. उ. तं. अ. ३९) |

Types of Visama Jwara and their relationship with tissues

Of such fevers, santata jwara involves rasa and rakta dhatus, anyedyuska jwara involves mamsa dhatu, tritiyaka jwara involves medas, chaturthaka jwara involves asthi and majja dhatus, which is a dreadful disease-complex and is even fatal. (32-33)

Symptoms of Santata and other types of Vishama Jwaras

सप्ताहं वा दशाहं वा द्वादशाहमथापि वा |
सन्तत्या योऽविसर्गी स्यात् सन्ततः स निगद्यते ||३४||
अहोरात्रे सततको द्वौ कालावनुवर्तते |
अन्येद्युष्कस्त्वहोरात्र एककालं प्रवर्तते ||३५||
तृतीयकस्तृतीयेऽह्नि, चतुर्थेऽह्नि चतुर्थकः |३६|
(सु. उ. तं. अ. ३९) |

Santata jwara is so named because the fever continues without remission for seven, ten, twelve or even more days.

Satataka jwara manifests twice in twenty four hours.

Anyedyuska jwara manifests once in twenty four hours.

Tritiyaka jwara manifests on alternative days.

Chaturthaka jwara manifests on every fourth day. (34-35)

केचिद्भूताभिषङ्गोत्थं ब्रुवते विषमज्वरम् ||३६||
(सु. उ. तं. अ. ३९) |

Some scholars opine that visama jwaras (intermittent fevers) are caused due to bhutabhisanga (bacterial infection). (36)

Tritiyaka Jwara

कफपित्तात्त्रिकग्राही पृष्ठाद्वातकफात्मकः |
वातपित्ताच्छिरोग्राही त्रिविधः स्यात्तृतीयकः ||३७||

Types of manifestation of Tritiyaka Jwara

Tritiyaka jwara manifests in three ways viz,

if kapha and pitta are increased, fever starts with catching pain in the lower

portion of the back,
if vāta and kapha are increased, the fever starts with pain in the upper portion of the back and
if vāta and pitta are increased, the fever starts with pain in the head. (37)

Chaturthaka Jwara

चतुर्थको दर्शयति प्रभावं द्विविधं ज्वरः ।
जङ्घाभ्यां श्लैष्मिकः पूर्वं शिरस्तोऽनिलसम्भवः ॥३८॥
(च. चि. अ. ३) ।

Types of manifestation of Chaturthaka Jwara
Chaturthaka also manifests in two ways,
if kapha is increased, fever starts with pain in the calf muscles and
if vata is increased it starts with pain in the head. (38)

Chaturthaka Viparyaya Jwara

विषमज्वर एवान्यश्चतुर्थकविपर्ययः ।
त्र्यहाद् द्वयहं ज्वरयति ह्यादावन्ते च मुञ्चति ॥३९॥
(च. चि. अ. ३) ।

There is yet another kind of visama jwara known as chaturthaka viparyāya jwara. In this condition, fever is not found on the first and fourth day but found on two days in the middle. (39)
Read - Ayurveda Home Remedy For Fever

Vata balasaka Jwara

नित्यं मन्दज्वरो रूक्षः शूनकस्तेन सीदति ।
स्तब्धाङ्गः श्लेष्मभूयिष्ठो भवेद्वातबलासकी ॥४०॥
(अ. सं. नि. अ. २) ।

Vata balasaka jwara is produced by increase of kapha and manifests as mild fever daily with dryness, oedema, debility and feeling of stiffness of the body. (40)

Pralepaka Jwara

प्रलिम्पन्निव गात्राणि घर्मेण गौरवेण च ।
मन्दज्वरविलेपी च सशीतः स्यात्प्रलेपकः ॥४१॥
सं. नि. अ. २) ।

Pralepaka jwara manifests with mild fever as though the skin is given a thin coating of heat, accompanied with a feeling of heaviness and cold. (41)

Ardhanga Santapayukta Jwara

विदग्धेऽन्नरसे देहे श्लेष्मपित्ते व्यवस्थिते |
तेनार्धं शीतलं देहमर्धमुष्णं प्रजायते ||४२||
काये दुष्टं यदा पित्तं श्लेष्मा चान्ते व्यवस्थितः |
तेनोष्णत्वं शरीरस्य शीतत्वं हस्तपादयोः ||४३||
काये श्लेष्मा यदा दुष्टः पित्तं चान्ते व्यवस्थितम् |
शीतत्वं तेन गात्राणामुष्णत्वं हस्तपादयोः ||४४||
सं. नि. अ. २) |

If the annarasa (nutrient portion of the food) gets vidagdha (overcooked due to increase of pitta during the process of digestion), there manifests a fever with half the body being hot and the other half being cold. When pitta gets increased in the trunk followed by kapha in the extremities, then the fever manifests with the trunk being hot and with hands and feet (extremities) cold. When kapha is increased in the trunk and pitta in the extremities, fever manifests with the trunk being cold and the hands and feet (extremities) hot.

Note: These fevers are called Ardhanga Santapa Jwara wherein the rise of heat is evident in half of the body (with coldness prevailing in the other half of the body). They are special types of Visama Jwara.

Shitapurva and Dahapurva Jwara

त्वक्स्थौ श्लेष्मानिलौ शीतमादौ जनयतो ज्वरे |
तयोः प्रशान्तयोः पित्तमन्ते दाहं करोति च ||४५||
करोत्यादौ तथा पित्तं त्वक्स्थं दाहमतीव च |
तस्मिन् प्रशान्ते त्वितरौ कुरुतः शीतमन्ततः ||४६||
द्वावेतौ दाहशीतादिज्वरौ संसर्गजौ स्मृतौ |
दाहपूर्वस्तयोः कष्टः कृच्छ्रसाध्यतमश्च सः ||४७||
(सु. उ. तं. अ. ३९) |

When the aggravated kapha and vāta lodged in the skin, there is a manifestation of cold (rigours) at the beginning of fever. Later when its bouts reduce, the patient experiences burning sensation (heat) due to pitta at the end of the fever.

Similarly, when the aggravated pitta is lodged in the skin, there is a manifestation of burning sensation (heat) at the beginning of the fever.

Later when its bouts reduce, the patient experiences cold (rigours) due to vata and kapha at the end of the fever.
These two types of fevers dāhapūrva (preceded by heat) and śītapūrva (preceded by cold) are samsargaja i.e. produced by the combination of two dosas. Among these fevers dāhapūrva is difficult to treat and is almost incurable. (42-47)

Dhatugata Jwara – fevers localised in the tissues

Rasa dhatu gata jwara
गुरुता हृदयोत्क्लेशः सदनं छर्द्यरोचकौ |
रसस्थे तु ज्वरे लिङ्गं दैन्यं चास्योपजायते ||४८||
Fever residing in rasa tissue:
The symptoms seen when jwara (fever) invades / resides in rasa dhatu (blood plasma) is - feeling of heaviness of the body, nausea, debility, vomiting, loss of appetite and timidity (feeling of helplessness). (48)

Rakta dhatu gata jwara
रक्तनिष्ठीवनं दाहो मोहश्छर्दनविभ्रमौ |
प्रलापः पिडका तृष्णा रक्तप्राप्ते ज्वरे नृणाम् ||४९||
Fever residing in blood tissue:
The symptoms evident when fever invades / resides in rakta dhatu (blood) is - haemoptysis, burning sensation, delusion, vomiting, dizziness, delirium, appearances of rashes (or small boils) on the skin and thirst. (49)

Mamsa dhatu gata jwara
पिण्डिकोद्वेष्टनं तृष्णा सृष्टमूत्रपुरीषता |
ऊष्माऽन्तर्दाहविक्षेपौ ग्लानिः स्यान्मांसगे ज्वरे ||५०||
Fever residing in muscle tissue:
The symptoms found when fever invades / resides in c(muscle tissue) is - pain in the calves, thirst, increased elimination of urine and faeces, high temperature, burning sensation inside, involuntary movements of the hands and feet and exhaustion manifest. (50)

Medo dhatu gata jwara
भृशं स्वेदस्तृषा मूर्छा प्रलापश्छर्दिरेव च |
दौर्गन्ध्यारोचकौ ग्लानिर्मेदःस्थे चासहिष्णुता ||५१||

Fever residing in fat tissue / adipose tissue:

The symptoms found when fever invades / resides in medo dhatu (fat / adipose tissue) is - profuse sweating, thirst, fainting, delirium, vomiting, bad smell from the body, loss of taste (anorexia), exhaustion and intolerance (irritability). (51)

Asthi dhatu gata jwara

भेदोऽस्थ्नां कूजनं श्वासो विरेकश्छर्दिरेव च |
विक्षेपणं च गात्राणामेतदस्थिगते ज्वरे ||५२||

Fever residing in bone tissue:

The symptoms found when fever invades / resides in asthi dhatu (bone tissue) is - splitting pain in the bones, low and indistinct sound from the throat (moaning), dyspnoea (increased respiration), diarrhoea, vomiting and throwing / involuntary movements of hands and feet. (52)

Majja dhatu gata jwara

तमःप्रवेशनं हिक्का कासः शैत्यं वमिस्तथा |
अन्तर्दाहो महाश्वासो मर्मच्छेदश्च मज्जगे ||५३||

Fever residing in bone marrow tissue:

The symptoms found when fever invades / resides in majja dhatu (bone marrow tissue) is - appearance of darkness before the eyes (feeling as if immersed in a zone of darkness), hiccough, cough, cold feeling, vomiting, burning sensation within the body, severe dyspnoea (greatly increased respiration) and cutting type of pain in the heart and other vital spots of the body. (53)

Shukra dhatu gata jwara

मरणं प्राप्नुयात्तत्र शुक्रस्थानगते ज्वरे |
शेफसः स्तब्धता मोक्षः शुक्रस्य तु विशेषतः ||५४||
(सु. उ. तं. अ. ३९) |

Fever residing in semen / reproductive tissue:

The symptoms found when fever invades / resides in shukra dhatu (semen tissue / reproductive tissue) is - constant erection of the penis and profuse discharge of semen followed by death. (54)

Prognosis of fevers residing in the tissues

(रसरक्ताश्रितः साध्यो मांसमेदोगतश्च यः |

अस्थिमज्जगतः कृच्छ्रो शुक्रस्थस्तु न सिध्यति) ||१||
(च. चि. अ. ३) |
Fever invading / residing in rasa and rakta (blood plasma and blood) tissues can be cured easily.
Similarly, the fevers residing in mamsa and medo dhatus (muscle and adipose / fat) tissues are also easily curable.
The fevers residing in asthi and majja (bones and bone marrow) tissues are difficult to cure.
The fever residing in shukra (semen, reproductive tissue) tissue does not respond to the treatment i.e. it is incurable). (54-1)

Fever based on Season
वर्षाशरद्वसन्तेषु वाताद्यैः प्राकृतः क्रमात् |
वैकृतोऽन्यः स दुःसाध्यः प्राकृतश्चानिलोद्भवः ||५५||
(वा. नि. अ. २) |
Prakrta (normal) and Vaikrta (abnormal) fevers explained on the basis of the seasonal relationship with the fevers
Fevers which manifest in varsa rutu (rainy season), Sarad rutu (autumn) and vasanta rutu (spring season) caused by vata, pitta and kapha respectively are considered as prakrta (normal / corresponding to the season). Apart from these fevers, the other fevers shall be considered as vaikrta (abnormal / not corresponding to the season). Prakrta fevers are easily curable. But vatika fever (fever caused by predominance of vata), though is prakrta (occurring in its normal season i.e., varsa rutu) cannot be easily treated. The fevers produced by vata are difficult to treat. Likewise, the Vaikrta fevers are also difficult to treat. (55)

Doshas and seasonal fevers
वर्षासु मारुतो दुष्टः पित्तश्लेष्मान्वितो ज्वरम् |
कुर्यात् पित्तं च शरदि तस्य चानुबलः कफः ||५६||
तत्प्रकृत्या विसर्गाच्च तत्र नानशनाद्भयम् |
कफो वसन्ते तमपि वातपित्तं भवेदनु ||५७||
(वा. नि. अ. २) |
In Varsa Ritu (rainy season) – the vitiated vata produces fever being associated with pitta and kapha.
In Sarad Ritu (autumn season) - pitta produces fever being associated with kapha.

Fasting or therapeutic starvation doesn't do harm in both these conditions because of the nature of associated doshas and nature of the season (visarga – cold predominant season).

Note: Reason behind administering fasting in rainy and autumn seasons - By nature pitta and kapha have fluid nature and can tolerate fasting. So, fasting can be readily recommended in Prakrata Vata fever occurring in the rainy season, especially when it is associated with pitta and kapha. The same rule is applicable in pitta fever associated with kapha occurring in Sharad Ritu also. Also – both these seasons (rainy and autumn) fall in visarga kala (cold predominant seasons) and hence fasting is recommended (the strength of the patients in these seasons is comparably good in comparison to heat predominant seasons).

In Vasanta Ritu (spring season) – the fever produced by vitiated kapha will probably have association and support of vata and pitta. (56-57)

Upashaya and Anupashaya

काले यथास्वं सर्वेषां प्रवृत्तिर्वृद्धिरेव वा |५८|

(वा. नि. अ. २) |

निदानोक्तानुपशयो विपरीतोपशायिता ||५८||

(वा. नि. अ. २) |

Upashaya (subsiding factors) and Anupashaya (aggravating factors) for fevers in relation to the causative dosas

It is only at that specified time / season during which the causative dosha is aggravated (powerful), we usually get to see the onset or exacerbation of the fevers.

Also, the factors (etiological factors) responsible for increasing a particular dosha also bring about an increase (onset or exacerbation) of the fever (caused by that particular dosha). On the other hand, the opposites (anything which is opposite to those mentioned amongst the etiological factors for that particular dosha) will be helpful and would mitigate the fever also.

Note: This means to tell that all fevers (usually) have their onset or exacerbation in accordance to their respective dosha aggravating time or season.

Upasaya and Anupasaya mentioned here can also be used as tools for identifying the dosha involved in the causation of a given fever. (58)

Antarvega and Bahirvega Jwaras

अन्तर्दाहोऽधिकस्तृष्णा प्रलापः श्वसनं भ्रमः ।
सन्ध्यस्थिशूलमस्वेदो दोषवर्चोविनिग्रहः ॥५९॥
अन्तर्वेगस्य लिङ्गानि ज्वरस्यैतानि लक्षयेत् ।
सन्तापो ह्यधिको बाह्यस्तृष्णादीनां च मार्दवम् ॥६०॥
बहिर्वेगस्य लिङ्गानि सुखसाध्यत्वमेव च ।६१।
(च. चि. अ. ३) ।

Antarvega Jwara (fevers predominantly manifesting from within or residing inside the body) – is diagnosed by the presence of symptoms including - feeling of burning sensation inside (the body), excessive thirst, delirium, dyspnoea, giddiness, pain in the joints and bones, absence of perspiration and non-elimination of doshas and faeces.

Bahirvega Jwara (fevers predominantly manifesting from without or residing / manifesting outside, on the surface of the body) – is diagnosed by the presence of very high temperature externally, but thirst and the other symptoms (mentioned in antarvega jwara) being mild. This condition is said to be easily curable. (59-60)

Ama jwara symptoms

लालाप्रसेको हृल्लासहृदयाशुद्ध्यरोचकाः ॥६१॥
तन्द्रालस्याविपाकास्यवैरस्यं गुरुगात्रता ।
क्षुन्नाशो बहुमूत्रत्वं स्तब्धता बलवान् ज्वरः ॥६२॥
आमज्वरस्य लिङ्गानि न दद्यात्तत्र भेषजम् ।
भेषजं ह्यामदोषस्य भूयो ज्वलयति ज्वरम् ॥६३॥
(शोधनं शमनीयं च करोति विषमज्वरम्) ।

The symptoms of ama jwara (unripe, early / first or initial stage of fever) are - profuse salivation, nausea, heaviness and oppression in the region of the heart (a strange discomfort in the cardiac region), loss of taste / appetite, drowsiness, laziness / lack of enthusiasm, indigestion, bad taste in the mouth (manifestation of abnormal tastes / opposite tastes in the mouth), feeling of heaviness of the body, loss of hunger, profuse urination, stiffness and high temperature.

During this stage of fever, treatment should not be given. If given, the medicines will cause an increase (in the severity) of fever. Also if sodhana (Panchakarma) and samana (palliative) therapies are administered in ama jwara, they will lead to Visama Jwara (irregular fevers). (61-63)

Pacyamana Jwara Symptoms

ज्वरवेगोऽधिकस्तृष्णा प्रलापः श्वसनं भ्रमः |
मलप्रवृत्तिरुत्क्लेशः पच्यमानस्य लक्षणम् ||६४||

The symptoms of Pachyamana Jwara (intermediate / middle stage or stage of ripening of the fever) are – severity in fever or bouts of fever, severe thirst, delirium, dyspnoea, giddiness, frequent elimination of faeces and nausea. (64)

Nirama Jwara Symptoms

क्षुत् क्षामता लघुत्वं च गात्राणां ज्वरमार्दवम् |
दोषप्रवृत्तिरष्टाहो निरामज्वरलक्षणम् ||६५||
(च. चि. अ. ३) |

The symptoms of Nirama Jwara (last stage of the fever / fever having absence of ama) are - appearance of hunger, slight emaciation and feeling of lightness of the body, decrease in intensity / temperature of the fever, elimination of dosas (and also feces, urine etc.) and fever entering into the eighth day are the symptoms of Nirama jwara (fully ripe or terminal stage of fever). (65)

Read - Ama Chikitsa: Treatment For Ama And Saama Conditions

Signs of curability

बलवत्स्वल्पदोषेषु ज्वरः साध्योऽनुपद्रवः |६६|
(च. चि. अ. ३) |

Fever affecting strong persons, produced by less dosas (dosas which are not severely aggravated) and having no complications are easily curable.

Signs of incurability

हेतुभिर्बहुभिर्जातो बलिभिर्बहुलक्षणः ||६६||
ज्वरः प्राणान्तकृद्यश्च शीघ्रमिन्द्रियनाशनः |
ज्वरः क्षीणस्य शूनस्य गम्भीरो दैर्घरात्रिकः ||६७||
असाध्यो बलवान् यश्च केशसीमन्तकृज्ज्वरः |
(च. चि. अ. ३) |

Fevers caused by many and powerful causes, manifesting with many and powerful symptoms, those which destroy the sense faculties (sense organs) in quick time will be life threatening and incurable. Similarly, strong (severe) fevers affecting persons who are very weak and afflicting those having oedema all over the body, which are deep seated (in the tissues), continuing for long periods (has become chronic) and those causing furrows in between the hairs of the head all of a sudden -are also difficult to treat or incurable. (66-67)

Gambhira Jwara

गम्भीरस्तु ज्वरो ज्ञेयो ह्यन्तर्दाहेन तृष्णया ||६८||
आनद्धत्वेन चात्यर्थं श्वासकासोद्गमेन च |
(सु. उ. तं. अ. ३९) |

The fever which manifests with burning sensation inside the body, thirst, severe distension of the abdomen, dyspnoea and cough is called as Gambhira Jwara. (68)

आरम्भाद्विषमो यस्तु यश्च वा दैर्घरात्रिकः ||६९||
क्षीणस्य चातिरूक्षस्य गम्भीरो यस्य [१] हन्ति तम् |
विसञ्ज्ञस्ताम्यते यस्तु शेते निपतितोऽपि वा ||७०||
शीतार्दितोऽन्तरुष्णश्च ज्वरेण म्रियते नरः |
यो हृष्टरोमा रक्ताक्षो हृदि सङ्घातशूलवान् ||७१||
वक्त्रेण चैवोच्छ्वसिति तं ज्वरो हन्ति मानवम् |
हिक्काश्वासतृषायुक्तं मूढं विभ्रान्तलोचनम् ||७२||
सन्ततोच्छ्वासिनं क्षीणं नरं क्षपयति ज्वरः |
हतप्रभेन्द्रियं क्षीणमरोचकनिपीडितम् ||७३||
गम्भीरतीक्ष्णवेगार्तं ज्वरितं परिवर्जयेत् |
(सु. उ. तं. अ. ३९) |

Fever which is irregular even from its commencement, is chronic (continuing for long periods) is incurable. Likewise, gambhira (and antardaha jwara) fever affecting persons who are weak or having dryness of the body is also incurable.

The patient will face death if the fever presents with loss of consciousness, darkness before the eyes, fainting – here the patient keeps laying down as he is not capable of getting up from that position, feeling cold externally and very hot internally (inside the body).

The fever is considered incurable and also tends to kill the person when it presents with frequent horripilation, redness of the eyes and pain as if injured by stone and similar other things in the region of the heart, patients breathing only through their mouth.

Fever associated with hiccough, increased respiration, thirst, delusion,

unsteady gaze, interrupted respirations (more expiration and fewer inspirations), severe emaciation will destroy the person (is incurable).
The patients of fever having loss of complexion and sensory activities, extreme debility, loss of appetite, deep seated fever, and having very high temperatures are to be refused treatment (because such a fever is incurable). (69-73)

Purvarupa of subsiding fever

दाहः स्वेदो भ्रमस्तृष्णा कम्पविड्भिदसञ्ज्ञता ।
कूजनं चास्यवैगन्ध्यमाकृतिर्ज्वरमोक्षणे ॥७४॥

Premonitory symptoms of subsiding fever
The symptoms of fever which is subsiding are - burning sensation, perspiration, giddiness, thirst, tremors, elimination of feces (diarrhea), loss of consciousness, making indistinct sounds (moaning) and bad smell from the mouth. (74)

Symptoms of relieved fever

स्वेदो लघुत्वं शिरसः कण्डूः पाको मुखस्य च ।
क्षवथुश्चान्नलिप्सा च ज्वरमुक्तस्य लक्षणम् ॥७५॥
(सु. उ. तं. अ. ३९) ।

The symptoms of the person who has been relieved from fever are - perspiration, feeling of lightness of the body, itching of the head, appearance of ulcers in the mouth, sneezing and desire for food. (75)

इति श्रीमाधवकरविरचिते माधवनिदाने ज्वरनिदानं समाप्तम् ॥२॥

Thus ends the chapter called 'Jwara Nidana' in the book Madhava Nidana, written by Acharya Madhavakara.

3

Madhava Nidana Chapter 3 Atisara Nidanam

Etiological Factors of Atisara - Diarrhoea

गुर्वतिस्निग्धरूक्षोष्णद्रवस्थूलातिशीतलैः |
विरुद्धाध्यशनाजीर्णैर्विषमैश्चापि भोजनैः ||१||
स्नेहाद्यैरतियुक्तैश्च मिथ्यायुक्तैर्विषैर्भयैः |
शोकाद्दुष्टाम्बुमद्यातिपानैः सात्म्यर्तुपर्ययैः ||२||
जलाभिरमणैर्वेगविघातैः क्रिमिदोषतः |
नृणां भवत्यतीसारो लक्षणं तस्य वक्ष्यते ||३||
(सु. उ. तं. अ. ४०) |

Over-indulgence in foods which are very heavy (hard to digest), very unctuous (fatty), very dry, very hot, very watery, very hard or very cold; foods which are mutually incompatible (antagonistic), taking foods in large quantities very frequently; foods which are not cooked or processed properly and taken at unusual times; excess or improper usage of therapies like oleation etc., consumption of poisons, fear, grief, drinking of polluted / contaminated water, consumption of excess of alcoholic drinks, changes in accustomed habits and abnormal changes in seasonal features (abnormal seasonal behaviors), over-indulgence in water sports, suppression of natural urges of the body and infestation by worms (intestinal parasites) – are the causative factors responsible for production of the disease atīsāra (diarrhoea). The symptoms of atisara are described herein. (1-3)

Samprapti – pathogenesis

संशम्यापान्धातुरग्निं प्रवृद्धः शकृन्मिश्रो वायुनाऽधः प्रणुन्नः |
सरत्यतीवातिसारं तमाहुर्व्याधिं घोरं षड्विधं तं वदन्ति |
एकैकशः सर्वशश्चापि दोषैः शोकेनान्यः षष्ठ आमेन चोक्तः ||४||
(सु. उ. तं. अ. ४०) |

Watery elements of the body undergo increase (following consumption of etiological factors). They then diminish / inactivate the digestive fire, get mixed with faeces, move downwards (out of the body through the rectum) by the action of vāta, in large quantities and very frequently producing the dreadful disease called Atīsāra. It is of six kinds, one from each dosha, one from the combination of the three doṣas together, fifth from grief and the sixth from āma (undigested food).(4)

Types:

- Vataja Atisara
- Pittaja
- Kaphaja
- Sannipataja Atisara
- Shokaja Atisra
- Amaja Atisara

Cycle of pathogenesis of Atisara -

Consumption of etiological factors of diarrhoea
Abnormal increase in watery elements in the body
Cause diminution / depletion of gastric fire (and weaken the digestion)
Gets mixed with faeces (increased watery elements get mixed with faeces)
Gets stimulated and propelled downwards by the action of vata (vata pushes water mixed faeces in the downward direction, towards the colon)
Excessive and frequent discharge of watery faeces (loose stools)
This disease is called as atisara – diarrhoea – it manifests in 6 different types

Notes – In Atisara types we can find that apart from those types formed by predominant aggravation of doshas there are 2 special forms. One is caused by ama. Ama is a by-product of sluggish digestion (caused by weak digestive fire – weak capacity of the stomach and intestine to digest the food). If not dealt with properly, this ama can cause different kinds of diseases including atisara. This also reflects that weak digestive power and subsequent formation of ama is one of the main causes for manifestation of atisara. This is called amatisara. The other type i.e. shokatisara is caused by excessive and constant grief. This reflects the psychological component of diarrhea. We also learn that a weak or imbalanced mind or emotional turmoil can cause or trigger the diseases or symptoms of the gastrointestinal system. Nervous diarrhoea is an example of this condition.

Purvarupa – premonitory symptoms

हृन्नाभिपायूदरकुक्षितोदगात्रावसादानिलसन्निरोधाः |
विट्सङ्ग आध्मानमथाविपाका भविष्यतस्तस्य पुरःसराणि ||५||
(सु. उ. तं. अ. ४०) |

The premonitory symptoms of diarrhoea include - pricking type of pain in the region of the heart, umbilicus, rectum, lower abdomen and flanks; weakness of the body, non-elimination of flatus, constipation, distension of the abdomen and indigestion of food. (5)

Symptoms of Vataja Atisara

अरुणं फेनिलं रूक्षमल्पमल्पं मुहुर्मुहुः |
शकृदामं सरुक्शब्दं मारुतेनातिसार्यते ||६||

Elimination of faeces which is slightly brown in colour, frothy, viscid, less in quantity but expelled very frequently and is accompanied with pain and noise are the symptoms of vātaja atīsāra (diarrhoea due to increase of vāta dosa).(6)

Symptoms of Pittaja Atisara

पित्तात् पीतं नीलमालोहितं वा तृष्णामूर्छादाहपाकोपपन्नम् |७|
(सु. उ. तं. अ. ४०) |

Faeces which are deep yellow, blue or red in colour; the patient having thirst, fainting, burning sensation and ulcerations (of the alimentary tract) are the symptoms of pittaja atīsāra (diarrhoea due to increase of pitta). (7)

Symptoms of Kaphaja Atisara

शुक्लं सान्द्रं श्लेष्मणा श्लेष्मयुक्तं विस्रं शीतं हृष्टरोमा मनुष्यः ||७||
(सु. उ. तं. अ. ४०) |

Faeces which is white, semi-solid, mixed with mucus and fat, cold and the patient having frequent horripilations (hairs standing on ends) are seen in kaphaja atīsāra (diarrhoea due to increase of kapha).(7)

Symptoms of Tridosaja Atisara

वराहस्नेहमांसाम्बुसदृशं सर्वरूपिणम् |
कृच्छ्रसाध्यमतीसारं विद्याद्दोषत्रयोद्भवम् ||८||

In tridoshaja atisāra (diarrhoea caused due to increase of all the three dosas together) there will be elimination of faeces resembling the fat of wild boar or water in which mutton is washed. The patient will also have the symptoms of all the three doṣas. This condition is difficult to cure. (8)

Symptoms of Shokaja Atisara

तैस्तैर्भावैः शोचतोऽल्पाशनस्य बाष्पोष्मा वै वह्निमाविश्य जन्तोः |
कोष्ठं गत्वा क्षोभयेत्तस्य रक्तं तच्चाधस्तात् काकणन्तीप्रकाशम् ||९||
निर्गच्छेद्वै विड्विमिश्रं ह्यविड्वा निर्गन्धं वा गन्धवद्वाऽतिसारः |
शोकोत्पन्नो दुश्चिकित्स्योऽतिमात्रं रोगो वैद्यैः कष्ट एष प्रदिष्टः ||१०||
(सु. उ. तं. अ. ४०) |

In persons who are very much afflicted with grief (due to loss of wealth, kith and kin, etc.,), who consume little food or no food at all, the heat of the tears (and also of the fluids of the nose, mouth, throat) increase in quantity. This enters into the alimentary tract and inactivates the digestive fire (digestive activity) and causes vitiation of the rakta dhātu (blood). This vitiated blood resembling the seed of kākaṇanti (guñjā – Abrus precatorius) gets expelled out of the body either mixed with faeces or alone (not mixed with faeces), with or without bad smell. This type of atisara – diarrhoea is known as śokātisāra. It is considered by physicians as difficult to cure.(9-10)

Symptoms of Amaja Atisara

अन्नाजीर्णात् प्रद्रुताः क्षोभयन्तः कोष्ठं दोषा धातुसङ्घान्मलांश्च |
नानावर्णं नैकशः सारयन्ति शूलोपेतं षष्ठमेनं वदन्ति ||११||
(सु. उ. तं. अ. ४०) |

In persons in whom the food is not properly digested, the dosas get increased by combining with undigested food. They travel in wrong channels and cause vitiation of koshta (abdominal cavity giving occupancy to many visceral organs, mainly stomach and colon), the dhātus (tissues) and malas (waste products) and cause elimination of faeces of many colours, frequently accompanied with pain in the abdomen. This is the sixth kind of atisara known as āmātisāra (diarrhoea due to indigestion).(11)

Ama and Pakva Atisara

**संसृष्टमेभिर्दोषैस्तु न्यस्तमप्स्ववसीदति |
पुरीषं भृशदुर्गन्धि पिच्छिलं चामसञ्ज्ञितम् ||१२||
एतान्येव तु लिङ्गानि विपरीतानि यस्य वै |
लाघवं च विशेषेण तस्य पक्वं विनिर्दिशेत् ||१३||
(सु. उ. तं. अ. ४०) |**

If the faeces associated with the vitiated doshas (and symptoms of aggravated dosas) has foul smell and is very sticky and if it sinks in the water, it (faeces) is said to be ama-mala i.e. faeces associated with ama (uncooked, inadequately processed hence abnormal). On the other hand if the faeces has opposite features of those mentioned above i.e. if it is not associated with foul smell and stickiness and floats on the water, it is said to be pakva mala (well formed, well processed and hence normal). (12-13)

Signs of incurability of atisara

**पक्वजाम्बवसङ्काशं यकृत्खण्डनिभं तनु |
घृततैलवसामज्जवेशवारपयोदधि ||१४||
मांसधावनतोयाभं कृष्णं नीलारुणप्रभम् |
मेचकं स्निग्धकर्बूरं चन्द्रकोपगतं घनम् ||१५||
कुणपं मस्तुलुङ्गाभं सुगन्धि कुथितं बहु |
तृष्णादाहतमःश्वासहिक्कापार्श्वास्थिशूलिनम् ||१६||
सम्मूर्छारतिसम्मोहयुक्तं पक्ववलीगुदम् |
प्रलापयुक्तं च भिषग्वर्जयेदतिसारिणम् ||१७||
असंवृतगुदं क्षीणं दूराध्मातमुपद्रुतम् |
गुदे पक्वे गतोष्माणमतिसारकिणं त्यजेत् ||१८||
(सु. उ. तं. अ. ४०) |
श्वासशूलपिपासार्तं क्षीणं ज्वरनिपीडितम् |
विशेषेण नरं वृद्धमतीसारो विनाशयेत् ||१९||
(सु. सू. अ. ३३) |
(शोथं शूलं ज्वरं तृष्णां कासं श्वासमरोचकम् |
छर्दिं मूर्छां च हिक्कां च दृष्टावातीसारिणं त्यजेत्) |**

Diarrhoea is said to be incurable if the faeces is having the colour of ripened fruit of jambū (jamun fruit), pieces of liver; which is very thin (like water), that which resembles ghee, oil, muscle-fat, marrow, mutton-broth, milk, curds, mutton-wash; which is black, blue, pink, brown or shining black in colour and appearance (like that of collyrium – black and dry); is unctuous (greasy, oily) and having many colors, containing shining particles (resembling the shining particles on the peacock feather), is heavy / scabelous, smells like that of a dead body, brain, putrefied matter or has even a sweet smell and large in quantity.

When the diarrhoea is incurable the patient also has thirst, burning sensation, darkness before the eyes, dyspnoea (difficulty in breathing), hiccough, pain in the flanks and bones, fainting, restlessness, delusion, suppuration in the layers of the anus and rectum (ulcers in the rectum) and delirium. In the presence of these symptoms the physician should reject (not treat) the patient of diarrhoea (because the disease would be incurable). Treatment should be refused to the patients of diarrhoea whose anal sphincters are unable to close, who are emaciated, who have highly distended abdomen, suppuration (ulceration) of the rectum and have very low body temperature.

Diarrhoea is going to kill patients who have increased / difficult respiration (dyspnoea), pain in the abdomen, thirst, emaciation, fever and who are of old age. Likewise, those who have oedema, pain in the abdomen, fever, thirst, cough, dyspnoea, loss of taste (appetite), vomiting, fainting and hiccoughs should also be rejected.(14-19)

Raktatisara

पित्तकृन्ति यदाऽत्यर्थं द्रव्याण्यश्नाति पैत्तिके |
तदोपजायतेऽभीक्ष्णं रक्तातीसार उल्बणः ||२०||

Patients suffering or have suffered from pittātisāra i.e. diarrhoea caused by predominant aggravation of pitta (or even others) who indulge in foods and activities causing increase of pitta, will develop quickly a dreaded disease-raktātisāra (diarrhoea in which heavy bleeding occurs). (20)

Pravahika

वायुः प्रवृद्धो निचितं बलासं नुदत्यधस्तादहिताशनस्य |
प्रवाहतोऽल्पं बहुशो मलाक्तं प्रवाहिकां तां प्रवदन्ति तज्ज्ञाः ||२१||
(सु. उ. तं. अ. ४०) |
प्रवाहिका वातकृता सशूला पित्तात् सदाहा सकफा कफाच्च |
सशोणिता शोणितसम्भवा च ताः स्नेहरूक्षप्रभवा मतास्तु |
तासामतीसारवदादिशेच्च लिङ्गं क्रमं चामविपक्वतां च ||२२||

In persons who indulge in unsuitable foods, vāta gets increased, and after getting associated with kapha produces the disease called by experts as pravāhikā. In this, the patient will eliminate little quantities of faeces mixed with mucus, frequently, only after straining.

Vātaja pravāhikā is characterized by elimination of faeces accompanied with pain.

Pittaja pravāhikā is characterized by elimination of faeces accompanied with burning sensation.

Kaphaja pravāhikā is characterized by elimination of faeces mixed with kapha (mucus).

Raktaja pravāhikā is characterized by elimination of faeces with admixture of blood with more moisture or little of it as the case may be.

The other symptoms of this disease and determination of āma (inadequately processed / unripe / unformed) and pakva (adequately processed / ripe / formed) state of faeces are the same as those of diarrhoea. (21-22)

Relieved Symptoms

यस्योच्चारं विना मूत्रं सम्यग्वायुश्च गच्छति |
दीप्ताग्नेर्लघुकोष्ठस्य स्थितस्तस्योदरामयः ||२३||
(सु. उ. तं. अ. ४०) |

Symptoms indicating that 'diarrhoea has been cured'

Atīsāra (diarrhoea) is said to have been cured when the patient is able to eliminate flatus and urine independent of expulsion of faeces (i.e. faeces is not eliminated while passing urine or expelling fart), when his digestion capacity increases (he has developed hunger) and lightness of the abdomen. (23)

Symptoms of Jwaratisara

(ज्वरातीसारयोरुक्तं निदानं यत् पृथक् पृथक् |
तत्स्याज्ज्वरातिसारस्य तेन नात्रोदितं पुनः) ||१||

Jwaratisara is caused by a combination of independent etiological factors of jwara (fever) and atisara (diarrhoea). Similarly the premonitory symptoms, symptoms, aggravating and relieving factors and pathogenesis explained individually in relation to fever and diarrhoea are mixed up (combined) in the clinical picture of jwaratisara. This is the reason that this condition has not been detailed in this context.

इति श्रीमाधवकरविरचिते माधवनिदानेऽतीसारनिदानं समाप्तम् ||३||

Thus ends the chapter called 'Atisara Nidana' in the book Madhava Nidana, written by Acharya Madhavakara.

4

Madhava Nidana Chapter 4 Grahani Roga Nidanam

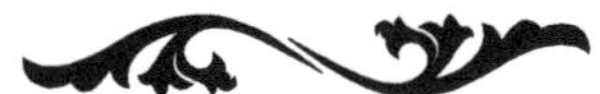

Samprapti – Pathogenesis of Grahani Roga

अतीसारे निवृत्तेऽपि मन्दाग्नेरहिताशिनः |
भूयः सन्दूषितो वह्निर्ग्रहणीमभिदूषयेत् ||१||
(सु. उ. तं. अ. ४०) |

Grahani disease occurs in persons who have been recently relieved of diarrhea but still have poor digestion (even others having poor digestion right from the beginning). When such persons indulge in unsuitable foods and activities, the doshas undergo increase. These doshas in turn affect the agni. This agni which has been contaminated by the doshas undergoes aggravation and affects the grahani (duodenum). (1)

एकैकशः सर्वशश्च दोषैरत्यर्थमूर्छितैः |
सा दुष्टा बहुशो भुक्तमाममेव विमुञ्चति ||२||
पक्वं वा सरुजं पूति मुहुर्बद्धं मुहुर्द्रवम् |
ग्रहणीरोगमाहुस्तमायुर्वेदविदो जनाः ||३||
(सु. उ. तं. अ. ४०) |

Thus, the grahani gets excessively affected by the doshas either individually or in combination (individual dosha or combination of doshas). Such affected duodenum causes expulsion of most of the consumed food in an undigested or digested form. In this condition the faeces is foul smelling, sometimes hard (constipated) and sometimes fluid (diarrhoea) in nature and is accompanied with pain in the abdomen. Scholars of Ayurveda call this disease as Grahani Roga.(2-3)

Grahani – chain of pathogenesis

Person who has just (recently) been relieved from atisara (diarrhoea) but still has weak digestion strength

Takes unsuitable foods and activities

Abnormal increase in doshas

Aggravated doshas afflict the agni (digestive fire)

Agni disturbed due to contamination / affliction by doshas will further contaminate (afflict) the grahani (duodenum)

Further the duodenum gets excessively affected by individual or combination of aggravated doshas

The affected duodenum expels the food either in an undigested form or digested formThe faeces smell foul and sometimes there is constipation and sometimes diarrhoea along with pain in the abdomen

This disease is called as Grahani

Note – These chains of events happen in a similar way even in those who haven't recovered from diarrhoea. These people have weak digestion from the beginning and in them the chronology of events of pathogenesis takes place in the same way explained here.

Purvarupa – premonitory symptoms of Grahani

पूर्वरूपं तु तस्येदं तृष्णाऽऽलस्यं बलक्षयः |
विदाहोऽन्नस्य पाकश्च चिरात् कायस्य गौरवम् ||४||
(च. चि. अ. १५) |

Premonitory symptoms of Grahani disease are - thirst, lack of enthusiasm, debility, improper digestion of food due to the action of weak digestive fire, delayed digestion of food and feeling of heaviness of the body.(4)

Vataja Grahani

कटुतिक्तकषायातिरूक्षसन्दुष्टभोजनः |
प्रमितानशनात्यध्ववेगनिग्रहमैथुनैः ||५||
मारुतः कुपितो वह्निं सञ्छाद्य कुरुते गदान् |
तस्यान्नं पच्यते दुःखं शुक्तपाकं खराङ्गता ||६||
कण्ठास्यशोषोऽक्षुत्तृष्णा तिमिरं कर्णयोः स्वनः |

पार्श्वोरुवङ्क्षणग्रीवारुगभीक्ष्णं विसूचिका ||७||
हृत्पीडाकार्श्यदौर्बल्यं वैरस्यं परिकर्तिका |
गृद्धिः सर्वरसानां च मनसः सदनं तथा ||८||
जीर्णे जीर्यति चाध्मानं भुक्ते स्वास्थ्यमुपैति च |
स वातगुल्महृद्रोगप्लीहाशङ्की च मानवः ||९||
चिरादुःखं द्रवं शुष्कं तन्वामं शब्दफेनवत् |
पुनः पुनः सृजेद्वर्चः कासश्वासार्दितोऽनिलात् ||१०||
(च. चि. अ. १५) |

Etiological factors, pathogenesis and symptoms of Vataja Grahani

Vata gets abnormally increased due to indulgence in foods which are pungent, bitter, astringent, dry, contaminated, and scanty or no food at all; too much of walk, suppression of natural urges of the body, excess sexual activities.

The vata thus increased destroys the agni – digestive fire and produces Vātaja Grahaṇi Roga. Vataja Grahani Roga.

In this type of Grahani, the food gets digested with difficulty and undergoes fermentation. There also occurs hardness of the body parts, dryness of the throat and mouth, increased hunger and thirst, darkness before the eyes, noise in the ears, constant pain in the flanks, thighs, groins and neck; vomiting and diarrhea occur together, pain in the region of the heart, emaciation, weakness, bad taste in the mouth, cutting pain in the rectum / anal region, desire for foods of all the tastes, mental depression, distension of the abdomen after the digestion of food and during the period of digestion and feeling of comfort on taking food.

The patient gets suspicious of getting vāta gulma , hrid roga (disease of the heart), plīhā (splenic disorder), in future. (Alternatively, we can tell that the symptoms very much resemble those of vāta gulma - abdominal tumour, hrid roga - disease of the heart, pleeha - splenic disorder, causing difficulty in diagnosis).

Such a patient having cough and breathing trouble (dyspnoea, difficulty in respiration) repeatedly voids faeces after a long time, which is watery or dry, thin, frothy, improperly processed, accompanied with pain and noise. (5-10)

Pittaja Grahani

कट्वजीर्णविदाह्यम्लक्षाराद्यैःपित्तमुल्बणम् |
आप्लावयद्धन्त्यनलंजलंतप्तमिवानलम् ||११||

सोऽजीर्णं नीलपीताभं पीताभः सार्यते द्रवम् |
पूत्यम्लोद्गारहृत्कण्ठदाहारुचितृडर्दितः ||१२||
(च. चि. अ. १५) |

Etiological factors, pathogenesis and symptoms of Pittaja Grahani

Pitta undergoes abnormal increase due to indulgence in foods which are pungent and uncooked, causing heartburn, sour and alkaline in nature. This increased pitta would activate the digestive fire just like the hot water poured over burning fire and produces pittaja grahaṇi roga.

In this condition the patient will be eliminating faeces which are inadequately processed, bluish yellow or deep yellow in colour, watery and fetid. The person will have bad, sour belching; burning sensation in the chest and throat, loss of taste or appetite and thirst. (11-12)

Kaphaja Grahani

गुर्वतिस्निग्धशीतादिभोजनदतिभोजनत् |
भुक्तमात्रस्य च स्वप्नाद्धन्त्यग्निं कुपितः कफः ||१३||
तस्यान्नं पच्यते दुःखं हृल्लासच्छर्द्यरोचकाः |
आस्योपदेहमाधुर्यं कासष्ठीवनपीनसाः ||१४||
हृदयं मन्यते स्त्यानमुदरं स्तिमितं गुरुः |
दुष्टो मधुर उद्गारः सदनं स्त्रीष्वहर्षणम् ||१५||
भिन्नामश्लेष्मसंसृष्टगुरुवर्चःप्रवर्तनम् |
अकृशस्यापि दौर्बल्यमालस्यं च कफात्मके ||१६||
(च. चि. अ. १५) |

Etiological factors, pathogenesis and symptoms of Kaphaja Grahani

Kapha gets abnormally increased due to indulgence in foods which are heavy (hard to digest), too unctuous (oily), cold and taken excessively (frequently); and sleeping immediately after midday meal. This aggravated kapha destroys (inactivates) the digestive fire and causes kaphaja grahani disease.

In these patients the food gets digested with difficulty. He also would have nausea, vomiting, loss of taste (appetite), coating in the mouth (on the tongue), sweet taste in the mouth, cough, expectoration, running in the nose, heaviness of the heart, feeling as if the abdomen is filled with dense fluids, hardness (devoid of movements, tight), and heaviness of the abdomen, bad and sweet smelling belchings, debility and lack of interest in sex. The faeces is semi-solid, inadequately processed (associated with ama), mucous mixed and heavy. The patient is debilitated though not emaciated and is non-enthusiastic. (13-16)

Tridosaja Grahani

पृथग्वातादिनिर्दिष्टहेतुलिङ्गसमागमे |
त्रिदोषं निर्दिशेदेवं, तेषां वक्ष्यामि भेषजम् ||१७||
(च. चि. अ. १५) |

Etiological factors, pathogenesis and symptoms of Tridosaja Grahani

The presence of causes and symptoms of all the three doshas together is found in case of tridosha grahani roga. (17)

This means to say that tridoshaja grahani is caused in those who consume the etiological factors responsible for aggravation of all vata, pitta and kapha together. In this condition, the symptoms mentioned in vataja, pittaja and kaphaja grahani are present in combination (mixed up).

Sangrahani Grahani

अन्त्रकूजनमालस्यं दौर्बल्यं सदनं तथा |
द्रवं शीतं घनं स्निग्धं सकटीवेदनं शकृत् |१|
आमं बहु सपैच्छिल्यं सशब्दं मन्दवेदनम् |
पक्षान्मासाद्दशाहाद्वा नित्यं वाऽप्यथ मुञ्चति ||२||
दिवा प्रकोपो भवति रात्रौ शान्तिं व्रजेच्च सा |
दुर्विज्ञेया दुश्चिकित्स्या चिरकालानुबन्धिनी ||३||
सा भवेदामवातेन सङ्ग्रहग्रहणी मता |
स्वपतः पार्श्वयोः शूलं गलज्जलघटीध्वनिः |
तं वदन्ति घटीयन्त्रमसाध्यं ग्रहणीगदम् ||४||

Sangrahani is marked by presence of gurgling sound in the intestines, laziness, weakness and malaise. In this condition the person excretes faeces which are liquid, cold, dense, and unctuous and associated with pain in the waist. The faeces which are inadequately processed (ama) is eliminated in large quantities, associated with slimy (sticky) material along with sounds and mild pain during excretion. These symptoms may appear once in 15, 30 or 10 days or even daily. The symptoms are pronounced during the day time and subside by night time. The nature of the disease cannot be understood easily, cannot be easily treated and persists for a long time. This condition is caused by vata associated with ama and is called sangraha grahani or samgrahani.

Ghatiyantra Grahani

This is also a variant of grahani disease. The person in this condition suffers from pain in the flanks while lying down and sounds resembling 'that produced when a pot is dipped in the water' are heard from the abdomen. This condition is incurable. (1-4)

Determination of ama and pakva states and signs of incurability of grahani

दोषं सामं निरामं च विद्यादत्रातिसारवत् ||१८||
लिङ्गैरसाध्यो ग्रहणीविकारो यैस्तैरतीसारगदो न सिध्येत् |
वृद्धस्य नूनं ग्रहणीविकारो हत्वा तनूं नैव निवर्तते च ||१९||

The determination of āma and pakva states of doshas and faeces in grahani disease shall be understood on the same lines as explained in the context of atisara (diarrhoea). The symptoms of incurability of grahani are the same as the symptoms of incurability of atisara. Grahaṇī roga does not leave the old people without killing them. (18-19)

Prognosis of grahani roga – age wise

(बालके ग्रहणी साध्या यूनि कृच्छ्रा समीरिता |
वृद्धे त्वसाध्या विज्ञेया मतं धन्वन्तरेरिदम्) ||१||

Grahaṇī roga is easily curable in children, cured with difficulty in the middle-aged persons and incurable in the senile - thus opines Dhanwantari). (1)

इति श्रीमाधवकरविरचिते माधवनिदाने ग्रहणीरोगनिदानं समाप्तम् ||४||

Thus ends the chapter called 'Grahani Roga NIdana' in the book Madhava Nidana, written by Acharya Madhavakara.

5

Madhava Nidana Chapter 5 Arshas Nidanam

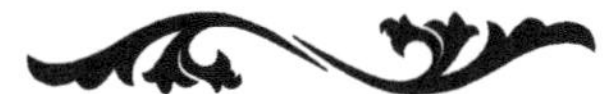

Types of Arshas – Piles

पृथग्दोषैः समस्तैश्च शोणितात् सहजानि च ।
अर्शांसि षट्प्रकाराणि विद्याद्गुदवलित्रये ॥१॥

Arshas (piles, haemorrhoids) is of six types, viz.,
one from each doṣa (vataja, pittaja and kaphaja),
fourth from the combination of all three doshas together (tridosaja, sannipataja),
fifth from rakta – blood (raktaja) and
the sixth which is sahaja (congenital / hereditary).
Piles will appear in the three folds of the rectum. (1)

Definition of Arsas

दोषास्त्वङ्मांसमेदांसि सन्दूष्य विविधाकृतीन् ।
मांसाङ्कुरानपानादौ कुर्वन्त्यर्शांसि तान् जगुः ॥२॥
(वा. नि. अ. ७) ।

The aggravated doshas contaminate the skin, muscle and adipose tissue (fat) and cause sprouts of muscle of different shapes in the rectum (anal region) and other places. These sprouts (Ankura) are called as Arśhas. (2)

Causes of Vataja Arshas

कषायकटुतिक्तानि रूक्षशीतलघूनि च |
प्रमिताल्पाशनं तीक्ष्णं मद्यं मैथुनसेवनम् ||३||
लङ्घनं देशकालौ च शीतौ व्यायामकर्म च |
शोको वातातपस्पर्शो हेतुर्वातार्शसां मतः ||४||
(च. चि. अ. १४) |

The causes for Vataja Arshas include over-indulgence in foods which are of astringent, pungent or bitter tastes, which are dry, cold, light (easily digestible), very scanty and non-nutritive; strong alcoholic drinks, excessive indulgence in sex, fasting / starvation, exposure to cold season, living in cold places, excessive physical activity, grief, exposure to heavy breeze and sunlight.(3-4)

Causes of Pittaja Arshas

कट्वम्ललवणोष्णानि व्यायामाग्न्यातपप्रभाः |
देशकालावशिशिरौ क्रोधो मद्यमसूयनम् ||५||
विदाहि तीक्ष्णमुष्णं च सर्वं पानान्नभेषजम् |
पित्तोल्बणानां विज्ञेयः प्रकोपे हेतुरर्शसाम् ||६||
(च. चि. अ. १४) |

The causes of Pittaja Arshas include:
Over-indulgence in foods which are pungent, sour, salt and hot;
physical exertion, too much exposure to fire and sunlight, hot season, living in hot places;
anger, excessive consumption of alcoholic drinks, jealousy, drinks, foods and medicines which cause heart-burn (corrosive),
penetrating (into the tissues) nature and heat producing and other causative factors which lead to increase of pitta. (5-6)

Causes of Kaphaja Arshas

मधुरस्निग्धशीतानि लवणाम्लगुरूणि च |
अव्यायामो दिवास्वप्नः शय्यासनसुखे रतिः ||७||
प्राग्वातसेवा शीतौ च देशकालावचिन्तनम् |
श्लैष्मिकाणां समुद्दिष्टमेतत् कारणमर्शसाम् ||८||
(च. चि. अ. १४) |

The causes of Kaphaja Arshas include - over-indulgence in foods which are sweet, fatty, cold, salty, sour and heavy (hard to digest); lack of physical activity, sleeping at daytime, very comfortably soft bed and seat, exposure to eastern breeze, cold season and places, not worrying and others causative factors which lead to increase of kapha. (7-8)

Dvandva and Tridosaja Arshas

हेतुलक्षणसंसर्गाद्विद्याद्द्वन्द्वोल्बणानि च |९|
सर्वो हेतुस्त्रिदोषाणां सहजैर्लक्षणं समम् ||९||
(च. चि. अ. १४) |

Dvandva arshas is produced by the causative factors of any two doshas. These types of arshas will have combined symptoms of aggravation of both those doshas.

Similarly, Tridoshaja arshas is produced by causative factors of all the three doshas. The symptoms of this type of arshas are similar to those of Sahaja arshas (arshas present right from the birth – congenital). (9)

Symptoms of Vataja Arsas

गुदाङ्कुरा बह्वनिलाः शुष्काश्चिमचिमान्विताः |
म्लानाः श्यावारुणाः स्तब्धा विशदाः परुषाः खराः ||१०||
मिथो विसदृशा वक्रास्तीक्ष्णा विस्फुटिताननाः |
बिम्बीखर्जूरकर्कन्धूकार्पासीफलसन्निभाः ||११||
केचित् कदम्बपुष्पाभाः केचित् सिद्धार्थकोपमाः |
शिरःपार्श्वांसकट्यूरुवङ्क्षणाद्यधिकव्यथाः ||१२||
क्षवथूद्गारविष्टम्भहृद्ग्रहारोचकप्रदाः |
कासश्वासाग्निवैषम्यकर्णनादभ्रमावहाः ||१३||
तैरार्तो ग्रथितं स्तोकं सशब्दं सप्रवाहिकम् |
रुक्फेनपिच्छानुगतं विबद्धमुपवेश्यते ||१४||
कृष्णत्वङ्नखविण्मूत्रनेत्रवक्त्रश्च जायते |
गुल्मप्लीहोदराष्ठीलासम्भवस्तत एव च ||१५||
(वा. नि. अ. ७) |

Sprouts (pile masses) are dry (doesn't exudate or bleed), have itching (tingling sensation), are shrunk (small in size, not developed properly),
blue or bluish pink in colour, stiff (hard), non-sticky (non-slimy),
dry, rough, furrowed, each one of different shape,
curved, pointed tip, cracked,
resemble fruits of bimbi (Cephalandra indica), kharjoora (date palm), karkandhu (Zizyphus ceroplia) and kaarpaasa (cotton seeds).
Some masses appear like kadamba flowers (having many sprouts), and some

others resemble mustard seeds (very small in size).|

The person complains of excessive pain in the head, flanks, shoulders, waist, thighs, groins, sneezing, belching, constipation, pain near the heart, anorexia, cough, difficult respiration (dyspnoea), irregular digestion, ringing in the ears and giddiness.

The patient eliminates faeces which is scrabulous, scanty, associated with noise, straining and pain; frothy and associated with slimy discharges and semi-solid in consistency or is constipated. There is blackish discoloration of skin, nails, faeces, urine, eyes and face. Gulma (abdominal tumour), pliha (spleen enlargement), udara (enlargement of abdomen) and asthila (enlargement of prostate) may appear as its complications. (10-15)

Symptoms of Pittaja Arshas

पित्तोत्तरा नीलमुखा रक्तपीतासितप्रभाः |
तन्वस्रस्राविणो विस्रास्तनवो मृदवः श्लथाः ||१६||
शुकजिह्वायकृत्खण्डजलौकोवक्त्रसन्निभाः |
दाहपाकज्वरस्वेदतृण्मूर्छारुचिमोहदाः ||१७||
सोष्माणो द्रवनीलोष्णपीतरक्तामवर्चसः |
यवमध्या हरित्पीतहारिद्रत्वङ्नखादयः ||१८||
(वा. नि. अ. ७) |

Sprouts (pile masses) are blue, red, yellow or black in colour. They will discharge thin blood, fetid smell, less in number (small in size), smooth to touch and suspended (flaccid, loose, hanging).

These masses resemble the parrot's tongue, piece of liver or mouth part of a leech. The patient complains of burning sensation, suppuration (ulceration), fever, perspiration, thirst, fainting (loss of consciousness), anorexia and delusion.

He eliminates faeces which are hot, watery, blue, yellow or red in colour and not properly processed (associated with ama). Some of these masses will resemble barley i.e. thick in the centre and thin / tapering towards the ends. The skin, nails, face, teeth, urine and faeces will get discoloured and will attain green, yellow or turmeric colour. (16-18)

Symptoms of Kaphaja Arsas

श्लेष्मोल्बणा महामूला घना मन्दरुजः सिताः |
उत्सन्नोपचितस्निग्धस्तब्धवृत्तगुरुस्थिराः ||१९||
पिच्छिलाः स्तिमिताः श्लक्ष्णाः कण्ड्वाढ्याः स्पर्शनप्रियाः |

करीरपनसास्थ्याभास्तथा गोस्तनसन्निभाः ||२०||
वङ्क्षणानाहिनः पायुबस्तिनाभिविकर्षिणः |
सश्वासकासहृल्लासप्रसेकारुचिपीनसाः ||२१||
मेहकृच्छ्रशिरोजाड्यशिशिरज्वरकारिणः |
क्लैब्याग्निमार्दवच्छर्दिरामप्रायविकारदाः ||२२||
वसाभसकफप्रायपुरीषाः सप्रवाहिकाः |
न स्रवन्ति न भिद्यन्ते पाण्डुस्निग्धत्वगादयः ||२३||
(वा. नि. अ. ७) |

Sprouts (pile masses) are deep rooted, hard (dense), with mild pain, and white in colour. These masses are elongated and elevated, big in size and circumference, unctuous / oily (smooth), stiff (not flabby – do not pit or get depressed when pressed), round in shape, heavy and fixed / stable. The masses are slimy / slippery, immobile (or damp, wet), smooth / shining, associated with severe itching and feels comfortable on touching.
They resemble karira (bamboo shoot/sprout), seed of panasa (jackfruit), or teet of cow udder.
The patient may have swelling or distension in the groins (hernia?), dragging sensation in the rectum, bladder, and umbilicus; difficulty in respiration, cough, nausea, salivation, anorexia, running in the nose, dysuria, heaviness of the head, fever with cold; impotency, indigestion, vomiting and other diseases which are caused by ama (undigested material). The faeces will resemble fat, mixed with mucus and is accompanied with straining. There will be no exudation (of mucus or blood) from the pile mass. There will also be no cracks and splits in spite of being subjected to friction by faeces. (19-23)

Symptoms of Tridosaja Arsas

सर्वैः सर्वात्मकान्याहुर्लक्षणैः सहजानि च |२४|

In case of Tridosaja arshas the symptoms of all the three dosas will be found together. (24)

Symptoms of Raktarsas (Rakta Arshas)

रक्तोल्बणा गुदेकीलाः पित्ताकृतिसमन्विताः ||२४||
वटप्ररोहसदृशा गुञ्जाविद्रुमसन्निभाः |
तेऽत्यर्थं दुष्टमुष्णं च गाढविट्कप्रपीडिताः ||२५||

स्रवन्ति सहसा रक्तं तस्य चातिप्रवृत्तितः |
भेकाभः पीड्यते दुःखैः शोणितक्षयसम्भवैः ||२६||
हीनवर्णबलोत्साहो हतौजाः कलुषेन्द्रियः |
(वा. नि. अ. ७) |

In case of raktarshas, (bleeding piles) all symptoms are similar to pittaja arshas. The sprouts (pile mass) resemble the shape and size of pittaja arshas. The sprouts will resemble the buds of vata (Ficus bengalensis), seeds of guñja (Abrus precatorius) or vidruma (coral).

There is continuous, frequent and heavy loss (bleeding) of dirty (contaminated) and hot blood from these masses due to the friction of hardened faeces on these masses. Due to heavy and excessive loss of blood, the skin of the patient appears (resembles) that of a monsoon frog (yellowish or greenish brown colour of frogs as evident in the rainy season). The person will suffer from various disorders due to excessive bleeding. This leads to loss of colour, strength, enthusiasm and ojas (essence of all the tissues) or valour. The senses (sense organs) become weak and the patient may later develop other diseases due to loss of blood. (24-26)

Dosha association in Raktarshas and related symptoms

(तत्रानुबन्ध्योद्विविधःश्लेष्मणोमारुतस्यच।)
विट् श्यावं कठिनं रूक्षमधोवायुर्न वर्तते ||२७||
तनु चारुणवर्णं च फेनिलं चासृगर्शसाम् |
कट्यूरुगुदशूलं च दौर्बल्यं यदि चाधिकम् ||२८||
तत्रानुबन्धो वातस्य हेतुर्यदि च रूक्षणम् |
शिथिलं श्वेतपीतं च विट् स्निग्धं गुरु शीतलम् ||२९||
यद्यर्शसां घनं चासृक् तन्तुमत् पाण्डु पिच्छिलम् |
गुदं सपिच्छं स्तिमितं गुरु स्निग्धं च कारणम् |
श्लेष्मानुबन्धो विज्ञेयस्तत्र रक्तार्शसां बुधैः ||३०||
(च. चि. अ. १४) |

There are two kinds of dosa associations with Raktarshas i.e. that of vata and kapha.

In case of vata association, the faeces will be black in colour, hard and dry. The flatus is not expelled out.

There occurs thin, red coloured, and frothy blood discharges from the pile mass. The patient would have pain in the waist, thighs and rectum and extreme weakness. Consumption of dry things (foods) are the causative

factors of vata aggravation in bleeding piles.
In case of kapha association, the faeces will be broken (semi-solid), whitish yellow in colour, unctuous, heavy and cold.
There will be exudation of thick, sticky, whitish yellow (pale) blood having thread like structures in it from the pile masses. The anal region of the patient will be sticky, and wet (as if covered by wet cloth). Consumption of heavy and unctuous things is the causative factor of kapha aggravation in bleeding piles. (27-30)

Purvarupa
विष्टम्भोऽन्नस्य दौर्बल्यं कुक्षेराटोप एव च |
कार्श्यमुद्गारबाहुल्यं सक्थिसादोऽल्पविट्कता ||३१||
ग्रहणीदोषपाण्ड्वर्तेराशङ्का चोदरस्य च |
पूर्वरूपाणि निर्दिष्टान्यर्शसामभिवृद्धये ||३२||
(च. चि. अ. १४) |
Purvaroopa – premonitory symptoms of arshas
The premonitory symptoms of arshas include - stasis of food in the stomach without digestion, debility / weakness, gurgling noise in the abdomen, emaciation, too many belchings, weakness of the thighs, scanty faeces, presence of symptoms resembling those of grahani dosha (sprue), pandu (anaemia) and udara (distension of abdomen) causing confusion in diagnosis. (31-32)

Involvement of dosha subtypes and folds of rectum in manifestation of arshas
पञ्चात्मा मारुतः पित्तं कफो गुदवलित्रयम् |
सर्व एव प्रकुप्यन्ति गुदजानां समुद्भवे ||३३||
तस्मादर्शांसि दुःखानि बहुव्याधिकराणि च |
सर्वदेहोपतापीनि प्रायः कृच्छ्रतमानि च ||३४||
(च. चि. अ. १४) |
In the manifestation of arsas vis-a-vis piles, all five subtypes (divisions) of vata, pitta and kapha and all three layers (folds) of rectum are vitiated (affected). All the five divisions of each of the doshas invade (vitiate) all the three layers (folds) of the rectum to produce arshas. So, arshas is a very painful disease and also gives rise to many other diseases. It affects and troubles the whole body and is difficult to cure. (33-34)

Prognosis

बाह्यायां तु वलौ जातान्येकदोषोल्बणानि च |
अर्शांसि सुखसाध्यानि न चिरोत्पतितानि च ||३५||
द्वन्द्वजानि द्वितीयायां वलौ यान्याश्रितानि च |
कृच्छ्रसाध्यानि तान्याहुः परिसंवत्सराणि च ||३६||
सहजानि त्रिदोषाणि यानि चाभ्यन्तरां वलिम् |
जायन्तेऽर्शांसि संश्रित्य तान्यसाध्यानि निर्दिशेत् ||३७||
(च. चि. अ. १४) |

Prognosis (curability and incurability) of arshas

Pile masses located in the external layer (fold) of the rectum, those manifested due to increase of any one dosha, and which are of recent onset are easily curable.

Arshas caused by increase of any two doshas together, located in the middle layer (fold) of the rectum and existing for more than a year, are difficult to cure.

The arshas which is congenital (hereditary), which is caused by simultaneous aggravation of all the three doshas, and located in the innermost layer (fold) of the rectum is incurable. (35-37)

Other signs of prognosis of arshas

शेषत्वादायुषस्तानि चतुष्पादसमन्विते |
याप्यन्ते दीप्तकायाग्नेः प्रत्याख्येयान्यतोऽन्यथा ||३८||
(च. चि. अ. १४) |

Patients who are fortunate to have a balance of lifespan (have the fortune of having long life), good services of all the four limbs of treatment (physician, medicine, nurse and patient), having good digestive capacity can hope to live on with arshas. On the other hand the persons in whom none of the above mentioned features are present shall be refused treatment (should not be treated because they are incurable). (38)

Incurability of arshas based on the associated complications

हस्ते पादे मुखे नाभ्यां गुदे वृषणयोस्तथा |
शोथो हृत्पार्श्वशूलं च यस्यासाध्योऽर्शसो हि सः ||३९||
हृत्पार्श्वशूलं सम्मोहश्छर्दिरङ्गस्य रुग्ज्वरः |
तृष्णा गुदस्य पाकश्च निहन्युर्गुदजातुरम् ||४०||
(च. चि. अ. १४) |

तृष्णा अरोचकशूलार्तमतिप्रस्रुतशोणितम् |
शोथातिसारसंयुक्तमर्शांसि क्षपयन्ति हि ||४१||
(सु. सू. अ. ३३) |

Appearance of oedema in the hands, feet, face, umbilicus, rectum and scrotum, pain in the region of the heart and flanks are symptoms of bad prognosis in arshas.

Pain in the region of the heart and flanks, delusion, vomiting, diffuse pain all over the body, fever, thirst, suppuration (ulceration) of the rectum -these symptoms kill the patients of arshas.

Thirst, anorexia, colic, heavy bleeding from the pile mass, generalized oedema and diarrhoea also kill the patient. (39-41)

Lingaja Arsas

मेढ्रादिष्वपि वक्ष्यन्ते यथास्वं, नाभिजानि च |
गण्डूपदास्यरूपाणि पिच्छिलानि मृदूनि च ||४२||
(वा. नि. अ. ७) |

Arsas (sprouts) also develop on the penis and other regions of the body including nose, eyes and ears. The symptoms of these conditions are found along with the disease manifesting in these structures. The arshas manifesting near the umbilicus have the resemblance of the mouth part of earthworm; are slippery and soft. (42)

Carmakila

व्यानो गृहीत्वा श्लेष्माणं करोत्यर्शस्त्वचो बहिः |
कीलोपमं स्थिरखरं चर्मकीलं तु तद्विदुः ||४३||
(वा. नि. अ. ७) |

Vyana (a division / subtype of vata) associated with kapha will invade the skin causing arshas on the skin. This arshas resembles a nail which is firm and rough (hard). This is also known as Carmakila (warts) (43)

Types and symptoms of Carmakila

वातेन तोदपारुष्यं पित्तादसितवक्त्रता |
श्लेष्मणा स्निग्धता चास्य ग्रथितत्वं सवर्णता ||४४||(वा. नि. अ. ७) |

The carmakila in which vata is predominant is painful and rough. The carmakila in which pitta is predominant would have a black coloured opening. The carmakila in which kapha is predominant is of the same colour of the skin, is unctuous (smooth) and is knotted. (44)

इति श्रीमाधवकरविरचिते माधवनिदानेऽर्शोनिदानं समाप्तम् ||५||

Thus ends the chapter on Arshas, in Madhava Nidana text written by Acharya Madhavakara.

6

Madhava Nidana Chapter 6 Agnimandya Ajeerna Visuchika Alasaka Vilambika Nidana

Jatharagni Types

Kinds of Jatharagni – digestive fire

मन्दस्तीक्ष्णोऽथ विषमः समश्चेति चतुर्विधः |
कफपित्तानिलाधिक्यात्तत्साम्याज्जाठरोऽनलः ||१||

The jatharaagni (gastric fire, digestive activity) is of four kinds, they are –
Mandagni (manda agni) – caused due to predominance of kapha
Tiksnagni (tiksna agni) – caused due to predominance of pitta
Visamagni (visama agni) – caused due to predominance of vata
Samagni (sama agni) – caused due to the normalcy of all the three doshas

Behaviour and functions of different kinds of agni

विषमो वातजान् रोगान् तीक्ष्णः पित्तनिमित्तजान् |
करोत्यग्निस्तथा मन्दो विकारान् कफसम्भवान् ||२||
समा समाग्नेरशिता मात्रा सम्यग्विपच्यते |
स्वल्पाऽपि नैव मन्दाग्नेर्विषमाग्नेस्तु देहिनः ||३||

कदाचित् पच्यते सम्यक्कदाचिन्न विपच्यते |
मात्राऽतिमात्राऽप्यशिता सुखं यस्य विपच्यते |
तीक्ष्णाग्निरिति तं विद्यात् समाग्निः श्रेष्ठ उच्यते ||४||

1. Mandagni – This type of agni dominated by kapha either partially digests the food (to a small extent) or is incapable of digesting even a small quantity of food. This type of agni causes kapha diseases.

2. Tikşngaani – This type of agni dominated by pitta digests the usual or even excess quantity of food without any difficulty. This agni is powerful and can digest the food within a short span of time. This type of agni causes pitta diseases.

3. Visamaagni – This type of agni dominated by vata sometimes digests the food properly and sometimes improperly. This erratic and fluctuant behaviour of the agni is due to the influence of vata. This type of agni causes vata diseases.

4. Samāgni – This type of agni is due to normalcy and balance of all the three doshas i.e., vata, pitta and kapha. This is a healthy state of digestive activity. This kind of agni digests the normal quantity of food without causing any difficulty,

Among these 4 kinds of agni, only samāgni is said to be ideal for good health. (2-4)

Types of Ajirna- Indigestion

There are basically three kinds of ajirna (indigestion) caused due to the predominance of one or the other type of dosha in each type. They are –

Ama ajeerṇa – caused by kapha excess

Vidagdha ajeerṇa – caused by pitta excess

Vistabdha ajeerṇa – caused by vata excess

Other types of ajeerṇa

आमं विदग्धं विष्टब्धं कफपित्तानिलैस्त्रिभिः |
अजीर्णं केचिदिच्छन्ति चतुर्थं रसशेषतः ||५|| (सु. सू. अ. ४६) |
अजीर्णं पञ्चमं केचिन्निर्दोषं दिनपाकि च |
वदन्ति षष्ठं चाजीर्णं प्राकृतं प्रतिवासरम् ||६||

Rasasesa ajeerna - Others include a fourth one the rasasesa ajīrna as fourth type of ajīrṇa. This type of indigestion is related to āhāra rasa (indigestion on a nutrient portion of food).

Dinapāki ajeerṇa – According to some others the fifth type of ajīrṇa is

dinapāki ajīrṇa. In this type of indigestion, the food is digested the next day but without causing any difficulty (delayed digestion).
Prativasara ajeerṇa - Yet others consider prativasara ajirna as the sixth type of ajirṇa. This type of indigestion is found every day, normally, immediately after taking the food i.e. until the taken food is digested. This is a normal state and the indigestion is temporary and not pathological. It goes away once the food is digested. (5-6)

Nidana

अत्यम्बुपानाद्विषमाशनाच्च सन्धारणात् स्वप्नविपर्ययाच्च |
कालेऽपि सात्म्यं लघु चापि भुक्तमन्नं न पाकं भजते नरस्य ||७||
ईर्ष्याभयक्रोधपरिप्लुतेन लुब्धेन रुग्दैन्यनिपीडितेन |
प्रद्वेषयुक्तेन च सेव्यमानमन्नं न सम्यक्परिपाकमेति ||८||
(सु. सू. अ. ४६) |
मात्रयाऽप्यभ्यवहृतं पथ्यं चान्नं न जीर्यति |
चिन्ताशोकभयक्रोधदुःखशय्याप्रजागरैः ||९|| (च. वि. अ. २) |

Nidana – etiological factors of ajīrṇa (indigestion)

The general causes of indigestion include drinking water in large quantities, taking large or small quantities of food at unusual times, suppression of natural urges of the body, erratic sleep patterns i.e., not sleeping during night times and excessive sleeping during daytime. These factors cause indigestion of food in spite of the person taking - normal quantity of food, foods which have been accustomed and foods at proper time.

Food does not get digested properly in a person who is afflicted with jealousy, fear, anger, greed, grief, humility and hatred feelings. (One would not digest the food properly in spite of taking normal food at proper time when he or she is afflicted with worry, grief, fear, anger, misery, (pain) or loss of sleep).(7-9)

Symptoms of Aamajirna

तत्रामे गुरुतोत्क्लेदः शोथो गण्डाक्षिकूटगः |
उद्गारश्च यथाभुक्तमविदग्धः प्रवर्तते ||१०||

The symptoms of āmājīrṇa are – heaviness (of the abdomen and whole body), nausea, swelling of the cheeks and eyes, belchings similar to those occurring soon after meals (non-acidic, not having burning sensation). (10)

Symptoms of Vidagdhajirna

विदग्धे भ्रमतृण्मूर्छाः पित्ताच्च विविधा रुजः |
उद्गारश्च सधूमाम्लः स्वेदो दाहश्च जायते ||११||

Symptoms of vidagdhajirna includes - giddiness, thirst, fainting, sour belching and belching with a feel of smoke being eliminated, perspiration, burning sensation inside and other symptoms of pitta increase. (11)

Vistabdhajirna and Rasasesajirna

विष्टब्धे शूलमाध्मानं विविधा वातवेदनाः |
मलवाताप्रवृत्तिश्च स्तम्भो मोहाऽङ्गपीडनम् ||१२||
रसशेषेऽन्नविद्वेषो हृदयाशुद्धिगौरवे |१३|

Symptoms of Vistabdhājīrṇa include - with pain in the abdomen (colic), tympanitis, non-movement of stools and flatus (stools and fart are not expelled naturally), stiffness, delusion (unconsciousness), pain in body parts and other symptoms of vāta (increase).

Symptoms of Rasasesajirna include - aversion to food, unpleasant feeling in the region of the heart (bad belching), and heaviness (in the region of the heart or the abdomen). (12)

Ajirna Upadrava - Complications of indigestion

मूर्छा प्रलापो वमथुः प्रसेकः सदनं भ्रमः |
उपद्रवा भवन्त्येते मरणं चाप्यजीर्णतः ||१३||
(सु. सू. अ. ४६) |

The complications of ajirna / indigestion include – fainting (unconsciousness), delirium, vomiting, excessive salivation, debility, giddiness and even death. (13)

Eating indiscipline and ajirna

अनात्मवन्तः पशुवद्भुञ्जते येऽप्रमाणतः |
रोगानीकस्य ते मूलमजीर्णं प्राप्नुवन्ति हि ||१४||

Persons who do not have self-control and eat large quantities (without even being concerned about the quantity of food they take) of food recklessly like cattle (eating with animal instinct), will develop this disease ajirna. This indigestion (ajirna) is the root cause of many other diseases. (14)

Origin of Visucika, Alasaka and Vilambika disorders

अजीर्णमामं विष्टब्धं विदग्धं च यदीरितम् |

विसूच्यलसकौ तस्माद्भवेच्चापि विलम्बिका ||१५||
(सु. उ. तं. अ. ५६) |

There are three diseases namely Visūcikā, Alasaka and Vilambikā. These diseases arise from three types of ajirna i.e., Amajirna, Vidagdhajirna and Vistabdhajirna. (These need not be respectively). (15)

Visucika

सूचीभिरिव गात्राणि तुदन् सन्तिष्ठतेऽनिलः |
यस्याजीर्णेन सा वैद्यैर्विसूचीति निगद्यते ||१६||
न तां परिमिताहारा लभन्ते विदितागमाः |
मूढास्तामजितात्मानो लभन्तेऽशनलोलुपाः ||१७||
(सु. उ. तं. अ. ५६) |
मूर्छाऽतिसारो वमथुः पिपासा शूलं भ्रमोद्वेष्टनजृम्भदाहाः |
वैवर्ण्यकम्पौ हृदये रुजश्च भवन्ति तस्यां शिरसश्च भेदः ||१८||
(सु. उ. तं. अ. ५६) |

The disease in which the patient suffers from pricking pain, as though pierced by needles, caused by vata aggravated due to ajirna (indigestion) is named as visūcikā by the physicians. The pain is also stable and localized. People who are well versed with Ayurveda and the principles related to consumption of food mentioned therein and also follow the dietetic rules and regulations promptly will not suffer from this condition.

This condition in fact occurs due to ajīrṇa manifesting in persons, who have mad craving for food and also eat recklessly without any limitation (without following the eating rules, regulations and etiquettes).

Symptoms of Visucika include - fainting, diarrhoea, vomiting, severe thirst, abdominal pain, giddiness, cramps / twitching, yawning, burning sensation all over, discolouration, tremors, pain in the region of the heart and headache.(16-18)

Alasaka

कुक्षिरानह्यतेऽत्यर्थं प्रताम्येत् परिकूजति |
निरुद्धो मारुतश्चैव कुक्षावुपरि धावति ||१९||
वातवर्चोनिरोधश्च यस्यात्यर्थं भवेदपि |
तस्यालसकमाचष्टे तृष्णोद्गारौ च यस्य तु ||२०||
(सु. उ. तं. अ. ५६) |

The symptoms of Alasaka include - severe distension of the abdomen, unconsciousness, makes some sounds from within the throat (crying helplessly), flatus gets blocked downwards (doesn't move downwards easily) and hence takes an abnormal route and start moving upwards (reaching the region of heart and throat), severe or complete obstruction (non expulsion) of flatus and faeces, thirst and belching. (19-20)

Vilambika

दुष्टं तु भुक्तं कफमारुताभ्यां प्रवर्तते नोर्ध्वमधश्च यस्य |
विलम्बिकां तां भृशदुश्चिकित्स्यामाचक्षते शास्त्रविदः पुराणाः ||२१||
(सु. उ. तं. अ. ५६) |

The disease in which the food contaminated by the vitiated kapha and vata does not move out of the body either in upward or downward direction is defined as vilambikā by the ancient Ayurveda scholars. This is either a very difficult condition to treat or is incurable. (21)

Disturbing effects of ama

यत्रस्थमामं विरुजेत्तमेव देशं विशेषेण विकारजातैः |
दोषेण येनावततं शरीरं तल्लक्षणैरामसमुद्भवैश्च ||२२||
(सु. उ. तं. अ. ५६) |

Ama gives rise to pain in whichever part of the body it resides (or gets localized). The same place also becomes the site for manifestation of many diseases, which are caused due to the action of the doshas travelling all over the body associated with āma. (22)

Symptoms of incurability of visucika and alasaka

यः श्यावदन्तौष्ठनखोऽल्पसञ्ज्ञो वम्यर्दितोऽभ्यन्तरयातनेत्रः |
क्षामस्वरः सर्वविमुक्तसन्धिर्यायान्नरः सोऽपुनरागमाय ||२३||
(सु. उ. तं. अ. ५६) |

The fatal signs of incurability of ajirna and associated diseases include - blackish discolouration of teeth, lips and nails, loss of consciousness, severe vomiting, in drawing of the eyes, feeble voice and looseness of all the joints of the body. (23)

Jirna Ahara Lakshanas – signs of proper digestion of food

उद्गारशुद्धिरुत्साहो वेगोत्सर्गो यथोचितः |
लघुता क्षुत्पिपासा च जीर्णाहारस्य लक्षणम् ||२४||

The signs of proper digestion of food are - pure belching (without bad smell or taste), enthusiasm, proper and timely elimination of urges (of faeces, flatus and urine), lightness of the body, appearance of hunger and thirst (desire for water) are the symptoms of proper digestion of food. (24)

Upadravas of Visucika

निद्रानाशोऽरतिः कम्पो मूत्राघातो विसञ्ज्ञता |
अमी ह्युपद्रवा घोरा विसूच्यां पञ्च दारुणाः ||२५||

The five difficult and dreadful complications of visūcikā are –
loss of sleep
restlessness
tremors
suppression of urine
loss of consciousness (25)

Ajirna – as the root of other diseases

प्रायेणाहारवैषम्यादजीर्णं जायते नृणाम् |
तन्मूलो रोगसङ्घातस्तद्विनाशाद्विनश्यति ||२६||

Probably Ajirṇa occurs due to irregularities of food. This Ajīrṇa in turn is the cause for other diseases. On the other hand, when ajirna is cured other diseases also get destroyed automatically. (26)

General symptoms of Ajirna

ग्लानिगौरवविष्टम्भभ्रममारुतमूढताः |
विबन्धो वा प्रवृत्तिर्वा सामान्याजीर्णलक्षणम् ||२७||

The general symptoms of ajirna (indigestion) are feeling of weakness (without physical exertion) heaviness of the body, absence of movement of the abdomen, giddiness, non-elimination of flatus, constipation or diarrhoea. (27)

इति श्रीमाधवकरविरचिते माधवनिदानेऽग्निमान्द्याजीर्णविसूचिकालसकविलम्बिकानिदानं समाप्तम् ||६||

Thus ends the chapter on Agnimandya, Ajirna, Visuchika, Alasaka, Vilambika Nidana, in Madhava Nidana text written by Acharya Madhavakara.

7

Madhava Nidana Chapter 7 Krimi Nidanam

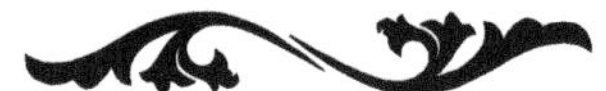

Krimi Bheda – types and origin of parasites

क्रिमयश्च द्विधा प्रोक्ता बाह्याभ्यन्तरभेदतः |
बहिर्मलकफासृग्विड्जन्मभेदाच्चतुर्विधाः ||१||
नामतो विंशतिविधा

Parasites are of two types - external and internal.

They are also counted as four kinds viz, arising from external dirt, kapha, rakta (blood) and purisa (faeces). They are totally twenty-four by name (and in number). (1)

Bahya Krimi – External parasites

बाह्यास्तत्र मलोद्भवाः | (वा. नि. अ. १४) |
तिलप्रमाणसंस्थानवर्णाः केशाम्बराश्रयाः ||२||
बहुपादाश्च सूक्ष्माश्च यूका लिक्षाश्च नामतः |
द्विधा ते कोठपिडकाकण्डूगण्डान् प्रकुर्वते ||३|| (वा. नि. अ. १४) |

External parasites which take their origin from excreta (mala) resemble tila (sesame seed) in size, features and colour, reside in hairs and clothes, have many legs and are small. They are of two kinds namely yūka and likṣa. They produce rashes, small pimples, itching and vesicles. (2-3)

Abhyantara Krimi Nidana – Causes of internal parasites

अजीर्णभोजी मधुराम्लनित्यो द्रवप्रियः पिष्टगुडोपभोक्ता |
व्यायामवर्जी च दिवाशयानो विरुद्धभुक् संलभते क्रिमींस्तु ||४||

Persons who indulge daily with foods which are raw (uncooked) or consume foods when previously consumed foods are not properly digested, sweet and sour, water and watery beverages or which are dry powders (flours) and jaggery: those who avoid physical exercise and those who sleep during day time and those who regularly consume incompatible (mutually antagonistic or unwholesome) foods become victims of krimiroga. (4)

Nidana – etiological factors of specific krimis

माषपिष्टाम्ललवणगुडशाकैः पुरीषजाः |
मांसमत्स्यगुडक्षीरदधिशुक्तैः कफोद्भवाः ||५||
विरुद्धाजीर्णशाकाद्यैः शोणितोत्था भवन्ति हि |
(सु. उ. तं. अ. ५४) |

Use of black gram, foods predominantly consisting of or prepared from flours, sour and salty foods, molasses and leafy vegetables give rise to growth of parasites in the faeces.

Use of mutton, fish, jaggery, milk, curds, fermented sugarcane juice, etc., gives rise to growth of parasites in kapha.

Indulgence in incompatible foods (mutually antagonistic foods), uncooked foods (or taking foods in the presence of indigestion of previously consumed foods) and leafy vegetables give rise to parasites in the blood. (5)

General symptoms of presence of internal parasites

ज्वरो विवर्णता शूलं हृद्रोगः सदनं भ्रमः ||६||
भक्तद्वेषोऽतिसारश्च सञ्जातक्रिमिलक्षणम् |
(सु. उ. तं. अ. ५४) |

Fever, discolouration, pain in the abdomen, disorders of (the region of) the heart, weakness, giddiness, aversion to food and diarrhoea are the symptoms of the presence of parasites inside the body. (6)

Kaphaja Krimi – size, shape, numbers, names and symptoms caused by these parasites

कफादामाशये जाता वृद्धाः सर्पन्ति सर्वतः ||७||
पृथुब्रध्ननिभाः केचित् केचिद्गण्डूपदोपमाः |
रूढधान्याङ्कुराकारास्तनुदीर्घास्तथाऽणवः ||८||

श्वेतास्ताम्रावभासाश्च नामतः सप्तधा तु ते |
अन्त्रादा उदारावेष्टा हृदयादा [१] महागुदाः ||९||
चुरवो दर्भकुसुमाः सुगन्धास्ते च कुर्वते |
हृल्लासमास्यस्रवणमविपाकमरोचकम् ||१०||
मूर्छाच्छर्दिज्वरा [३] नाहकार्श्यक्षवथुपीनसान् |
(वा. नि. अ. १४) |

The Kaphaja Krimis take their origin from the stomach due to the excess of kapha (excess kapha in the stomach is an ideal environment for these krimis to manifest). The parasites arising from kapha reside in the stomach and move all over the alimentary tract (they move in the upward as well as downward direction). Some resemble a thick leather strip and some are long, resembling earthworms. Some others look like the fresh sprouts of grains; are thin, long, and small or round, white or coppery in colour. They are of seven kinds and are known as antrada, udaravesta, hrdayada, mahaguda, curava, darbhakusuma and sugandha.

They produce nausea, excess salivation, indigestion, anorexia, fainting, vomiting, fever, constipation or blocks in stomach due to ama or in colon due to faeces (enlargement of abdomen), emaciation, too many sneezes and running in the nose. (7-10)

Raktaja Krimi – size, shape, numbers, names and symptoms caused by these parasites

रक्तवाहिसिरास्थानरक्तजा जन्तवोऽणवः ||११||
अपादा वृत्तताम्राश्च सौक्ष्म्यात् केचिददर्शनाः |
केशादा रोमविध्वंसा रोमद्वीपा उदुम्बराः |
षट् ते कुष्ठैककर्माणः सहसौरसमातरः ||१२||
(वा. नि. अ. १४) |

Parasites arising from rakta (blood) are found in all the organs / channels of blood i.e. raktavaha srotas (liver, spleen, arteries, veins and blood itself). They are very minute, devoid of legs, round in shape and have coppery colour. Among these many are very minute (microscopic) and hence cannot be visible (invisible) to the naked eyes. They are of six kinds and known as kesada,

romavidhvamsa, romadvipa, udumbara, sourasa and matara. All these parasites cause kushta

(leprosy, skin disorders) or many other diseases / symptoms which resemble kushta. (11-12)

Purishaja Krimi
पक्वाशये पुरीषोत्था जायन्तेऽधोविसर्पिणः |
प्रवृद्धाः स्युर्भवेयुश्च ते यदाऽऽमाशयोन्मुखाः ||१३||
तदाऽस्योद्गारनिःश्वासा विड्गन्धानुविधायिनः |
पृथुवृत्ततनुस्थूलाः श्यावपीतसितासिताः ||१४||
ते पञ्च नाम्ना क्रिमयः ककेरुकमकेरुकाः |
सौसुरादाः सशूलाख्या लेलिहा जनयन्ति हि ||१५||
विड्भेदशूलविष्टम्भकार्श्यपारुष्यपाण्डुताः |
रोमहर्षाग्निसदनं गुदकण्डूर्विमार्गगाः ||१६||
(वा. नि. अ. १४) |

Purishaja Krimi – size, shape, numbers, names and symptoms caused by these parasites

Parasites arising from purisa (faeces) are found in the large intestine. These parasites usually travel downwards. But when their numbers increase, they can even travel upwards towards the stomach. When they move upwards, they cause faecal smell in the mouth, belching and breath. They are big, round, thin or thick; blue, yellow, white or black in colour. They are of five kinds known as kakeruka makeruka, sausurada, sasula and leliha.

They produce diarrhoea, pain in the abdomen, constipation, emaciation, dryness, pallor (whitish-yellow discolouration), horripilations, poor digestion and itching in the anus. They even move into other places (organs nearby). (13-16)

इति श्रीमाधवकरविरचिते माधवनिदाने क्रिमिनिदानं समाप्तम् ||७||

Thus ends the chapter on Krimi Roga in Nidana Madhava Nidana text written by Acharya Madhavakara.

8

Madhava Nidana Chapter 8 Panduroga Kamala Kumbhakamala Halimaka Nidanam

Pandu Roga Types

पाण्डुरोगाः स्मृताः पञ्च वातपित्तकफैस्त्रयः |
चतुर्थः सन्निपातेन पञ्चमो भक्षणान्मृदः ||१||
(च. चि. अ. १६) |

Pānduroga (anaemia, disease characterized by pallor) is of five kinds - one each from (each dosa) vāta, pitta, kapha; fourth from the combination of all three doshas and fifth from eating mud.(1)

Pānduroga (anaemia, disease characterized by pallor) is of five kinds - one each from (each dosa) vāta, pitta, kapha; fourth from the combination of all three doshas and fifth from eating mud.(1)

Panduroga Nidana

व्यायाममम्लं लवणानि मद्यं मृदं दिवास्वप्नमतीव तीक्ष्णम् |
निषेवमाणस्य प्रदूष्य रक्तं दोषास्त्वचं पाण्डुरतां नयन्ति ||२||
(सु. उ. तं. अ. ४४) |

Over-exertion or strenuous physical exercises, sour and salty foods, alcoholic drinks, eating mud, sleeping during daytime, use of very irritating / strong / pungent substances (spices, etc.,) are the causative factors of Panduroga.

In persons who are excessively indulged in the above said causative factors, the dosas get excessively aggravated and produce whitish yellow discolouration of the skin by vitiating the rakta. This disease is called panduroga. (2)

Pandu Purvarupa

त्वक्स्फोटनष्ठीवनगात्रसादमृद्भक्षणप्रेक्षणकूटशोथाः |
विण्मूत्रपीतत्वमथाविपाको भविष्यतस्तस्य पुरःसराणि ||३||
(सु. उ. तं. अ. ४४) |

Premonitory symptoms of Panduroga - cracking of the skin, expectoration, debility, desire for eating earth (mud), oedema of the eye sockets (around the eyes), yellow discolouration of faeces and urine and indigestion. (3)

Vataja Pandu Symptoms

त्वङ्मूत्रनयनादीनां रूक्षकृष्णारुणाभताः |
वातपाण्ड्वामये तोदकम्पानाहभ्रमादयः ||४||

Symptoms of vataja pāṇdu (pandu disease caused by predominant vitiation of vata) are dryness, blackish-red discolouration of the skin, urine, eyes, etc., pricking / throbbing pain (of the body), tremors, enlargement of abdomen, giddiness, etc. (4)

Pittaja Pandu Symptoms

पीतमूत्रशकृन्नेत्रो दाहतृष्णाज्वरान्वितः |
भिन्नविट्कोऽतिपीताभः पित्तपाण्ड्वामयी नरः ||५||

Symptoms of pittaja pāndu (pandu disease caused by predominant vitiation of pitta) – are yellowish discolouration of urine, faeces, eyes; burning sensation, thirst, fever and deep yellow discoloration of the body and watery faeces (diarrhoea). (5)

Kaphaja Pandu Symptoms

कफप्रसेकश्वयथुतन्द्रालस्यातिगौरवैः |
पाण्डुरोगी कफाच्छुक्लैस्त्वङ्मूत्रनयनाननैः ||६||

Symptoms of kaphaja pandu (pandu disease caused by predominant vitiation of kapha) – are watery discharges (from mouth, nose, eyes etc.), oedema, drowsiness, lack of enthusiasm, excessive heaviness of the body and white discolouration of the skin, urine, eyes and face.(6)

Tridoshaja Pandu Symptoms

ज्वरारोचकहृल्लासच्छर्दितृष्णाक्लमान्वितः |
पाण्डुरोगी त्रिभिर्दोषैस्त्याज्यः क्षीणो हतेन्द्रियः ||७||

Symptoms of Tridosaja Pandu (pandu disease caused by predominant vitiation of kapha) – are fever, loss of taste (appetite), nausea, vomiting, thirst, tiredness / weakness. The person having the above-mentioned symptoms along with emaciation and loss of perception in the sense organs shall be considered as unfit for treatment and shall be refused treatment because this condition is incurable. (7)

Mrid Bhakshana Janya Pandu

मृत्तिकादनशीलस्य कुप्यत्यन्यतमो मलः |
कषाया मारुतं, पित्तमूषरा, मधुरा कफम् ||८|
कोपयेन्मृद्रसादींश्च रौक्ष्याद्भुक्तं च रूक्षयेत् |
पूरयत्यविपक्वैव स्रोतांसि निरुणद्ध्यपि ||९||
इन्द्रियाणां बलं हत्वा तेजो वीर्यौजसी तथा |
पाण्डुरोगं करोत्याशु बलवर्णाग्निनाशनम् ||१०||
(च. चि. अ. १६) |

The doshas get increased in persons who have the habit of eating mud. Astringent mud increases vāta. Salty mud increases pitta. Sweet mud increases kapha.

The mud contaminates and vitiates the rasa and other tissues of the body. The mud is dry in nature and by its extreme dryness causes dryness of the food also. Mud doesn't get digested in the body (gut). Being dry and indigestible, the mud fills up the passages of the body (mainly that of rasa dhatu) and blocks them. This leads to debility of sense organs, loss of physical strength, lustre (complexion), potency and ojas. They quickly cause pänduroga which brings about destruction of strength, normal colour and digestive fire. Since this condition is caused by eating mud, it is called mrud bhakshana janya pandu roga. (8-10)

शूनाक्षिकूटगण्डभ्रूः शूनपान्नाभिमेहनः |
क्रिमिकोष्ठोऽतिसार्येत मलं सासृक्कफान्वितम् ||११||

(च. चि. अ. १६) |

Mrud bhakshana janya pandu lakshanas – Symptoms of pandu roga caused due to eating of mud

Such persons have oedema of the eye sockets, cheek bones, brows, feet (legs), umbilicus and genital organs; parasites develop inside their alimentary tract, eliminate watery faeces mixed with blood and mucus. (11)

Signs of incurability

पाण्डुरोगश्चिरोत्पन्नः खरीभूतो न सिध्यति |
कालप्रकर्षाच्छूनानां यो वा पीतानि पश्यति ||१२||
बद्धाल्पविट् सहरितं सकफं योऽतिसार्यते |
दीनः श्वेतातिदिग्धाङ्गश्छर्दिमूर्छातृडर्दितः ||१३||
स नास्त्यसृक्क्षयाद्यश्च पाण्डुः श्वेतत्वमाप्नुयात् |
(च. चि. अ. १६) |
पाण्डुदन्तनखो यस्तु पाण्डुनेत्रश्च यो भवेत् |
पाण्डुसङ्घातदर्शी च पाण्डुरोगी विनश्यति ||१४||
(सु. सू. अ. ३३) |
अन्तेषु शूनं परिहीणमध्यं म्लानं तथाऽन्तेषु च मध्यशूनम् ||
गुदे च शेफस्यथ मुष्कयोश्च शूनं प्रताम्यन्तमसञ्ज्ञकल्पम् |
विवर्जयेत्पाण्डुकिनं यशोऽर्थी तथाऽतिसारज्वरपीडितं च ||१५||
(सु. उ. तं. अ. ४४) |

Pandu Roga Asadhya Lakshanas –

Pandu roga is incurable if it is of long duration (has become chronic), and has existed for long enough to get deep seated.

It is also incurable in those people who have oedema for a long time (long standing), who sees all objects yellow (everything he sees appears yellow in colour), in those having constipation or less stools or diarrhea with green coloured faeces mixed with mucus, who are very weak, whose body is very white / pale (due to loss of blood) i.e., the body appears as if coated in white, have vomiting, fainting and thirst. The person whose body becomes white due to excessive loss of blood will not survive.

Persons whose teeth, nails, eyes have become pale (yellowish white) and who sees everything around him as being pale (yellowish white) are going to die of panduroga.

Patients (of pandu roga) who have oedema of the extremities i.e. the limbs and head are swollen but the middle part of the body (trunk) is emaciated

or patients who have swelling of the trunk while the limbs and head are not swollen should be considered as incurable.
Those who have swelling of rectum, penis and scrotum, who faint often and have loss of consciousness, who are having diarrhoea and fever are also to be refused treatment (because these conditions will be incurable). (12-15)

Kamala Roga
Nidana, Samprapti
पाण्डुरोगी तु योऽत्यर्थं पित्तलानि निषेवते |
तस्य पित्तमसृङ्मांसं दग्ध्वा रोगाय कल्पते ||१६||
Nidana, Samprapti of Kamala Roga – Etiological factors and pathogenesis of Jaundice
In such patients of pandu roga, who indulge in foods and habits which increase pitta, the pitta would get abnormally increased. This pitta on getting increased burns up the rakta (blood) and mamsa (muscle tissue) and produces the disease known as kamala. (16)

Symptoms of Kamala, Kumba Kamala
हारिद्रनेत्रःसभृशंहारिद्रत्वङ्गखाननः।
रक्तपीतशकृन्मत्रोभेकवर्णोहतेन्द्रियः।।१७।।
दाहाविपाकदौर्बल्यसदनारुचिकर्षितः।
कामलाबहुपित्तैषाकोष्ठशाखाश्रयामता।।१८।। (च. चि. अ. १६)
कालान्तरात् खरीभूता कृच्छ्रा स्यात् कुम्भकामला |१९| (च. चि. अ. १६) |
Symptoms of Kamala, Manifestation of Kumbha-kamala
The symptoms of kamala (jaundice) include - deep turmeric (yellow) colouration of the eyes, skin, nails and face, reddish-yellow faeces and urine, skin colour resembling that of frog (greenish, brown, or brownish yellow), weakness of sense organs, burning sensation, indigestion, weakness, debility, anorexia are the symptoms of kamala (jaundice). It involves both the kostha (alimentary tract) and also the shaka (rakta - blood and other tissues). If left untreated kamala makes the organs rough (dry) / hard and turns into a difficult disease called kumbha-kamala. (17-18)

Signs of incurability
कृष्णपीतशकृन्मूत्रो भृशं शूनश्च मानवः ||१९||
सरक्ताक्षिमुखच्छर्दिविण्मूत्रो यश्च ताम्यति |
दाहारुचितृडानाहतन्द्रामोहसमन्वितः ||२०||

नष्टाग्निसञ्ज्ञः क्षिप्रं हि कामलावान् विपद्यते |
(च. चि. अ. १६) |
छर्द्यरोचकहृल्लासज्वरक्लमनिपीडितः ||२१||
नश्यति श्वासकासार्तो विड्भेदी कुम्भकामली |२२|
Signs of incurability of Kamala and Kumbha-kamala
The patient suffering from Kamala – jaundice will die soon if he has these symptoms – blackish-yellow faeces and urine, profound oedema, bleeding in the eyes and mouth; vomitus, faeces and urine also mixed with blood; loss of consciousness (fainting), burning sensation, anorexia, thirst, constipation or blockages caused in the stomach by ama or colon by impacted faeces, stupor, delusion, loss of digestion capacity and unconsciousness with.
The patient of kumbha kamala also dies if he has vomiting, anorexia, nausea, fever, debility, dyspnoea (increased / difficult respiration), cough or diarrhoea. (19-21)

Halimaka Symptoms
यदा तु पाण्डोर्वर्णः स्याद्धरितः श्यावपीतकः ||२२||
बलोत्साहक्षयस्तन्द्रा मन्दाग्नित्वं मृदुज्वरः |
स्त्रीष्वहर्षोऽङ्गमर्दश्च [१] दाहस्तृष्णाऽरुचिर्भ्रमः |
हलीमकं तदा तस्य विद्यादनिलपित्ततः ||२३||
When the colour of the skin (or nails, eyes, urine etc) of the patient of Pandu roga turns into yellow, green or blackish yellow colour, has loss of strength and enthusiasm, stupor, poor digestion, mild fever, disinterestedness in women (sex), pain in the body, burning sensation, thirst, anorexia, giddiness - the disease is to be known as halimaka (chlorosis) which is due to increased vata and pitta. (22-23)

Symptoms of Panaki
सन्तापो भिन्नवर्चस्त्वं बहिरन्तश्च पीतता |
पाण्डुता नेत्रयोर्यस्य पानकीलक्षणं भवेत्) |
(च. चि. अ. १६) |
(Fever, diarrhoea, yellow colouration both externally and internally and pale eyes - these are the symptoms of the disease called 'Panaki'.)
Thus ends the chapter on Panduroga, Kamala, etc.

इति श्रीमाधवकरविरचिते माधवनिदाने पाण्डुरोगकामलाकुम्भकामलाहलीमकनिदानं

समाप्तम् ||८||

Thus ends the chapter on Panduroga Kamala Kumbhakamala Halimaka Nidanam in Madhava Nidana text written by Acharya Madhavakara.

9

Madhava Nidana Chapter 9 Raktapitta Nidanam

Nidana and Samprapti – Etiological factors and pathogenesis of Raktapitta

घर्मव्यायामशोकाध्वव्यवायैरतिसेवितैः |
तीक्ष्णोष्णक्षारलवणैरम्लैः कटुभिरेव च ||१||
पित्तं विदग्धं स्वगुणैर्विदहत्याशु शोणितम् |
ततः प्रवर्तते रक्तमूर्ध्वं चाधो द्विधाऽपि वा ||२||
(सु. उ. तं. अ. ४५) |
ऊर्ध्वं नासाक्षिकर्णास्यैर्मेढ्रयोनिगुदैरधः |
कुपितं रोमकूपैश्च समस्तैस्तत्प्रवर्तते ||३||

Etiological factors of raktapitta include excessive exposure to sunlight, physical exercise, grief, walking long distances, excessive sexual intercourse; consumption of foods which are hot, alkaline, salty, sour and pungent.

Pathogenesis - All the above said causative factors when consumed lead to abnormal increase of pitta in its vidagdha state (by its uşna, tīksna properties). This aggravated pitta afflicts rakta – blood and quickly causes increase of blood and causes it to flow out of the body through upper or lower orifices or through both these orifices, viz, nostrils, eyes, ears and mouth being the upper passages and the urethra, vagina, rectum being the lower passages. In severe conditions, blood comes out of the hair follicles of the skin also.(1-3)

Purvarupa

सदनं शीतकामित्वं कण्ठधूमायनं वमिः ।
लोहगन्धिश्च निःश्वासो भवत्यस्मिन् भविष्यति ।।४।।
(सु. उ. तं. अ. ४५) ।

Weakness, desire for cold things (food, drink, places, etc.,) feeling as though hot fumes are coming out of the throat, vomiting, smell of iron in the breath – are the premonitory symptoms of Raktapitta. (4)

Dosha association in Raktapitta

सान्द्रं सपाण्डु सस्नेहं पिच्छिलं च कफान्वितम् ।५। (च. चि. अ. ४) ।
श्यावारुणं सफेनं च तनु रूक्षं च वातिकम् ।।५।। (च. चि. अ. ४) ।
रक्तपित्तं कषायाभं कृष्णं गोमूत्रसन्निभम् ।
मेचकागारधूमाभमञ्जनाभं च पैत्तिकम् ।।६।। (च. चि. अ. ४) ।
संसृष्टलिङ्गं संसर्गात्त्रिलिङ्गं सान्निपातिकम् । (च. चि. अ. ४) ।

If kapha is associated, the blood coming out will be thick, yellowish, white, greasy and sticky.

If vāta is associated, the blood will be blackish red, frothy, thin and viscid.

If pitta alone is the cause, the blood coming out will be black resembling decoction of drugs, cow's urine, and black pigment of a cymbal, chimney soot or antimony.

If there is a combination of two or three doshas their specific symptoms are also found together. (5-6)

ऊर्ध्वगं कफसंसृष्टमधोगं पवनानुगम् ।
द्विमार्गं कफवाताभ्यामुभाभ्यामनुवर्तते ।।७।। (च. चि. अ. ४) ।

Dosha association in raktapitta having upward (urdhwaga) and downward (adhoga) course

The Urdhwaga Raktapitta (having upward course with bleeding from upward orifices) is by association of kapha

The Adhoga Raktapitta (having downward course and bleeding occurring from downward orifices) is by association of vāta.

Kapha and Väta together will cause for both the upward and downward movement (bleeding) of raktapitta.(7)

- Urdhwaga Raktapitta - Kapha dominant

- Adhoga Raktapitta - Vata dominant|
- Ubhayaga - Kapha and Vata dominant.

Prognosis

ऊर्ध्वं साध्यमधो याप्यमसाध्यं युगपद्गतम् |८| (सु. उ. तं. अ. ४५) |
एकमार्गं बलवतो नातिवेगं नवोत्थितम् ||८||
रक्तपित्तं सुखे काले साध्यं स्यान्निरुपद्रवम् | (च. चि. अ. ४) |

Upward one (raktapitta having upward course) is easy to cure.
Downward one (raktapitta having downward course) is manageable i.e. persists all through life and can be handled with effective treatments and medicines from time to time.
Raktapitta having its course in both directions is incurable.
Raktapitta is easy to treat, if bleeding occurs from any one passage, in persons who are strong, if bleeding is not large, if it is of recent origin, if seen in good season (favourable season for its cure) and if not associated with other complications. (8)

एकदोषानुगं साध्यं द्विदोषं याप्यमुच्यते ||९||
यत्त्रिदोषमसाध्यं [१] स्यान्मन्दाग्नेरतिवेगवत् |
व्याधिभिः क्षीणदेहस्य वृद्धस्यानश्नतश्च यत् ||१०||
(च. चि. अ. ४) |

Raktapitta is easy to treat if only one dosha is associated, is manageable (persists for life) if two doshas are associated and incurable if all the three doshas are involved. Likewise in persons having poor digestive functions where bleeding is copious; in persons debilitated by other diseases, who are of advanced age and who do not take any food, raktapitta is incurable. (9-10)

Upadrava – complications of raktapitta

दौर्बल्यश्वासकासज्वरवमथुमदाः पाण्डुतादाहमूर्छा,
भुक्ते घोरो विदाहस्त्वधृतिरपि सदा हृद्यतुल्या च पीडा |
तृष्णा कोष्ठस्य भेदः शिरसि च तपनं पूतिनिष्ठीवनत्वं,
भक्तद्वेषाविपाकौ विकृतिरपि भवेद्रक्तपित्तोपसर्गाः ||११||
(सु. उ. तं. अ. ४५) |

Debility, dyspnoea (increased / difficult respiration), cough, fever, vomiting, intoxication, pallor (yellowish-white discoloration), burning sensation, fainting, severe heart-burn after consumption of food, constant anxiety, severe pain near the heart, thirst, tearing pain in the abdomen, headache, bad smelling sputum coming out, aversion to food and indigestion and abnormal colour of the blood, are the complications of raktapitta. (11)

Signs of incurability

मांसप्रक्षालनाभं कुथितमिव च यत् कर्दमाम्भोनिभं वा,
मेदःपूयास्रकल्पं यकृदिव यदि वा पक्वजम्बूफलाभम् |
यत् कृष्णं यच्च नीलं भृशमतिकुणपं यत्र चोक्ता विकारा
स्तद्वर्ज्यं रक्तपित्तं सुरपतिधनुषा यच्च तुल्यं विभाति ||१२||(सु. उ. तं. अ. ४५) |

Patients in whom the blood coming out resembles water in which mutton has been washed, a decoction, muddy water with lot of silt, fat, pus, pieces of liver, ripe fruit of jambu (Eugenia jambolana), which is black or blue in color, which smells like a cadaver, or resembles a rainbow and who have one or more of the complications cited above - are to be refused treatment (i.e. in the presence of the above mentioned signs, raktapitta is considered as incurable and hence the physician shall refuse treating such patients). (12)

येन चोपहतो रक्तं रक्तपित्तेन मानवः |
पश्येद्दृश्यं वियच्चापि तच्चासाध्यमसंशयम् ||१३||
(च. नि. अ. २) |
लोहितं छर्दयेद्यस्तु बहुशो लोहितेक्षणः |
लोहितोद्गारदर्शी च म्रियते रक्तपैत्तिकः ||१४||
(सु. सू. अ. ३३) |

If the patient (of raktapitta) sees everything visible (visible objects) and invisible (space, sky etc and those which doesn't have any colour) as red in colour, raktapitta should be considered as incurable.

If the patient of raktapitta vomits blood in large quantity, who sees everything as red, who gets belching accompanied with bleeding (or gets belching having the smell of iron) is going to die (i.e., such raktapitta conditions are definitely incurable and would lead to death). (13-14)

इति श्रीमाधवकरविरचिते माधवनिदाने रक्तपित्तनिदानं समाप्तम् ||९||

Thus ends the chapter on Raktapitta Nidanam in Madhava Nidana text written by Acharya Madhavakara.

10

Madhava Nidana Chapter 10 Rajayakshma Kshatakshina Nidanam

4 main causes of Rajayakshma

वेगरोधात् क्षयाच्चैव साहसाद्विषमाशनात् |
त्रिदोषो जायते यक्ष्मा गदो हेतुचतुष्टयात् ||१||

Yakshma is a disease caused by all the three doshas together. Below mentioned are the four important factors which would produce yakshma

1. Suppression of natural urges
2. Loss or deficiency of tissues
3. Over-exertion and
4. Indulgence in unhealthy foods (1)

Samprapti – pathogenesis of Yakshma

कफप्रधानैर्दोषैस्तु रुद्धेषु रसवर्त्मसु |
अतिव्यवायिनो वाऽपि क्षीणे रेतस्यनन्तराः |
क्षीयन्ते धातवः सर्वे ततः शुष्यति मानवः ||२||

Pathogenesis of Yakshma

There are two pathways in which Yakshma develops

When the rasavaha srotas become obstructed by the tridoshas among which kapha is predominant or
In persons who indulge in excessive sexual intercourse leading to the loss of semen
When these events occur, they cause deficiency of all the other dhātus – tissues of the body making the person too emaciated. Such a disease is called Yakshma or rajayakshma. (2)

Purvarupa

श्वासाङ्गमर्दकफसंस्रवतालुशोषवम्यग्निसादमदपीनसकासनिद्राः |
शोषे भविष्यति भवन्ति स चापि जन्तुः शुक्लेक्षणो भवति मांसपरो रिरंसुः ||३||
(सु. उ. तं. अ. ४१) |
स्वप्नेषु काकशुकशल्लकिनीलकण्ठा गृध्रास्तथैव कपयः कृकलासकाश्च |
तं वाहयन्ति स नदीर्विजलाश्च पश्येच्छुष्कांस्तरून् पवनधूमदवार्दितांश्च ||४||
(सु. उ. तं. अ. ४१) |

The premonitory symptoms of rajayakshma include - dyspnoea (breathlessness, increased / difficult respiration), pain in the body, expectoration of sputum, dryness of the palate, vomiting, poor digestion, intoxication, running nose, cough, excessive sleep, eyes becoming bright white; person craves for meat and sexual intercourse. In his dreams he sees himself being carried away by the crow, parrot, porcupine, peacock vultures, monkey and chameleon, sees rivers without water, trees without leaves, breeze, smoke and forest fires. (3-4)

Symptoms of Rajayakshma

अंसपार्श्वाभितापश्च सन्तापः करपादयोः |
ज्वरः सर्वाङ्गगश्चेति लक्षणं राजयक्ष्मणः ||५|| (च. चि. अ. ८) |
(भक्तद्वेषो ज्वरः श्वासः कासः शोणितदर्शनम् |
स्वरभेदश्च जायेत षड्रूपं राजयक्ष्मणि) |६|

Discomfort (pain) in the scapular region (shoulders) and flanks, feeling of warmth (mild burning sensation) in the hands and feet, fever all over the body are the symptoms of rājavaksmā.(5)
(According to other opinions - aversion to food, fever, dyspnoea or increased / difficult respiration, cough appearance of blood in the sputum and hoarseness of voice are the six symptoms of rajayakshma.)

Ekadasha Lakshanas

स्वरभेदोऽनिलाच्छूलं सङ्कोचश्चांसपार्श्वयोः |
ज्वरो दाहोऽतिसारश्च पित्ताद्रक्तस्य चागमः ||६|| (सु. उ. तं. अ. ४१) |
शिरसः परिपूर्णत्वमभक्तच्छन्द एव च |
कासः कण्ठस्य चोद्ध्वंसो विज्ञेयः कफकोपतः ||७|| (सु. उ. तं. अ. ४१) |

Symptoms caused by Vata predominance are 3 in number - Hoarseness of voice, pain in the shoulders, constriction (deformity) of shoulders and flanks.
Symptoms caused by Pitta predominance are 4 in number - Fever, burning sensation, diarrhoea and blood in the sputum (haemoptysis).
Symptoms caused by Kapha predominance are 4 in number - Feeling of fullness of the head, aversion to food, cough and irritation in the throat.
These are the (eleven) important symptoms of Rajayakshma. (6-7)

6 symptoms, 3 symptoms, Prognosis

एकादशभिरेभिर्वा षड्भिर्वाऽपि समन्वितम् |
कासातीसारपार्श्वार्तिस्वरभेदारुचिज्वरैः ||८||
त्रिभिर्वा पीडितं लिङ्गैः कासश्वासासृगामयैः |
जह्याच्छोषार्दितं जन्तुमिच्छन् सुविमलं यशः ||९||
(सु. उ. तं. अ. ४१) |
सर्वैरर्धैस्त्रिभिर्वाऽपि लिङ्गैर्मांसबलक्षये |
युक्तो वर्ज्यश्चिकित्स्यस्तु सर्वरूपोऽप्यतोऽन्यथा ||१०||
महाशनं क्षीयमाणमतीसारनिपीडितम् |
शूनमुष्कोदरं चैव यक्ष्मिणं परिवर्जयेत् ||११||
शुक्लाक्षमन्नद्वेष्टारमूर्ध्वश्वासनिपीडितम् |
कृच्छ्रेण बहुमेहन्तं यक्ष्मा हन्तीह मानवम् ||१२||

Presence of all the eleven symptoms (enumerated above) or the six symptoms viz., cough diarrhoea, pain in the flanks, hoarseness of voice, anorexia and fever or even the three symptoms viz., cough, dyspnoea (increased / difficult respiration and appearance of blood in the sputum - calls for refusal of such patients by physicians desiring a good reputation.
This means to say that in the presence of all these symptoms together will indicate bad prognosis and hence the doctor can deny treating such conditions by the physicians who want to keep away from getting a bad name and reputation.
Appearance of all the symptoms (11 symptoms), or half of it (six – approximately half of eleven) or of even three, in persons who have loss

of muscles (wasting of muscles) and strength are also indications of bad prognosis and hence should be refused by a wise physician.

Patients of yakshma who eat large quantities of food but still undergo wasting; who are having diarrhoea, swelling of the scrotum and abdomen are also to be avoided (denied treatment).

Yakshma kills such persons who have whiteness of eyes, aversion to food, heavy and troublesome expirations and who eliminate large quantities of urine with difficulty. (8-12)

Conditions for treating the patients of Rajayakshma

ज्वरानुबन्धरहितं बलवन्तं क्रियासहम् |
उपक्रमेदात्मवन्तं दीप्ताग्निमकृशं नरम् ||१३||
(सु. उ. तं. अ. ४१) |

Treatment can be given to patients of yakshma who do not have fever, who are strong, able to withstand the discomforts of treatments, of strong will, good (strong) digestive capacity and who are not emaciated.(13)

Types of Shosha

व्यवायशोकवार्धक्यव्यायामाध्वप्रशोषितान् |
व्रणोरःक्षतसञ्ज्ञौ च शोषिणौ लक्षणैः शृणु ||१४||
(सु. उ. तं. अ. ४१) |

Shosha (consumption, wasting, emaciation) is of 7 types. They are caused due to –

sexual intercourse
grief
old age
physical exertion,
walking long distances,
ulcers and
injury to the chest

Henceforth the symptoms of the persons afflicted with above mentioned types of shoshas are described. (14)

Vyavaya Shosha Lakshanas

व्यवायशोषी शुक्रस्य क्षयलिङ्गैरुपद्रुतः |
पाण्डुदेहो यथापूर्वं क्षीयन्ते चास्य धातवः ||१५||
(सु. उ. तं. अ. ४१) |

Vyavaya Shosha Lakshanas – Symptoms of wasting caused due to excessive indulgence in sexual intercourse

In persons who indulge in excessive sexual intercourse, symptoms of deficiency of semen and yellowish white discolouration of the body (pallor) and subsequent wasting of the other tissues of the body are seen. (15)

Shoka Shosha, Jara Shosha Lakshanas

प्रध्यानशीलः स्रस्ताङ्गः शोकशोष्यपि तादृशः |१६| (सु. उ. तं. अ. ४१) |
जराशोषी कृशो मन्दवीर्यबुद्धिबलेन्द्रियः ||१६||
कम्पनोऽरुचिमान् भिन्नकांस्यपात्रहतस्वरः |
ष्ठीवति श्लेष्मणा हीनं गौरवारतिपीडितः ||१७||
सम्प्रस्रुतास्यनासाक्षिः शुष्करूक्षमलच्छविः |
(सु. उ. तं. अ. ४१) |

Symptoms of wasting caused due to grief & ageing

In people whose body is wasted due to excessive grief, too much of worry, looseness and weakness of the body are seen.

The symptoms of persons wasted due to senility (old age) include - emaciation, decrease of vigour, intellect, strength and capacity of sense organs; shaking of the body parts and anorexia. The voice of such a person would be husky, feeble and broken as that of a piece of broken bronze vessel. The patient tries hard to expectorate but brings out little sputum or no sputum. The other symptoms are heaviness of the body, restlessness, fluid oozing out of mouth, nose and eyes, loss of complexion and dryness (of faeces).(16-17)

Adhwa Shosha Lakshanas

अध्वशोषी च स्रस्ताङ्गः सम्भृष्टपरुषच्छविः ||१८||
प्रसुप्तगात्रावयवः शुष्कक्लोमगलाननः |
(सु. उ. तं. अ. ४१) |

Symptoms of wasting due to constant long-distance walking

Persons wasted due to constant long-distance walking will be having weakness, hardness and loss of sensation of body parts, dryness of klomā, throat and mouth. (18)

Note – Kloma is an organ whose description has not been detailed in Ayurveda texts. As per this context and kloma being one of the roots of 'water transporting channels' in the body, it can be considered as pharynx or palate (roof of the inside of the mouth).

Vyayama Shosha

व्यायामशोषी भूयिष्ठमेभिरेव समन्वितः |
लिङ्गैरुरःक्षतकृतैः संयुक्तश्च क्षतं विना ||१९||
(सु. उ. तं. अ. ४१) |

Symptoms of wasting caused due to excessive physical exertion

Persons wasted due to excess physical exertion will also have the same symptoms as above and symptoms of injury to the chest without of course an actual tear. (19)

Vrana Shosha

रक्तक्षयाद्वेदनाभिस्तथैवाहारयन्त्रणात् |
व्रणितस्य भवेच्छोषः स चासाध्यतमो मतः ||२०||
(सु. उ. तं. अ. ४१) |

Symptoms of wasting caused due to ulcer / wound

Wasting due to ulcer is caused by loss of blood, pain and control over food by the person. This condition is difficult to treat.(20)

Urah Kshata - Nidana, Lakshanas

धनुषाऽऽयस्यतोऽत्यर्थं भारमुद्वहतो गुरुम् |
युध्यमानस्य बलिभिः पततो विषमोच्चतः ||२१||
वृषं हयं वा धावन्तं दम्यं वाऽन्यं निगृह्णतः |
शिलाकाष्ठाश्मनिर्घातान् क्षिपतो निघ्नतः परान् ||२२||
अधीयानस्य वाऽत्युच्चैर्दूरं वा व्रजतो द्रुतम् |
महानदीर्वा तरतो हयैर्वा सह धावतः ||२३||
सहसोत्पततो दूरं तूर्णं वाऽपि प्रनृत्यतः |
तथाऽन्यैः कर्मभिः क्रूरैर्भृशमभ्याहतस्य वा ||२४||
विक्षते वक्षसि व्याधिर्बलवान् समुदीर्यते |
स्त्रीषु चातिप्रसक्तस्य रूक्षाल्पप्रमिताशिनः ||२५||
उरो विभज्यतेऽत्यर्थं भिद्यतेऽथ विरुज्यते |
प्रपीड्यते ततः पार्श्वे शुष्यत्यङ्गं प्रवेपते ||२६||
क्रमाद्वीर्यं बलं वर्णो रुचिरग्निश्च हीयते |
ज्वरो व्यथा मनोदैन्यं विड्भेदाग्निवधावपि ||२७||
दुष्टः श्यावः सुदुर्गन्धः पीतो विग्रथितो बहुः |
कासमानस्य चाभीक्ष्णं कफः सासृक् प्रवर्तते ||२८||

स क्षती क्षीयतेऽत्यर्थं तथा शुक्रौजसोः क्षयात् |
(च. चि. अ. १६) |

Causes and symptoms of 'chest injury'

Chest injury (tear inside the lungs) is caused due to one or more of - excessive indulgence in archery, carrying heavy loads on the head, combating / wrestling with strong persons, falling from a height recklessly, forcibly trying to stop a mighty bull or horse which is running, or taming wild animals, throwing heavy stones, wooden rafters or catapults, fighting with enemies (using weapons),reading loudly with high pitch, running fast for long distances, swimming mighty rivers, running along with horses, sudden jumping, strenuous dancing and such other acts of violence and excessive sexual intercourse, partaking of dry, scanty and non-nutritious foods.

As a result, the patient will have cut or pricking pain in the chest and flanks, followed by emaciation, tremors; loss of vigour, strength, complexion, interest and digestive capacity. There also occurs the appearance of fever, grief, helplessness, diarrhoea, indigestion, cough with bad, black, fetid, yellowish pellets of sputum in large quantities coming out often mixed with blood. This condition is known as 'uraksata'. This condition causes quick loss of sukra (semen) and ojas (essence of all the tissues) and leads to severe emaciation.(20-28)

Purvarupa

अव्यक्तं लक्षणं तस्य पूर्वरूपमिति स्मृतम् ||२९||

Premonitory symptoms

The very symptoms of this disease itself are seen in mild form during the premonitory period. (29)

Difference between Ksata and Ksina

उरोरुक् शोणितच्छर्दिः कासो वैशेषिकः क्षते |
क्षीणे सरक्तमूत्रत्वं पार्श्वपृष्ठकटीग्रहः ||३०||
(च. चि. अ. १६) |

Pain in the chest, vomiting of blood, cough is prominent if ksata - trauma (tear) is present. On the other hand, if only emaciation is present, urine mixed with blood, catching pain in the flanks, back and waist (hips) are predominant. (30)

Prognosis

अल्पलिङ्गस्य दीप्ताग्नेः साध्यो बलवतो नवः |
परिसंवत्सरो याप्यः सर्वलिङ्गं तु वर्जयेत् ||३१||
(च. चि. अ. १६) |

Uraksata which has mild symptoms, manifesting in strong persons, is of recent origin and occurring in whom the digestive capacity is good is curable.

Uraksata which has remained over one year (one year old), does persist throughout life, and that which has all the symptoms is incurable. (31)

इति श्रीमाधवकरविरचिते माधवनिदाने राजयक्ष्मक्षतक्षीणनिदानं समाप्तम् ||१०||

Thus ends the chapter on RājayaksmāNidanam in Madhava Nidana text written by Acharya Madhavakara.

11

Madhava Nidana Chapter 11 Kasa Nidanam

Kasa Nidana, Samprapti

धूमोपघाताद्रसतस्तथैव व्यायामरूक्षान्ननिषेवणाच्च |
विमार्गगत्वाच्च हि भोजनस्य वेगावरोधात् क्षवथोस्तथैव ||१||
प्राणो ह्युदानानुगतः प्रदुष्टः स भिन्नकांस्यस्वनतुल्यघोषः |
निरेति वक्त्रात् सहसा सदोषो मनीषिभिः कास इति प्रदिष्टः ||२||
(सु. उ. तं. अ. ५२) |

Smoke entering the nose, mouth and throat and harming these organs
Dust entering the nose, mouth and throat and harming these organs
Excessive indulgence in exercises (strenuous physical activities)
Excessive consumption of foods which are dry in nature
Entry of the consumed food into wrong passages (respiratory passages – trachea etc.)
Suppression of natural urges of the body
Suppression / forcibly controlling the sneezing urge

Pathogenesis of Kasa

The prana vata aggravated due to the above said etiological factors gets mixed (associated) with udana vata and comes out of the mouth suddenly, along with the other doshas (pitta and kapha), producing a sound resembling that made by obstructing (or hitting against) a broken piece of bronze. This disease is called kāsa. (1-2)

Kasa Bheda

पञ्च कासाः स्मृता वातपित्तश्लेष्मक्षतक्षयैः ।
क्षयायोपेक्षिताः सर्वे बलिनश्चोत्तरोत्तरम् ॥३॥
(अ. हृ. नि. अ. ३) ।

Types of coughs

Kāsa is of five kinds –

Vataja kasa – caused by predominant vitiation of vata
Pittaja kasa – caused by predominant aggravation of pitta
Kaphaja kasa – caused by predominant aggravation of kapha
Kshataja kasa – caused due to the chest injury
Kshayaja kasa – caused due to loss of tissues

The first four types of kasa if neglected will lead to kshaya (dhātukshaya-wasting of the tissues). These five types of kasa are stronger (dangerous, damaging, harmful) in the successive order. (3)

Note – Going with strength of kasa as mentioned in the above said context –

Pittaja Kasa is stronger than Vataja Kasa.
Kaphaja Kasa is stronger than Pittaja Kasa.
Kshataja Kasa is stronger than Kaphaja Kasa.
Kshayaja Kasa is stronger than Kshataja Kasa.

Therefore, Kshayaja Kasa is more powerful and troublesome amongst all the kasa and Vataja Kasa is the least troublesome one. The prognosis of kasa also will follow the same chronology.

Purvarupa

पूर्वरूपं भवेत्तेषां शूकपूर्णगलास्यता ।
कण्ठे कण्डूश्च भोज्यानामवरोधश्च जायते ॥४॥
(च. चि. अ. २२) ।

Premonitory symptoms of cough

Premonitory symptoms (of cough) are - feeling as if the throat and mouth are filled with thorns / spikes and (pricking inside these organs), itching sensation inside the throat and obstruction to inward movement of food (swallowing). (4)

Vataja Kasa symptoms

हृच्छङ्खमूर्धोदरपार्श्वशूली क्षामाननः क्षीणबलस्वरौजाः ।

प्रसक्तवेगस्तु समीरणेन भिन्नस्वरः कासति शुष्कमेव ||५||
(सु. उ. तं. अ. ५२) |
In Vatika Kasa, the person suffers from - pain in the region of the heart, temples, head, abdomen and flanks; dry face (mouth), loss of strength, voice and ojas. The person will have continuous bouts of husky (small) and dry cough, and cracked voice due to aggravation of vata. (5)

Pittaja Kasa symptoms

उरोविदाहज्वरवक्त्रशोषैरभ्यर्दितस्तिक्तमुखस्तृषार्तः |
पित्तेन पीतानि वमेत् कटूनि कासेत् सपाण्डुः परिदह्यमानः ||६||
(सु. उ. तं. अ. ५२) |
In pittaja kasa, the person will have a burning sensation in the chest, fever, dryness of the mouth, bitter taste in the mouth, severe thirst, and bitter taste in the mouth, severe thirst, vomiting with the contents appearing yellow in colour and bitter in taste, anaemia and burning sensation inside the body. (6)

Kaphaja Kasa symptoms

प्रलिप्यमानेन मुखेन सीदन् शिरोरुजार्तः कफपूर्णदेहः |
अभक्तरुग्गौरवकण्डुयुक्तः कासेद्भृशं सान्द्रकफः कफेन ||७||
(सु. उ. तं. अ. ५२) |
The symptoms of kaphaja kasa are – inside of the mouth is coated with thick secretions (saliva), weakness, headache, accumulation of kapha in the entire body, anorexia / tastelessness, heaviness, itching, heavy cough along with expectoration of thick sputum. (7)

Kshataja Kasa causes, symptoms

अतिव्यवायभाराध्वयुद्धाश्वगजविग्रहैः |
रूक्षस्योरःक्षतं वायुर्गृहीत्वा कासमाचरेत् ||८||
स पूर्वं कासते शुष्कं ततः ष्ठीवेत् सशोणितम् |
कण्ठेन रुजताऽत्यर्थं विरुग्णेनेव चोरसा ||९||
सूचीभिरिव तीक्ष्णाभिस्तुद्यमानेन शूलिना |
दुःखस्पर्शेन शूलेन भेदपीडाभितापिना ||१०||
पर्वभेदज्वरश्वासतृष्णावैस्वर्यपीडितः |
पारावत इवाकूजन् [१] कासवेगात् क्षतोद्भवात् ||११||
(सु. उ. तं. अ. ५२) |

Etiological Factors – Excessive indulgence in sexual intercourse, carrying heavy weights, walking long distances, wrestling, taming or fighting with horses and elephants (forcibly trying to stop the running of horses and elephants) etc. are the causative factors of kshataja kasa.

Pathogenesis – The above-mentioned etiological factors cause injury in the chest (tear in the lungs) in a person who is dry (weak). The aggravated vata reaches the site of injury and produces cough.

Symptoms

Initially the person suffers from dry cough. Later this is followed by expectoration of blood mixed sputum.

The other symptoms include –

Severe pain in the throat

Severe pain in the chest

The person feels as if he is pricked by sharp needles in the chest (and throat) / cutting or gnawing pain

Intolerance to touch (the patient resists others from touching the afflicted area, painful area) / tenderness,

Splitting pain and pain associated with burning sensation

Splitting pain in the small joints of the hands and feet (interphalangeal joints),

Fever

Dyspnoea

Severe thirst

Hoarseness (change of) of voice

Makes sounds from the throat resembling that of a pigeon (8-11)

Kshayaja Kasa causes, symptoms

विषमासात्म्यभोज्यातिव्यवायाद्वेगनिग्रहात् |
घृणिनां शोचतां नृणां व्यापन्नेऽग्नौ त्रयो मलाः |
कुपिताः क्षयजं कासं कुर्युर्देहक्षयप्रदम् ||१२||
स गात्रशूलज्वरदाहमोहान् प्राणक्षयं चोपलभेत कासी |
शुष्यन् विनिष्ठीवति दुर्बलस्तु प्रक्षीणमांसो रुधिरं सपूयम् |
तं सर्वलिङ्गं भृशदुश्चिकित्स्यं चिकित्सितज्ञाः क्षयजं वदन्ति ||१३||
(सु. उ. तं. अ. ५२) |

Etiological factors - Indulgence in irregular and untimely meals, unaccustomed foods, indulgence in excessive sex, suppression of bodily urges, too much jealousy, grief, etc.

Pathogenesis – Due to the above said etiological factors, the digestive fire gets contaminated. This fire in turn causes aggravation of all the three doshas. These aggravated dosas produce kshayaja kasa which would cause destruction of the body (wasting of body tissues).
Symptoms – Kshayaja Kasa would present with symptoms including pain in the body parts (all over the body), fever, burning sensation, delusion & threat to life. There occurs severe dryness / wasting of the body, extreme weakness, deterioration (destruction) of strength and muscles, and the patient expectorates blood with pus as he coughs. This form of cough having all the symptoms (symptoms caused by all three doshas) and is difficult to cure is called by the name Kshayaja Kasa by the clinical experts who are well versed in the knowledge of treatment principles (of Ayurveda). This cough would kill the weak ones. (12-14)

Prognosis

साध्यो बलवतां वा स्याद्याप्यस्त्वेवं क्षतोत्थितः ||१४||
नवौ कदाचित्सिध्येतामपि पादगुणान्वितौ |
स्थविराणां जराकासः सर्वो याप्यः प्रकीर्तितः |
त्रीन् पूर्वान् साधयेत् साध्यान् पथ्यैर्याप्यांस्तु यापयेत् ||१५||
(सु. उ. तं. अ. ५२) |

In strong people this cough (kshayaja) is sometimes curable and sometimes manageable.
Similarly, the kshataja kasa caused by chest injury is curable in weak and emaciated patients. It is sometimes curable and sometimes manageable in strong patients.
Kshayaja or Kshataja Kasa of recent origin are sometimes curable if the four limbs of treatment (physician, patient, medicines and attendants) are bestowed with good qualities and are operational towards cure of the disease.
All kinds of kasa caused due to ageing (and natural depletion of tissues occurring in the old age) are manageable in older persons if the four limbs of treatment are bestowed with good qualities.
The first three kinds of kasa (i.e., vataja, pittaja and kaphaja) are easily curable. Therefore, they shall be treated. The manageable kinds (chronic) of kasa shall be controlled by using a suitable diet etc. (15)

इति श्रीमाधवकरविरचिते माधवनिदाने कासनिदानं समाप्तम् ||११||

Thus ends the chapter on Kāsa Nidanam in Madhava Nidana text written by Acharya Madhavakara.

12

Madhava Nidana Chapter 12 Hikka Shwasa Nidanam

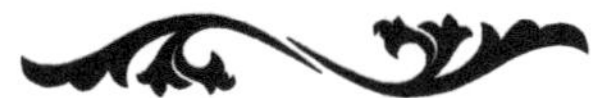

Hikka Swasa Nidanam

विदाहिगुरुविष्टम्भिरूक्षाभिष्यन्दिभोजनैः ।
शीतपानाशनस्थानरजोधूमातपानिलैः ॥१॥
व्यायामकर्मभाराध्ववेगाघातापतर्पणैः ।
हिक्का श्वासश्च कासश्च नृणां समुपजायते ॥२॥
(सु. उ. तं. अ. ५०) ।

Etiological factors of hiccough and dyspnoea

Excessive indulgence in foods which are corrosive (produce heartburn), heavy (difficult to digest), which could cause constipation, dry in nature and which cause blockages in the pores of the tissues or channels of transportation,

Excessive consumption of very cold water (or other beverages) and foods,

Starvation,

Living in cold places

Exposure to dust, smoke, sunlight and breeze,

Excessive physical exercise / exertion

Indulgence in activities beyond one's capacity,

Lifting or carrying heavy weights,

Walking long distances,

Suppression of natural urges and

Malnutrition
The person who indulges in the above-mentioned etiological factors becomes victim of hikkā (hiccough), śwāsa (dyspnoea / difficult respiration) and kasa (cough).(1-2)

Definition/Meaning of Hikka

मुहुर्मुहुर्वायुरुदेति सस्वनो यकृत्प्लीहान्त्राणि मुखादिवाक्षिपन् |
स घोषवानाशु हिनस्त्यसून् यतस्ततस्तु हिक्केत्यभिधीयते बुधैः ||३||
(सु. उ. तं. अ. ५०) |

The aggravated Vāyu (udana along with prana vata) comes out of the mouth with immense velocity (speed), repeatedly, as if throwing the liver, spleen and intestines out of the mouth (the patient feels as if these organs are coming out of the mouth), it produces hik-hik sounds. Making the sounds in this way the vayu tends to cause harm to the life in quick time. Wise physicians call this disease as hikka (compared to hiccough). (3)

Types of Hikka

अन्नजां यमलां क्षुद्रां गम्भीरां महतीं तथा |
वायुः कफेनानुगतः पञ्च हिक्काः करोति हि ||४||
(सु. उ. तं. अ. ५०) |

Vāta associated with kapha produces hikkā. This hikka is of 5 types, they are –

- Annajā hikka
- Yamalā hikka
- Kshudrā hikka
- Gambhīrā hikka and
- Mahatī hikka (4)

Hikka Purvarupa

कण्ठोरसोर्गुरुत्वं च वदनस्य कषायता |
हिक्कानां पूर्वरूपाणि कुक्षेराटोप एव च ||५||
(च. चि. अ. २१) |

Premonitory symptoms of Hikka

Premonitory symptoms of hikkā are heaviness of throat and chest, astringent taste in the mouth and gurgling noise in the abdomen. (5)

Annaja Hikka

पानान्नैरतिसंयुक्तैः सहसा पीडितोऽनिलः |
हिक्कयत्यूर्ध्वगो भूत्वा तां विद्यादन्नजां भिषक् ||६||
(सु. उ. तं. अ. ५०) |

This type of hikka is caused by excessive consumption of foods and drinks too quickly. Such foods and drinks taken in excess immediately impart pressure on vata. Thus, vata gets aggravated and moves in upward direction and causes hikka. Such a hikka caused by anna (foods and drinks) is called as Annajā hikkā. (6)

Yamala Hikka

चिरेण यमलैर्वेगैर्या हिक्का सम्प्रवर्तते |
कम्पयन्ती शिरोग्रीवं यमलां तां विनिर्दिशेत् ||७||
(सु. उ. तं. अ. ५०) |

Yamala means two. Yamalā hikkā (its bouts) occur in pairs.

The hikka which occurs while causing shaking of head and neck, continues for a long time (repeatedly occurs, after breaks, intermittently) and occurs in pairs (produces two sounds of hik at a time, one after the other) is called Yamala hikka.(7)

Kshudra Hikka

प्रकृष्टकालैर्या वेगैर्मन्दैः समभिवर्तते |
क्षुद्रिका नाम सा हिक्का जत्रुमूलात् प्रधाविता ||८||
(सु. उ. तं. अ. ५०) |

Kshudrā hikkā is that which occurs occasionally (after long gaps), whose bouts are mild in intensity, and starts only from the base of the neck (junction of neck and chest). (8)

Gambhira Hikka

नाभिप्रवृत्ता या हिक्का घोरा गम्भीरनादिनी |
अनेकोपद्रववती गम्भीरा नाम सा स्मृता ||९||
(सु. उ. तं. अ. ५०) |

Gambhirā hikkā, which starts from deep inside the umbilicus, is very powerful, makes heavy sound and is accompanied with many complications. (9)

Maha Hikka

मर्माण्युत्पीडयन्तीव सततं या प्रवर्तते |
महाहिक्केति सा ज्ञेया सर्वगात्रविकम्पिनी ||१०||
(सु. उ. तं. अ. ५०) |

Mahāhikkā is that which produces powerful feeling as though all the vital organs are being pulled out of the body, continuously persists without giving a break, and causes tremors / shaking of the whole body.(10)

Symptoms of incurability of Hikka

आयम्यते हिक्कतो यस्य देहो दृष्टिश्चोर्ध्वं नाम्यते यस्य नित्यम् |
क्षीणोऽन्नद्विट् क्षौति यश्चातिमात्रं तौ द्वौ चान्त्यौ वर्जयेद्धिक्कमानौ ||११||

Patients of hikkā who have developed excessive stretching of the entire body, has gaze fixed in upward direction (or gets constricted) and the body always bent, is emaciated, has aversion towards food, has many bouts of sneezing and who has the last two types of hikka i.e., gambhira and mahati. These people shall be refused treatment (because this condition is incurable). (11)

अतिसञ्चितदोषस्य भक्तच्छेदकृशस्य च |
व्याधिभिः क्षीणदेहस्य वृद्धस्यातिव्यवायिनः ||१२||
आसां या सा समुत्पन्ना हिक्का हन्त्याशु जीवितम् |
यमिका च प्रलापार्तिमोहतृष्णासमन्विता ||१३||

The patient of hikka will succumb to death in quick time when there is excessive increase of all the doshas, he is unable to take food and hence has become emaciated, has become weak and debilitated as an effect of long-standing diseases, is aged, indulged in excessive sexual intercourse, who has yamala type of hikka, has delirium, pain, delusion and severe thirst. (12-13)

अक्षीणश्चाप्यदीनश्च स्थिरधात्विन्द्रियश्च यः |
तस्य साधयितुं शक्या यमिका हन्त्यतोऽन्यथा ||१४||
(च. चि. अ. २१) |

Yamalā hikkā is curable in those who are not emaciated (physically strong), who have strong mind, whose tissues and senses are good (and in a state of health), whereas it kills others (those who are weak physically and mentally, whose tissues and senses are not in a good state of health).(14)

Types of Swasa (dyspnoea)

महोर्ध्वच्छिन्नतमकक्षुद्रभेदैस्तु पञ्चधा |
भिद्यते स महाव्याधिः श्वास एको विशेषतः ||१५||
(सु. उ. तं. अ. ५१) |

Swasa which is counted as a mahāvyādhi (powerful disease) is a single entity (disease). But based on the different forms of its manifestation and on the basis of different kinds of etiological factors and symptoms swasa is mentioned to be of five kinds.
The five kinds of swasa are –

1. Mahatī Swasa
2. Urdhwa Swasa
3. Chinna Swasa
4. Tamaka Swasa and
5. Kshudra Swasa (15)

Dosha relationship with different kinds of swasa

(वाताधिको भवेत् क्षुद्रस्तमकस्तु कफोद्भवः |
कफवाताधिकश्चैव संसृष्टश्छिन्नसञ्ज्ञकः |
श्वासो मारुतसंसृष्टो महानूर्ध्वस्तथा(तो) मतः) |
(सु. उ. तं. अ. ५१) |

In Kshudra Swasa – vata is predominant (vataja)
In Tamaka Swasa – kapha is predominant (kaphaja)
In Chinna Swasa – Kapha and Vata are predominant (kapha-vataja)
In Mahat and Urdhva Swasa – Vata is predominant (vataja)
(Along with these, the other doshas are also associated – pitta)

Swasa Purvarupa

प्राग्रूपं तस्य हृत्पीडा शूलमाध्मानमेव च |
आनाहो वक्त्रवैरस्यं शङ्खनिस्तोद एव च ||१६||

The premonitory symptoms of Swasa are – pain in the region of the heart, abdominal colic and distension (tympanitis) and enlargement of abdomen / flatulence, bad taste in the mouth and pricking (throbbing) pain in the temples. (16)

Swasa Samprapti

यदा स्रोतांसि संरुध्य मारुतः कफपूर्वकः |
विष्वग्व्रजति संरुद्धस्तदा श्वासान् करोति सः ||१७||
(सु. उ. तं. अ. ५१) |

The vata being obstructed by kapha, travelling in abnormal directions causes obstruction of the channels carrying prana – vital air (passages inside the lungs) and begins to move in all directions producing the disease swasa. (17)

उद्धूयमानवतो यः शब्दवद्दुःखितो नरः |
उच्चैः श्वसिति संरुद्वो मत्तर्षभ इवानिशम् ||१८||
प्रनष्टज्ञानविज्ञानस्तथा विभ्रान्तलोचनः |
विवृताक्ष्याननो बद्धमूत्रवर्चा विशीर्णवाक् ||१९||
दीनः प्रश्वसितं चास्य दूराद्विज्ञायते भृशम् |
महाश्वासोपसृष्टस्तु क्षिप्रमेव विपद्यते ||२०||
(च. चि. अ. २१) |

Vata, having increased greatly moves upwards constantly and produces this condition called Maha swasa.

The patient afflicted by this condition would constantly breathe in producing heavy sounds resembling those produced by a mad or tired and intoxicated bull tied firmly to a peg, huffing and puffing along with pain.

The patient loses awareness and intellect; eyes begin to roll, with terrified looks and wide-open mouth. There will be obstruction to passage (excretion) of faeces and urine. The patient will have a broken voice (pronounces broken words with difficulty) and would feel helpless. The sounds of his breathing can be heard from a long distance. These are the symptoms of Maha Swasa. The person suffering from Maha Swasa will die soon. (18-20)

Symptoms of Urdhva Swasa

ऊर्ध्वं श्वसिति यो दीर्घं न च प्रत्याहरत्यधः |
श्लेष्मावृतमुखस्रोताः क्रुद्धगन्धवहार्दितः ||२१||
ऊर्ध्वदृष्टिर्विपश्यंस्तु विभ्रान्ताक्ष इतस्ततः |
प्रमुहृयन् वेदनार्तश्च शुक्लास्योऽरतिपीडितः ||२२||
ऊर्ध्वश्वासे प्रकुपिते हृयधःश्वासो निरुध्यते |

मुह्यतस्ताम्यतश्चोर्ध्वं श्वासस्तस्यैव हन्त्यसून् ||२३||
(च. चि. अ. २१) |

The person suffering from Urdhva Swasa will have long expiration (breathes out for a longer duration) but will be unable to breathe in (inspiration) easily.

The mouth and other passages will be filled up with sputum. The other symptoms will be produced by vata which has undergone severe aggravation.

The person looks with an upward gaze i.e., the eyes are fixed up. The eyeballs roll in different directions. He will faint repeatedly and suffers from pain. There is whitish discoloration of the face and the patient will get restless.

The expiration gets deep and exacerbated while the inspiration gets obstructed. Due to this the person gets repeatedly restless and experiences loss of consciousness. These are the features of Urdhva Swasa and this also kills the patient. (21-23)

Symptoms of Chinna Swasa

यस्तु श्वसिति विच्छिन्नं सर्वप्राणेन पीडितः |
न वा श्वसिति दुःखार्तो मर्मच्छेदरुगर्दितः ||२४||
आनाहस्वेदमूर्छार्तो दह्यमानेन बस्तिना |
विप्लुताक्षः परिक्षीणः श्वसन् रक्तैकलोचनः ||२५||
विचेताः परिशुष्कास्यो विवर्णः प्रलपन्नरः |
छिन्नश्वासेन विच्छिन्नः स शीघ्रं विजहात्यसून् ||२६||
(च. चि. अ. २९) |

Chinna means interrupted or broken. In Chinna Swasa the respiration (breathing pattern) is often interrupted in the middle. It takes immense effort for the person to breathe in this condition. In spite of all efforts the person is in distress because he breathes with interruptions. In this condition there will be severe pain in all the vital organs. Due to this pain the person will not be capable of breathing properly. Also, due to fear of the pain getting worsened, the person would not attempt at respiration.

The person also would suffer from abdominal distension (flatulence), perspiration and fainting (loss of consciousness), burning sensation in the urinary bladder, eyes filled with tears, emaciation, redness of one eye, loss of consciousness, dryness of the mouth, discolouration and delirium. These are the symptoms of Chinna Swasa. This condition also kills the patient in a quick time. (24-26)

Pathogenesis, Symptoms of Tamaka Swasa

प्रतिलोमं यदा वायुः स्रोतांसि प्रतिपद्यते |
ग्रीवां शिरश्च सङ्गृह्य श्लेष्माणं समुदीर्य च ||२७||
करोति पीनसं तेन रुद्धो घुर्घुरकं तथा |
अतीव तीव्रवेगं च श्वासं प्राणप्रपीडकम् ||२८||
प्रताम्यति स वेगेन तृष्यते सन्निरुध्यते |
प्रमोहं कासमानश्च स गच्छति मुहुर्मुहुः ||२९||
श्लेष्मण्यमुच्यमाने तु भृशं भवति दुःखितः |
तस्यैव च विमोक्षान्ते मुहूर्तं लभते सुखम् ||३०||
तथाऽस्योद्ध्वंसते कण्ठः कृच्छ्राच्छक्नोति भाषितुम् |
न चापि लभते निद्रां शयानः श्वासपीडितः ||३१||
पार्श्वे तस्यावगृह्णाति शयानस्य समीरणः |
आसीनो लभते सौख्यमुष्णं चैवाभिनन्दति ||३२||
उच्छ्रिताक्षो ललाटेन स्विद्यता भृशमार्तिमान् |
विशुष्कास्यो मुहुः श्वासो मुहुश्चैवावधम्यते ||३३||
मेघाम्बुशीतप्राग्वातैः श्लेष्मलैश्च विवर्धते |
स याप्यस्तमकः श्वासः साध्यो वा स्यान्नवोत्थितः ||३४||
(च. चि. अ. २१) |

Pathogenesis – The aggravated vata moves in the opposite direction i.e., upwards and enters the channels of transportation of prana (vital air). On reaching these passages vata grasps the head and neck and further aggravates the kapha therein. On aggravating the kapha and finding its association, vata (along with kapha) causes pinasa (running nose). The movements of vata are also blocked by kapha. This vata which is obstructed by kapha (in the respiratory passages) will produce bubbling sounds in the throat. This ultimately produces severe bouts of increased respirations (in number and intensity) which pose a threat to life. This condition is called Tamaka Swasa.

Symptoms

The person suffers from darkness in front of the eyes (feels as if he is surrounded by darkness), severe thirst, and becomes motionless.

The person loses consciousness and faints as an effect of continuous bouts of cough.

The patient remains restless and worried until the sputum is expelled. He

keeps trying hard to expel that sputum by coughing repeatedly. When due to repeated coughing the sputum gets expelled, the person finds momentary relief.
He would experience itching (obstruction) in the throat. He would be able to speak with great difficulty while putting constant effort. He will not be able to sleep when he lies down due to severe catching of breath (dyspnoea). This is also because the vayu (located in the flanks) creates severe pain in the flanks when he sleeps. He finds comfort when he comes back to sitting posture. (This is the only posture in which he finds relief).
He desires hot / warm comforts and when given he finds relief.
His eyes are wide open (swelling of eyes, upward gaze), there is sweating on the forehead and severe pain (in the chest).
There is dryness of the mouth.
He breathes in repeatedly and later breathes out putting all efforts and straining all his body parts with great difficulty and sounds.
The symptoms get increased during cloudy days, by use of cold water, getting exposed to the breeze flowing from the east and other kapha aggravating causative factors.
These are the symptoms of tamaka swasa. The disease is said to be yapya i.e., manageable (persists throughout life in spite of administering suitable treatment). This condition might also get cured if it is of very recent onset. (27-34)

Pratamaka Swasa

ज्वरमूर्छापरीतस्य विद्यात् प्रतमकं तु तम् |
उदावर्तरजोऽजीर्णक्लिन्नकायनिरोधजः ||३५||

When this disease i.e., tamaka swasa manifests along with fever and fainting (loss of consciousness), it will be called as Pratamaka Swasa.
Upward movement of vata in many channels (abdomen – alimentary tract) / reverse peristalsis,
Inhalation / exposure to dust
Indigestion (indigested foods, ama etc)
Increase of wetness or dampness of the body / excessive consumption of foods soaked in water
Suppression of urges of the body (35)

Santamaka Swasa

तमसा वर्धतेऽत्यर्थं शीतैश्चाशु प्रशाम्यति |
मज्जतस्तमसीवास्य विद्यात् सन्तमकं तु तम् ||३६||
(च. चि. अ. २१) |

When Tamaka Swasa is caused or gets increased (triggered) by tamas (darkness, contaminant of mind, inactivity, cloudy weather etc), makes the patient to go into a zone of darkness (the person feels as if he is entering into darkness or surrounded by darkness) and the symptoms get quickly subsided (patient gets comfort) by use of cold things, it is called as Santamaka Swasa. (36)

Symptoms of Kshudra Swasa

रूक्षायासोद्भवः कोष्ठे क्षुद्रो वात उदीरयन् |
क्षुद्रश्वासो न सोऽत्यर्थं दुःखेनाङ्गप्रबाधकः ||३७||
हिनस्ति न स गात्राणि न च दुःखो यथेतरे |
न च भोजनपानानां निरुणद्ध्युचितां गतिम् ||३८||
नेन्द्रियाणां व्यथां नापि काञ्चिदापादयेद्रुजम् |
स साध्य उक्तो, बलिनः सर्वे चाव्यक्तलक्षणाः ||३९||
(च. चि. अ. २१) |

Causes – Kshudra Swasa is caused due to consumption of dry foods and physical exertion.

Vata getting aggravated by above said etiological factors moves upwards and causes difficulty in respiration. Kshudra means less. Since this condition is caused by less causative factors and has less symptoms (of lesser strength and severity) it is called as kshudra swasa.

Symptoms – The symptoms and bouts are mild in nature. It does not trouble the patient like other kinds of swasa (explained above). It doesn't pose a threat to the life of the patient.

This swasa doesn't cause any obstruction in the passage of food and respiration (the person can swallow food and water easily). It doesn't interfere with the functioning of the sense organs (the power of perception of sense organs remains intact, and is not disturbed). It doesn't produce any other disease or pain in the form of complications.

Kshudra Swasa is curable.

The other kinds of swasa are curable when they manifest in strong persons and when the symptoms manifest in an unclear / incomplete way (are mild or when in earlier stages of manifestation). (37-39)

Prognosis of Swasa

क्षुद्रः साध्यो मतस्तेषां तमकः कृच्छ्र उच्यते |
त्रयः श्वासा न सिध्यन्ति तमको दुर्बलस्य च ||४०||
(सु. उ. तं. अ. ५१) |

Kshudra Swasa is curable. Tamaka Swasa is difficult to treat. The other three types of swasa are incurable. Tamaka Swasa occurring in weak persons is incurable. (40)

Dangerous nature of Swasa and Hikka

कामं प्राणहरा रोगा बहवो न तु ते तथा |
यथा श्वासश्च हिक्का च हरतः प्राणमाशु च ||४१||
(च. चि. अ. २१) |

There are many dreadful diseases which take away life, but no disease is as quick as swasa and hikka in taking away the life of the patients. (41)

इति श्रीमाधवकरविरचिते माधवनिदाने हिक्काश्वासनिदानं समाप्तम् ||१२||

Thus ends the chapter on Śwāsa-hikkā Nidanam in Madhava Nidana text written by Acharya Madhavakara.

13

Madhava Nidana Chapter 13 Swara Bheda Nidanam

Swara Bheda Nidana, Samprapti, Bheda – Etiological factors, pathogenesis and types of hoarseness of voice

अत्युच्चभाषणविषाध्ययनाभिघातसन्दूषणैः प्रकुपिताः पवनादयस्तु |
स्रोतःसु ते स्वरवहेषु गताः प्रतिष्ठां हन्युः स्वरं भवति चापि हि षड्विधः सः ||१||
(सु. उ. तं. अ. ५३) |
(वातादिभिः पृथक् सर्वैर्मेदसा च क्षयेण च) |

Etiological factors - Speaking in high pitch, effect of (consumption of) poisons, studying or reading loudly, injury and such other causes are considered to be the etiological factors of swara bheda – hoarseness of vata.

Types

Types – Swarabheda is of six kinds, one from each dosha (vata, pitta and kapha), one from combination of all the three doshas (tridoshaja / sannipataja), the fifth type caused by medas (adipose tissue) and the sixth form of swarabheda is caused by ksaya (depletion of body tissues).(1)

The six types of Swarabheda are –

1. Vataja Swarabheda
2. Pittaja Swarabheda
3. Kaphaja Swarabheda
4. Sannipataja Swarabheda

5. Ksayaja Swarabheda
6. Medoja Swarabheda

Symptoms

वातेन कृष्णनयनाननमूत्रवर्चा भिन्नं शनैर्वदति गर्दभवत् खरं च |२|
(सु. उ. तं. अ. ५३) |
पित्तेन पीतनयनाननमूत्रवर्चा ब्रूयाद्गलेन स च दाहसमन्वितेन ||२||
(सु. उ. तं. अ. ५३) |
ब्रूयात् कफेन सततं कफरुद्धकण्ठः स्वल्पं शनैर्वदति चापि दिवा विशेषात् |३|
(सु. उ. तं. अ. ५३) |
सर्वात्मके भवति सर्वविकारसम्पत् तं चाप्यसाध्यमृषयः स्वरभेदमाहुः ||३||
(सु. उ. तं. अ. ५३) |

Vataja Swarabheda Symptoms – The patient would have blackish discolouration of eye, face, urine and faeces. His voice is broken and he speaks slowly, with a harsh voice resembling that of a donkey.

Pittaja Swarabheda Symptoms – The patient would have yellowish discoloration of the eyes, face, urine and faeces. He would experience a burning sensation in the throat.

Kaphaja Swarabheda Symptoms – In this condition the throat of the patient is always obstructed by kapha (sputum, thick fluid). Due to this, the patient speaks slowly (indistinct, in low pitch). He can speak a little clearly during day time (the speech and voice are slightly better).

Tridoshaja / Sannipataja Swarabheda Symptoms – In this condition, all the symptoms of all the doshas coexist. According to the opinion of the great sages, this condition is incurable. (2-3)

Symptoms of Ksayaja and Medoja Swarabheda

धूप्येत वाक् क्षयकृते क्षयमाप्नुयाच्च वागेष चापि हतवाक् परिवर्जनीयः |४|
(सु. उ. तं. अ. ५३) |
अन्तर्गतस्वरमलक्ष्यपदं चिरेण मेदोऽन्वयाद्वदति दिग्धगलस्तृषार्तः ||४||(सु. उ. तं. अ. ५३) |

Ksayaja Swarabheda Symptoms - In this type of hoarseness of voice, the patient feels as if hot fumes are coming out of the throat and nose, andas an impact of ksaya (depletion of tissues and destruction of nerves supplying the throat) the voice is completely destroyed. Such a patient who has completely lost his voice shall not be treated because it is incurable.

Medoja Swarabheda Symptoms – In this type of hoarseness of voice, the patient will have a coating of fat inside the throat or over the vocal nerves. As a result, the voice appears to be stuck within the throat (appears as though coming from great depth, from deep inside the throat). Whatever the person speaks is not clear. Some words (syllables) are clear and some are not clear and the person speaks slowly. The person will suffer from severe thirst in this condition. (4)

Prognosis of Swarabheda

क्षीणस्य वृद्धस्य कृशस्य वाऽपि चिरोत्थितो यश्च सहोपजातः |
मेदस्विनः सर्वसमुद्भवश्च स्वरामयो यो न स सिद्धिमेति ||५||(सु. उ. तं. अ. ५३) |

Swarabhedam is incurable in persons who are very weak, aged and emaciated. Also, swarabheda which is long standing or congenital, or that which occurs in persons who are obese and that which is produced by all the three doshas together (tridoshaja or sannipataja swarabheda) is incurable.(5)

इति श्रीमाधवकरविरचिते माधवनिदाने स्वरभेदनिदानं समाप्तम् ||१३||

Thus ends the chapter on Swarabheda Nidanam in Madhava Nidana text written by Acharya Madhavakara.

14

Madhava Nidana Chapter 14 Arochaka Nidanam

Causes

वातादिभिः शोकभयातिलोभक्रोधैर्मनोघ्नाशनरूपगन्धैः|
अरोचकाः स्युः ... |१|
(च. चि. अ. २६) |

Arochaka (anorexia) is produced by the three doshas (vata, pita, kapha), excessive grief, fear, greed, anger and foods, the sight and smell of which are very unpleasant to the mind. (1)

Symptoms of Arochak

... परिहृष्टदन्तः कषायवक्त्रश्च मतोऽनिलेन ||१||
(च. चि. अ. २६) |
कट्वम्लमुष्णं विरसं च पूति पित्तेन विद्यात् ... |२|
(च. चि. अ. २६) |
... लवणं च वक्त्रम् |
माधुर्यपैच्छिल्यगुरुत्वशैत्यविबद्धसम्बद्धयुतं कफेन ||२||
(च. चि. अ. २६) |

Vataja Arochaka – presents with tingling in the teeth (and gums) & manifestation of astringent taste in the mouth.

Pittaja Arochaka – presents with manifestation of bitter and sour taste, warmth and bad smell in the mouth.

Kaphaja Arochaka – presents with manifestation of salty or sweet taste, stickiness, heaviness, coldness, stiffness and thick coating of kapha inside the mouth. (2)

Agantuja Arochaka

अरोचके शोकभयातिलोभक्रोधाद्यहृद्याशुचिगन्धजे स्यात् |
स्वाभाविकं चास्यमथारुचिश्च ... |३| (च. चि. अ. २६) |
... त्रिदोषजे नैकरसं भवेत्तु ||३|| (च. चि. अ. २६) |

Agantuja Arochaka is that which is caused due to grief, fear, excessive greed, excessive fear, anger and other mental affections, things unpleasant to mind (foods etc), unclean and dirty and foul-smelling things (foods). In this condition the taste of the mouth is normal. In spite of that, the person suffers from arochaka – anorexia.

Tridoshaja Arochaka

In tridosaja type of anorexia, the patient experiences many kinds of tastes (mixture of different tastes mentioned in doshaja types). (3)

Specific Dosha symptoms of Arochaka

हृच्छूलपीडनयुतं पवनेन, पित्तात्तृड्दाहचोषबहुलं, सकफप्रसेकम् |
श्लेष्मात्मकं, बहुरुजं बहुभिश्च विद्याद्वैगुण्यमोहजडताभिरथापरं च ||४|| (च. चि. अ. २६) |

Pain in the region of the heart is found in vātaja arochaka.
Thirst, burning sensation and local heat are found in pittaja arochaka.
In Kaphaja arochaka, excessive secretions / exudation from mouth, nose etc are found.
In tridoshaja type of arochaka many kinds of pain and discomforts are experienced.
Confused state of mind, delusion / fainting and dullness of the mind are the symptoms which are predominantly found in arochaka caused due to grief etc causes (agantuja arochaka). (4)

इति श्रीमाधवकरविरचिते माधवनिदाने अरोचकनिदानं समाप्तम् ||१४||

Thus ends the chapter on Arochaka Nidanam in Madhava Nidana text written by Acharya Madhavakara.

15

Madhava Nidana Chapter 15 Chardi Nidanam

Types

दुष्टैर्दोषैः पृथक् सर्वैर्बीभत्सालोचनादिभिः |
छर्दयः पञ्च विज्ञेयास्तासां लक्षणमुच्यते ||१||

Chardi (vomiting) is of five types. They are - one from each dosha, fourth from the combination of all the three together and fifth from the sight of unpleasant things, etc. (1)|

The five kinds of chardi are –
Vataja Chardi
Pittaja Chardi
Kaphaja Chardi
Tridoshaja (sannipataja) Chardi
Agantuja Chardi (that occurring from sight of unpleasant things)

Causes for Chardi

अतिद्रवैरतिस्निग्धैरहृद्यैर्लवणैरति |
अकाले चातिमात्रैश्च तथाऽसात्म्यैश्च भोजनैः ||२||
श्रमाद्भयात्तथोद्वेगादजीर्णात् क्रिमिदोषतः |
नार्याश्चापन्नसत्त्वायास्तथाऽतिद्रुतमश्नतः ||३||
बीभत्सैर्हेतुभिश्चान्यैर्द्रुतमुत्क्लेशितो बलात् |
छादयन्नाननं वेगैरर्दयन्नङ्गभञ्जनैः |

अत्यन्तमपरीतस्य च्छर्दवै सम्भवो ध्रुवम् |
निरुच्यते छर्दिरिति दोषो वक्त्रं प्रधावितः ||४||
(सु. उ. तं. अ. ४९) |

Indulgence in foods which are very watery, very unctuous (fatty), unpleasant and very salty;
Taking meals at odd time, in excess quantity and of unaccustomed food
Excessive physical exertion
Fear, sudden emotions / anxiety,
Indigestion
Infection by worms
Pregnancy in women
Eating foods very quickly
Sight of terrific, fearsome, ugly and such other unpleasant things

Definition and Pathogenesis

The above said causes and similar others cause sudden increase of doshas. These doshas fill the mouth of the patient (with the contents of the stomach which have moved upwards) and come out forcibly through the mouth, causing immense discomfort (pain in different parts and organs of the body). This is called Chardi – vomiting. (2-4)

Purvarupa of Chardi

हृल्लासोद्गाररोधौ च प्रसेको लवणस्तनुः |
द्वेषोऽन्नपाने च भृशं वमीनां पूर्वलक्षणम् ||५||
(सु. उ. तं. अ. ४९) |

Premonitory symptoms of vomiting - The premonitory symptoms of vomiting are – nausea (oppression in the chest), obstruction of belching, thin (watery) and salty salivation and aversion to foods and drinks. (5)

Vataja Chardi Symptoms

हृत्पार्श्वपीडामुखशोषशीर्षनाभ्यर्तिकासस्वरभेदतोदैः |
उद्गारशब्दप्रबलं सफेनं विच्छिन्नकृष्णं तनुकं कषायम् |
कृच्छ्रेण चाल्पं महता च वेगेनार्तोऽनिलाच्छर्दयतीह दुःखम् ||६||
(च. चि. अ. २३) |

The symptoms of vataja chardi include - pain in the region of the heart and flanks, dryness of the mouth, pain / discomfort in head and umbilicus, cough, hoarseness of voice, and pricking sensation / pain all over the body. The vomiting occurs with great sounds during belching, mixed with froth, with less of fluids, composed of blackish material, thin, astringent in taste, brought out (vomited) with difficulty, scanty, severe bouts and severely troublesome (accompanied with pain all over the body). (6)

Pittaja Chardi Symptoms

मूर्छापिपासामुखशोषमूर्धताल्वक्षिसन्तापतमोभ्रमार्तः |
पीतं भृशोष्णं हरितं सतिक्तं धूम्रं च पित्तेन वमेत् सदाहम् ||७||
(च. चि. अ. २३) |

The symptoms of pittaja chardi are – fainting (loss of consciousness), severe thirst, dryness of mouth, burning sensation in the head, palate and eyes: darkness before the eyes & dizziness. In the vomiting, yellowish, greenish or black with reddish tinge, very hot, bitter material is expelled along with burning sensation. (7)

Kaphaja Chardi Symptoms

तन्द्रास्यमाधुर्यकफप्रसेकसन्तोषनिद्रारुचिगौरवार्तः |
स्निग्धं घनं स्वादु कफाद्विशुद्धं सरोमहर्षोऽल्परुजं वमेत्तु ||८||
(च. चि. अ. २३) |

The symptoms of Kaphaja Chardi are - stupor / drowsiness, sweet taste in the mouth, excessive salivation, a feeling of happiness (which is abnormal) or contentment (no desire to eat food anymore), feeling sleepy, anorexia, and feeling of heaviness of the body. While vomiting, the patient brings out unctuous, thick, sweet tasting, and white coloured material, accompanied with horripilations and little or no pain. (8)

Tridoshaja Chardi Symptoms

शूलाविपाकारुचिदाहतृष्णाश्वासप्रमोहप्रबला प्रसक्तम् |
छर्दिस्त्रिदोषाल्लवणाम्लनीलसान्द्रोष्णरक्तं वमतां नृणां स्यात् ||९||
(च. चि. अ. २३) |

The symptoms of tridoshaja chardi are - pain in the abdomen, indigestion, anorexia, burning sensation, thirst, dyspnoea (increased / difficult respirations), and delusions, being severe and constant. The vomited material would be salty or sour, blue or red in colour, semisolid and hot. (9)

Symptoms of incurability

विट्स्वेदमूत्राम्बुवहानि वायुः स्रोतांसि संरुध्य यदोर्ध्वमेति |
उत्सन्नदोषस्य समाचितं तं दोषं समुद्धूय नरस्य कोष्ठात् ||१०||

विण्मूत्रयोस्तत्समगन्धवर्णं तृट्श्वासहिक्कार्तियुतं प्रसक्तम् ।
प्रच्छर्दयेद्दुष्टमिहातिवेगात्तयाऽर्दितश्चाशु विनाशमेति ॥११॥
(च. चि. अ. २३) ।

When the aggravated vayu moves in upward direction and blocks the channels of faeces, sweat, urine and water (body fluids) in a person in whom the other doshas (pitta and kapha) have already undergone severe aggravation, it brings with it the doshas accumulated in the koshta (visceral organs, stomach and intestines) in the upward direction. In this case the person vomits the material which would have the smell and colour similar to those of faeces and urine. Apart from this, the patient will also suffer from severe thirst, dyspnoea (increased or difficult respiration) and hiccough which are constant. The person would have vomiting with continuous bouts occurring with great force associated with severe discomfort. Such type of vomiting is incurable and the person will face death in quick time. (10-11)

Agantuja and Krimija Chardi Symptoms

बीभत्सजा दौर्हृदजाऽऽमजा च ह्यसात्मजा च क्रिमिजा च या हि ।
सा पञ्चमी तां च विभावयेच्च दोषोच्छ्रयेणैव यथोक्तमादौ ॥१२॥
(सु. उ. तं. अ. ४९) ।
शूलहृल्लासबहुला क्रिमिजा च विशेषतः ।
क्रिमिहृद्रोगतुल्येन लक्षणेन च लक्षिता ॥१३॥
(सु. उ. तं. अ. ४९) ।

Agantuja Chardi Symptoms

The fifth kind of vomiting occurs due to sight and contact of things which are unpleasant, pregnancy, indigestion (caused due to excessive build-up of ama), unaccustomed foods and parasitic infections (worms). This is called agantuja chardi. Even in this type of vomiting, the symptoms of doshas (described earlier) shall be considered.

Krimija Chardi Symptoms

In krimija chardi (vomiting caused by parasitic infection) pain in the abdomen and nausea are prominent. Apart from this, the symptoms of krimija hrdroga (heart disease produced by worms) will also be found. (12-13)

Symptoms of incurability of chardi

क्षीणस्य या छर्दिरतिप्रसक्ता सोपद्रवा शोणितपूययुक्ता ।

सचन्द्रिकां तां प्रवदेदसाध्यां साध्यां चिकित्सेन्निरुपद्रवां च ||१४||
(च. चि. अ. २३) |
Vomiting is incurable when it occurs in emaciated persons, when the vomiting is continuous with too many bouts, is associated with complications and when the vomited material consists of blood, pus and white shining particles. The vomiting devoid of complications shall be considered as curable and should be treated promptly. (14)

Chardi Upadrava
कासः श्वासो ज्वरो हिक्का तृष्णा वैचित्त्यमेव च |
हृद्रोगस्तमकश्चैव ज्ञेयाश्छर्देरुपद्रवाः ||१५||
Complications of vomiting - (The complications of vomiting are – cough, dyspnoea (increased / difficult respiration), fever, hiccough, thirst, mental torpidity, heartache (heart disease) and feeling of being in darkness (darkness in front of the eyes or feeling as if enveloped by darkness).

इति श्रीमाधवकरविरचिते माधवनिदाने छर्दिनिदानं समाप्तम् ||१५||
Thus ends the chapter on Chardi Nidanam in Madhava Nidana text written by Acharya Madhavakara.

16

Madhava Nidana Chapter 16 Trishna Nidanam

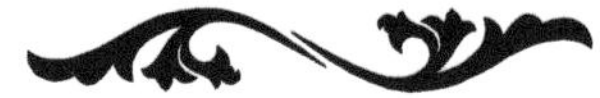

Trishna Samprapti

भयश्रमाभ्यां बलसङ्क्षयाद्वा ह्यूर्ध्वं चितं पित्तविवर्धनैश्च |
पित्तं सवातं कुपितं नराणां तालुप्रपन्नं जनयेत् पिपासाम् |
स्रोतस्स्वपांवाहिषु दूषितेषु दोषैश्च तृट् सम्भवतीह जन्तोः ||१||

Pathogenesis of Trishna - Pitta which has undergone increase due to its etiological factors (pitta aggravating factors like excessive consumption of pungent, hot, corrosive foods, anger, consumption of alcohol etc) gets association of vata which has undergone increase due to fear, physical exhaustion (fatigue) and loss of strength. Now, this pitta along with vata reaches the palate, gets lodged therein and produces severe thirst. This condition is called Trishna .

Also, Trishna – thirst may be manifested when the vitiated doshas contaminate the channels transporting water (organs controlling the water balance and supply in the body). (1)

Pathway of pathogenesis of Trishna

Pitta aggravated by its own etiological factors

Finds association of vata which has undergone aggravation due to fear, physical exertion and loss ofphysical strength

Both doshas reach and get lodged in the palate (or contaminate the water transporting channels) and

Cause severe thirst – this condition is called as Trishna

Trisna Purvarupa, Rupa

ताल्वोष्ठ कण्ठास्य विशेष दाह सन्ताप मोह भ्रम प्रविलापाः ।
पूर्वाणि रूपाणि भवन्ति तासामुप्तत्ति काले तु विशेषतो हि ॥

Premonitory symptoms and symptoms of Trishna – The premonitory symptoms of Trisna are – dryness and also burning sensation of the palate, lips, throat and mouth, increased temperature in the entire body, dizziness, and delirium.

Rupa / Lakshanas – When the same symptoms mentioned in the premonitory symptoms clearly manifest in a stronger way they become the lakshanas or symptoms of Trisna disease.

Types of Trishna

तिस्रः स्मृतास्ताः क्षतजा चतुर्थी क्षयात्तथा ह्यामसमुद्भवा च |
भक्तोद्भवा सप्तमिकेति तासां निबोध लिङ्गान्यनुपूर्वशस्तु ||२||
(सु. उ. तं. अ. ४८) |

Trishna is of seven kinds, one from each dosa, the fourth from injury (ulcerations), the fifth one due to the depletion (loss) of body tissues, the sixth one from ama (excessive accumulation of undigested materials formed due to sluggish digestion in the stomach) and the seventh one is caused by food (consumption of bad foods). The symptoms of all these types of Trishna will be described further. (2)

The 7 types of Trishna are –

- Vataja Trishna
- Pittaja Trishna
- Kaphaja Trishna
- Kshataja Trishna
- Kshayaja Trishna
- Amaja Trishna
- Bhaktodbhava Trishna

Symptoms

Vataja Trisna

क्षामास्यता मारुतसम्भवायां तोदस्तथा शङ्खशिरःसु चापि |
स्रोतोनिरोधो विरसं च वक्त्रं शीताभिरद्भिश्च विवृद्धिमेति ||३||
(सु. उ. तं. अ. ४८) |

The symptoms of Vataja Trishna are - pinched or dry face, pricking pain in the temples and head, obstruction of the channels of transportation of nutrition and water, manifestation of bad tastes in the mouth and increase of thirst on drinking cold water. (3)

Pittaja Trisna

मूर्छान्नविद्वेषविलापदाहा रक्तेक्षणत्वं प्रततश्च शोषः |
शीताभिनन्दा मुखतिक्तता च पित्तात्मिकायां परिदूयनं च ||४||
(सु. उ. तं. अ. ४८) |

The symptoms of pittaja trishna are – fainting (loss of consciousness), aversion to food, delirium, burning sensation, reddish eyes, constant dryness (due to immense thirst all the tissues of the body dry up continuously), liking towards cold things / cold comforts, manifestation of bitter taste in the mouth, feel of discomfort in the entire body or smoke (hot fumes) being eliminated from the entire body, and yellowish discoloration of faeces, urine, eyes skin etc. (4)

Kaphaja Trushna

बाष्पावरोधात् कफसंवृतेऽग्नौ तृष्णा बलासेन भवेत्तथा तु |
निद्रा गुरुत्वं मधुरास्यता च तृष्णार्दितः शुष्यति चातिमात्रम् ||५||
(सु. उ. तं. अ. ४८) |

Pathogenesis of kaphaja trishna – The kapha which has been aggravated due to its own causes (etiological factors causing aggravation of kapha) envelopes (destroys, puts off) the digestive fire. This leads to obstruction of heat in the channels of transportation of water. This will further lead to manifestation of trsna. Such a thirst caused by kapha is called kaphaja trsna. **The symptoms of kaphaja trishna** are – excessive sleep, heaviness of the body, manifestation of sweet taste in the mouth and excessive emaciation (quick emaciation) of the body of the patient. (5)

Symptoms of Ksataja and Ksayaja Trishna

क्षतस्य रुक्शोणितनिर्गमाभ्यां तृष्णा चतुर्थी क्षतजा मता तु |६| **(सु. उ. तं. अ. ४८) |**
रसक्षयाद्या क्षयसम्भवा सा तयाऽभिभूतश्च निशादिनेषु ||६||
पेपीयतेऽम्भः स सुखं न याति तां सन्निपातादिति केचिदाहुः |

रसक्षयोक्तानि च लक्षणानि तस्यामशेषेण भिषग्व्यवस्येत् ||७|| (सु. उ. तं. अ. ४८) |

Ksataja Trishna – This type of thirst manifests as a result of excessive bleeding and pain caused due to injury.

Ksayaja Trishna – This type of thirst manifests due to loss of rasa tissue (the first and predominantly watery tissue of the body). The person suffering from this type of thirst repeatedly drinks water during day time and also at night but the thirst is not relieved by any amount of water intake. Along with this, the symptoms of rasa ksaya (symptoms of decrease of rasa tissue including pain, tremors, feeling of dryness and emptiness in the region of heart, dryness of the mouth, skin etc) are also manifested.

Some authorities consider this type of Trishna (ksayaja Trishna) as sannipātaja (caused by all three doses together). (6-7)

Amaja Trishna

त्रिदोषलिङ्गाऽऽमसमुद्भवा च हृच्छूलनिष्ठीवनसादकर्त्री |८| (सु. उ. तं. अ. ४८) |

In this type of thirst, the combined symptoms of all the three doshas are seen.

Apart from this, pain in the region of the heart, excessive spitting of sputum and weakness (always lying down) are found as specific symptoms.

Bhaktodbhava Trishna

स्निग्धं तथाऽम्लं लवणं च भुक्तं गुर्वन्नमेवाशु तृषां करोति ||८|| (सु. उ. तं. अ. ४८) |

Bhaktodbhava / Annaja Trishna – This kind of thirst is produced by excessive consumption of unctuous (fatty), sour, salty and heavy foods. (8)

Upasargaja Trishna

दीनस्वरः प्रताम्यन् दीनः संशुष्कवक्त्रगलतालुः |
भवति खलु योपसर्गात्तृष्णा सा शोषिणी कष्टा ||९||

Signs of thirst manifested as a complication of other diseases

It is very difficult to treat patients of thirst in whom there is manifestation of –

Suppression of voice / feeble voice

Repeated fainting (goes into state of unconsciousness repeatedly)

Tiredness / restless (feel of helplessness)

Dryness of mouth, throat and palate

Excessive emaciation

This type of thirst caused as a complication of other diseases is called as upasargaja Trishna. (9)

Complications of Trishna

ज्वरमोहक्षयकासश्वासाद्युपसृष्टदेहानाम् |१०| (च. चि. अ. २२) |
सर्वास्त्वतिप्रसक्ता रोगकृशानां वमिप्रयुक्तानाम् |
घोरोपद्रवयुक्तास्तृष्णा मरणाय विज्ञेयाः ||१०|| (च. चि. अ. २२) |

Fever, delusion, emaciation, cough, dyspnoea (increased / difficult respiration) are the complications of Trishna . (According to others these are the causes of upasargaja Trishna mentioned above i.e., people suffering from these diseases can develop upasargaja trishna).

Any type of Trishna , which is very severe and persists for long (continuously present) is incurable. Thirst manifesting in persons who have been debilitated or emaciated by other diseases, in those who have continuous bouts of vomiting and those associated with complications will definitely cause death. (10-11)

इति श्रीमाधवकरविरचिते माधवनिदाने तृष्णानिदानं समाप्तम् ||१६||

Thus ends the chapter on Trishna Nidanam in Madhava Nidana text written by Acharya Madhavakara.

17

Madhava Nidana Chapter 17 Murcha Bhrama Nidra Tandra Sanyasa Nidanam

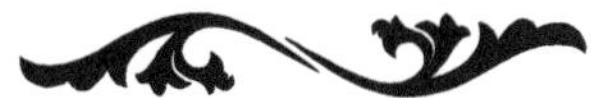

Nidana and Samprapti of Murcha

क्षीणस्य बहुदोषस्य विरुद्धाहारसेविनः |
वेगाघातादभिघाताद्धीनसत्त्वस्य वा पुनः ||१||
करणायतनेषूग्रा बाह्येष्वाभ्यन्तरेषु च |
निविशन्ते यदा दोषास्तदा मूर्छन्ति मानवाः ||२||

Nidana: Casues of murcha – The aggravated doshas cause murcha – fainting in persons who are emaciated (debilitated), in whom the doshas have undergone profound increase, those who indulge in incompatible foods and suppression of urges, those who are injured and those who are mentally weak.

Samprapti: Due to the above said factors the doshas undergo severe aggravation. These doshas get entry into and lodged in the external and internal organs related to the mind and cause the disease murcha – fainting. (1-2)

How does murcha develop? – extended pathogenesis & types of murcha

सञ्ज्ञावहासु नाडीषु पिहितास्वनिलादिभिः |
तमोऽभ्युपैति सहसा सुखदुःखव्यपोहकृत् ||३||

सुखदुःखव्यपोहाच्च नरः पतति काष्ठवत् |
मोहो मूर्छेति तामाहुः षड्विधा सा प्रकीर्तिता ||४||
वातादिभिः शोणितेन मद्येन च विषेण च |
षट्स्वप्येतासु पित्तं तु प्रभुत्वेनावतिष्ठते ||५||
(सु. उ. तं. अ. ४६) |

When the sajnavaha srotas (channels that carry sensations) are blocked by the increased vata and other doshas, the person experiences darkness in front of his eyes (goes into deep darkness). Due to this, the person will not be able to differentiate between pleasure and pain. He falls on the ground like a dry log of wood and becomes unconscious.

This condition is known as moha or murcha.

Types of Murcha

Murcha is of 6 kinds, one from each dosha, one from rakta (blood), one from madya (alcoholic beverages), and another from visa (poisons). Pitta will be the predominant dosha in all these types of murcha. (3-5)

Murcha Purvarupa

हृत्पीडा जृम्भणं ग्लानिः सञ्ज्ञादौर्बल्यमेव च |
सर्वासां पूर्वरूपाणि, यथास्वं ता विभावयेत् ||६||
(सु. उ. तं. अ. ४६) |

Premonitory symptoms of fainting

The premonitory symptoms of all types of murcha are – pain in the heart, excessive yawning, and weakness, improper or inadequate knowledge (inability of sense organs to perceive their respective sense objects leading to inadequate knowledge of things around us). These are the general premonitory symptoms of all types of murcha. Along with this the premonitory symptoms of the other types of murcha shall be understood by seeing the presence of their symptoms along with these general symptoms.

Example – if along with these premonitory symptoms, the symptoms of vataja type of murcha are present, they shall be considered as the premonitory symptoms of vataja murcha. (6)

Murcha Symptoms

नीलं वा यदि वा कृष्णमाकाशमथवाऽरुणम् |
पश्यंस्तमः प्रविशति शीघ्रं च प्रतिबुध्यते ||७||
वेपथुश्चाङ्गमर्दश्च प्रपीडा हृदयस्य च |
कार्श्यं श्यावाऽरुणा छाया मूर्छाये वातसम्भवे ||८||

(च. सू. अ. २४) |

In **vataja murcha** – while fainting (going into unconsciousness) the person sees the sky (or his surroundings) in blue, black or crimson colours, goes into darkness (experiences darkness in front of his eyes), falls down unconscious but regains consciousness quickly. He would also have tremors, pain all over the body, and severe pain in the heart, emaciation, blackish red discoloration of the body. (7-8)

Pittaja Murcha Symptoms

रक्तं हरितवर्णं वा वियत् पीतमथापि वा |
पश्यंस्तमः प्रविशति सस्वेदश्च प्रबुध्यते ||९||
(सपिपासः ससन्तापो रक्तपीताकुलेक्षणः) |
जातमात्रे पतति च शीघ्रं च प्रतिबुध्यते |
सम्भिन्नवर्चाः पीताभो मूर्छाये पित्तसम्भवे ||१०||
(च. सू. अ. २४) |

In **pittaja murcha** – while fainting (going into unconsciousness), the person sees the sky and surroundings in red, green or yellow colours. The person faints and goes into unconsciousness and would sweat a lot when he regains consciousness (gains consciousness along with sweating). (In this stage the person would experience thirst, increase in temperature of the body, red or yellow colour of the eyes, would go into a state of unconsciousness along with these symptoms and quickly regain consciousness). Diarrhoea and yellowish discolouration of the body are the other symptoms of pittaja type of murcha. (9-10)

Kaphaja Murcha Symptoms

मेघसङ्काशमाकाशमावृतं वा तमोघनैः |
पश्यंस्तमः प्रविशति चिराच्च प्रतिबुध्यते ||११||
गुरुभिः प्रावृतैरङ्गैर्यथैवार्द्रेण चर्मणा |
सप्रसेकः सहृल्लासो मूर्छाये कफसम्भवे ||१२||
(च. सू. अ. २४) |

In **kaphaja mūrchā** - while fainting (going into unconsciousness), the person sees the sky covered with thick clouds, falls unconscious. In this condition, the person regains consciousness after a long time. He feels as though his body is covered with heavy moist leather. Excessive salivation and nausea are the other symptoms of kaphaja type of murcha. (11-12)

Symptoms of Sannipataja Murcha

सर्वाकृतिः सन्निपातादपस्मार इवागतः |
स जन्तुं पातयत्याशु विना बीभत्सचेष्टितैः ||१३||
(च. सू. अ. २४) |

In **sannipātaja mūrchā** (caused by all the doṣhas together) there will be manifestation of all the symptoms (of all the doshas) together. Leaving out 'bibhatsa chesta – disgusting or loathsome activities' the person would have all the other symptoms of apasmara disease (epilepsy, memory disorders). The bouts of fainting will be similar to those seen or experienced in apasmara. In this condition the person will faint (go into a state of unconsciousness) very quickly. (13)

Raktaja Murcha Symptoms

पृथिव्यापस्तमोरूपं रक्तगन्धस्तदन्वयः |
तस्माद्रक्तस्य गन्धेन मूर्छन्ति भुविमानवाः ||१४||
द्रव्यस्वभाव इत्येके दृष्ट्वा यदभिमुह्यति |
(सु. उ. तं. अ. ४६) |

The prthvi and ap bhutas (earth and water elements) are predominant in tamo guna. The smell of blood is also predominant in prthvi and ap bhutas and hence predominant in tamo guna (the disease murcha is also predominant in tamo guna).

This is the reason that some persons who are predominant in tamo guna (in their constitution) become unconscious and faint, falling to the ground when they smell (and also sight) the blood. Some consider this to be the specific property of the blood. (14)

गुणास्तीव्रतरत्वेन स्थितास्तु विषमद्ययोः ||१५||
त एव तस्मात्ताभ्यां तु मोहौ स्यातां यथेरितौ |
(सु. उ. तं. अ. ४६) |

The properties (qualities) of poison and alcoholic drinks are very intense / sharp and damaging in comparison to any other things having intense / sharp quality. Therefore, the vishaja and madhyaja murcha are produced due to the effect of these qualities. In murcha caused by poisons and alcoholic drinks the symptoms are very profound.

Symptoms of Raktaja, Madhyaja and Vishaja Murcha

स्तब्धाङ्गदृष्टिस्त्वसृजा गूढोच्छ्वासश्च मूर्छितः ||१६||
मद्येन विलपंश्छेते नष्टविभ्रान्तमानसः |
गात्राणि विक्षिपन् भूमौ जरां यावन्न याति तत् ||१७||
वेपथुस्वप्नतृष्णाः स्युस्तमश्च विषमूर्छिते |
वेदितव्यं तीव्रतरं यथास्वं विषलक्षणैः ||१८||
(सु. उ. तं. अ. ४६) |

Raktaja Murcha - In raktaja murcha stiffness of the body, fixed gaze and deep (difficult) breathing – severe dyspnoea is seen.

Madyaja (alcoholic) Murcha – In Madyaja Murcha inconsistent (irrelevant) speech (delirium), falling on the ground with loss of consciousness and mental activities are seen. The person makes in-coordinated movements of the body parts (throwing of hands and feets), falls unconscious and stays in that state until the alcohol is digested in the body. (This means to tell that the symptoms of this type of murcha disappear once the alcohol gets digested).

Vishaja (due to poison) Murcha – In Visaja Murcha there are tremors (rigors), sleep, thirst and feeling of darkness (in front of the eyes). Apart from this, the other symptoms specific to the particular (specific) poisons too will be present. The symptoms will be specific to the poison and can be mild, severe or harmful depending on the sharpness and intensity of the poison involved. (15-18)

Dosha predominance

मूर्छा पित्ततमःप्राया रजःपित्तानिलाद्भ्रमः |
तमोवातकफात्तन्द्रा निद्रा श्लेष्मतमोभवा ||१९||
(सु. शा. अ. ४) |

Dosha predominance in murcha, bhrama, tandra and nidra

Mürcha (fainting, unconsciousness) is caused by predominance of pitta and tamas.

Bhrama (giddiness) is caused by predominance of rajas, pitta and vata.

Tandra (stupor) is caused by predominance of tamas, vata and kapha.

Nidra (sleep) is caused by predominance of kapha and tamas. (19)

Bhrama

(चक्रवद्भ्रमतो गात्रं भूमौ पतति सर्वदा |
भ्रमरोग इति ज्ञेयो रजःपित्तानिलात्मकः) |

The body reeling like a turning (spinning) wheel and the person falling on the ground (repeatedly) always is known as bhrama roga (giddiness). It is caused due to predominance of rajas, pitta and vata.

Tandra

इन्द्रियार्थेष्वसंवित्तिर्गौरवं जृम्भणं क्लमः |
निद्रार्तस्येव यस्येहा तस्य तन्द्रां विनिर्दिशेत् ||२०||
(सु. शा. अ. २४) |

The symptoms of tandra (stupor) include - non-perception of the sense objects by their related sense organs, feeling of heaviness (of the body), excessive yawning, weakness / fatigue (even without physical work) and the person appearing as though sleeping. (20)

Mada, Murcha Sanyasa - Difference

दोषेषु मदमूर्छायाः कृतवेगेषु देहिनाम् |
स्वयमेवोपशाम्यन्ति सन्न्यासो नौषधैर्विना ||२१||
(च. सू. अ. २४) |

In cases of mada and all types of mürcha, etc. the person recovers soon after the bouts produced by doshas are over and even without medicines. On the other hand, sanyasa (another similar disease – compared to coma) does not subside without appropriate treatment. (21)

Sanyasa

वाग्देहमनसां चेष्टामाक्षिप्यातिबला मलाः |
सन्न्यस्यन्त्यबलं जन्तुं प्राणायतनमाश्रिताः ||२२||
स ना सन्न्याससन्न्यस्तः काष्ठीभूतो मृतोपमः |
प्राणैर्विमुच्यते शीघ्रं मुक्त्वा सद्यःफलां क्रियाम् ||२३||
(च. सू. अ. २४) |

The doshas which have become very powerful invade the chief seat of prana and obstruct the functions of speech, body and mind and makes a debilitated person unconscious and fall on the ground. This condition is known as sanyasa (coma). In this condition the person falls down on the ground like a dry log of wood or like a dead person. If this condition is not addressed immediately and if proper and quick restorative treatment is not given the person will surely die. (22-23)

इति श्रीमाधवकरविरचिते माधवनिदाने मूर्छाभ्रमनिद्रातन्द्रासन्न्यासनिदानं समाप्तम्

||१७||
Thus ends the chapter on Murchā Nidanam in Madhava Nidana text written by Acharya Madhavakara.

18

Madhava Nidana Chapter 18 Panatyaya Paramada Panajirna Panavibhrama Nidanam

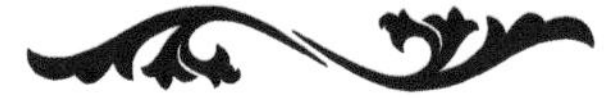

Alcoholic Intoxication

ये विषस्य गुणाः प्रोक्तास्तेऽपि मद्ये प्रतिष्ठिताः ।
तेन मिथ्योपयुक्तेन भवत्युग्रो मदात्ययः ॥१॥

Relationship between madya and visha (alcohol and poison)

All the qualities and properties present in poisons are also found in madya (alcoholic beverages). Hence, indiscriminate use of madya – alcohol causes madatyaya (alcoholic intoxication). (1)

Properties of Madya: Alcoholic drinks

किन्तु मद्यं स्वभावेन यथैवान्नं तथा स्मृतम् ।
अयुक्तियुक्तं रोगाय युक्तियुक्तं यथाऽमृतम् ॥२॥
प्राणाः प्राणभृतामन्नं तदयुक्त्या हिनस्त्यसून् ।
विषं प्राणहरं तच्च युक्तियुक्तं रसायनम् ॥३॥
(च. चि. अ. २४) ।

By nature, alcoholic drinks are considered to be similar to food. When

it is used improperly it causes many diseases. On the other hand, when it is used properly it acts like nectar. Food sustains life. But if the same food is taken improperly (violating the basic rules and regulations of food consumption, in terms of quality, quantity and time of eating) it takes away life. Similarly, the basic nature of the poison is to take away the life but when used judiciously it acts like a rejuvenator.
(2-3)

विधिना मात्रया काले हितैरन्नैर्यथाबलम् |
प्रहृष्टो यः पिबेन्मद्यं तस्य स्यादमृतोपमम् ||४||
(च. चि. अ. २४) |
स्निग्धैस्तदन्नैर्मांसैश्च भक्ष्यैश्च सह सेवितम् |
भवेदायुःप्रकर्षाय बलायोपचयाय च ||५||
काम्यता मनसस्तुष्टिस्तेजो विक्रम एव च |
विधिवत्सेव्यमाने तु मद्ये सन्निहिता गुणाः ||६||
(सु. उ. तं. अ. ४७) |
Alcohol is considered to be similar to (acts like) nectar when it is taken in accordance with proper procedure (of consumption), dose & time (of intake), with right combinations of food and in accordance to one's physical strength. This type of consumption of alcohol gives happiness (joy) to the person.
Alcohol taken with unctuous foods (fatty foods), meats or other nurturing foods brings about an increase of lifespan, strength and development of the body.
The alcohol taken judiciously bestows beauty (good looking body), happiness of (pleasantness) of mind, physical strength and valour. (4-6)

Symptoms
Effects of first stage of alcoholism
Symptoms of prathama mada
बुद्धिस्मृतिप्रीतिकरः सुखश्च पानान्ननिद्रारतिवर्धनश्च |
सम्पाठगीतस्वरवर्धनश्च प्रोक्तोऽतिरम्यः प्रथमो मदो हि ||७||
In the first stage of the alcoholic effect, there is an increase of intelligence, memory, pleasantness / desire and happiness (pleasure). It enhances desire towards drinks, foods and sleep. It enhances the capacity and interest in reading, singing and the quality of voice (speech). Thus, the first stage is said to provide a very pleasant experience. (7)

Second stage of alcoholism
Symptoms of Madhya / Dvitiya mada
अव्यक्तबुद्धिस्मृतिवाग्विचेष्टः सोन्मत्तलीलाकृतिरप्रशान्तः |
आलस्यनिद्राभिहतो मुहुश्च मध्येन मत्तः पुरुषो मदेन ||८|

Effects of second (intermediary) stage of alcoholism- intellect, memory and speech of the person becomes heavily disturbed (opposite, abnormal). His activities and appearance appear like those of an insane person. He becomes uncontrollable, becomes lazy and sleeps frequently. (8)

Third stage of alcoholism
Symptoms of Trtiya Mada
गच्छेदगम्यान्न गुरूंश्च मन्येत् खादेदभक्ष्याणि च नष्टसञ्ज्ञः |
ब्रूयाच्च गुह्यानि हृदि स्थितानि मदे तृतीये पुरुषोऽस्वतन्त्रः ||९||

In the third stage of alcoholic effect - the person indulges in forbidden acts and things, does not care for (disrespect) elders, eats things which are not to be eaten, having lost control speaks out secrets hidden in his mind.(9)

Symptoms of Chaturtha Mada
चतुर्थे तु मदे मूढो भग्नदार्विव निष्क्रियः |
कार्याकार्यविभागज्ञो मृतादप्यपरो मृतः ||१०||
को मदं तादृशं गच्छेदुन्मादमिव चापरम् |
बहुदोषमिवामूढः कान्तारं स्ववशः कृती ||११||
Fourth stage of alcoholism

In the fourth stage of alcoholic effect - the person falls to the ground and stays inactive (unconsciousness) just like a cut tree or dry log of wood. The person will not know the difference between activity and inactivity (confused so as to what to do and what not to, becomes incapable of doing any activity) and his condition becomes worse than a dead body.

Which intelligent person would wish to be in such a worst intoxicated condition which almost makes the man insane? Which person would develop a strange desire to enter and stroll in a dense forest which is inhabited (by the fear of) by many cruel animals like lion etc.

Note – Here the fearful forest inhabited animals are compared to the 4th stage of alcoholic intoxication. Just like a person entering into the jungle becomes a prey for these animals and would not come back, the person entering into the 4th stage of alcoholic intoxication too becomes a victim of this condition and would not return back. (10-11)

Effects of taking alcohol in an unmethodical way

निर्भक्तमेकान्तत एव मद्यं निषेव्यमाणं मनुजेन नित्यम् |
आपादयेत्कष्टतमान्विकारानापादयेच्चापि शरीरभेदम् ||१२||
(स. उ. अ. ४७) |

Only such a person who drinks (alcoholic beverages) on empty stomach and in solitude daily becomes a victim of very difficult diseases. This can also cause loss of life (death). (12)

Other causative factors which are responsible for Madhya vikaras (diseases caused due to alcoholic intoxication)

क्रुद्धेन भीतेन पिपासितेन शोकाभितप्तेन बुभुक्षितेन |
व्यायामभाराध्वपरिक्षतेन वेगावरोधाभिहतेन चापि ||१३||
अत्यम्बुभक्षावततोदरेण साजीर्णभुक्तेन तथाऽबलेन |
उष्णाभितप्तेन च सेव्यमानं करोति मद्यं विविधान्विकारान् ||१४||
(सु. उ. तं. अ. ४७) |

Alcoholic drinks produce many diseases in persons afflicted with anger, fear, thirst, grief and hunger. Similarly, it produces many diseases in those debilitated by physical exercises, lifting heavy weights, too much of walking (travelling), and those who suppress natural urges of the body, those drinking large quantities of water, eating too much quantity of food or eating foods while having indigestion (before the previously taken food is digested), those who are very weak and those who are very much exposed to the heat. (13-14)

Diseases caused due to unmethodical consumption of alcohol

पानात्ययं परमदं पानाजीर्णमथापि वा |
पानविभ्रममुग्रं च तेषां वक्ष्यामि लक्षणम् ||१५||
(सु. उ. तं. अ. ४७) |

Pānātyaya, paramada, pānājīrna and pānavibhrama are diseases caused due to excessive consumption of alcohol in an unmethodical way. The symptoms of these conditions will be described further. (15)

Symptoms of dosha predominant alcoholic intoxication

हिक्काश्वासशिरःकम्पपार्श्वशूलप्रजागरैः |

विद्याद्बहुप्रलापस्य वातप्रायं मदात्ययम् ||१६||
तृष्णादाहज्वरस्वेदमोहातीसारविभ्रमैः |
विद्याद्धरितवर्णस्य पित्तप्रायं मदात्ययम् ||१७||
छर्द्यरोचकहृल्लासतन्द्रास्तैमित्यगौरवैः |
विद्याच्छीतपरीतस्य कफप्रायं मदात्ययम् |
ज्ञेयस्त्रिदोषजश्चापि सर्वलिङ्गैर्मदात्ययः ||१८||
(च. चि. अ. २४) |

Vataja Madatyaya

Hiccough, dyspnoea (increased respiration), shaking of the head, pain in the flanks, excessive awakening (loss of sleep) and excessive talking (delirium) are symptoms of pānātyaya in which vata is the predominant dosha.

Pittaja Madatyaya

Thirst, burning sensation, fever, excessive sweating, delusion, diarrhoea, giddiness and greenish discoloration of the body are symptoms of paanaatyaya in which pitta is dominant.

Kaphaja Madatyaya

Vomiting, anorexia, nausea, stupor, feeling as if the body has been wrapped with wet cloth (laziness), feeling of heaviness and cold are symptoms of paanaatyaya in which kapha is predominant.

Tridoshaja Madatyaya

Presence of all the symptoms together (symptoms of all the three doshas) is found in tridoshaja pānātyaya. (16-18)

Symptoms of Paramada

श्लेष्मोच्छ्रयोऽङ्गगुरुता विरसास्यता च विण्मूत्रसक्तिरथ तन्द्रिररोचकश्च |
लिङ्गं परस्य च मदस्य वदन्ति तज्ज्ञास्तृष्णा रुजा शिरसि सन्धिषु चापि भेदः ||१९||
(सु. उ. तं. अ. ४७) |

According to experts paramada is a type of madatyaya in which the below mentioned symptoms are seen –

increase of kapha (seen as excess salivation, running in the nose, etc.)
feeling of heaviness of the body,
bad taste in the mouth (manifestation of abnormal tastes in the mouth),
non-elimination of faeces and urine;
stupor,
anorexia,
thirst,pain in the head and joints. (19)

Panajirna Symptoms

आध्मानमुग्रमथ चोद्गिरणं विदाहः पानेऽजरां समुपगच्छति लक्षणानि |२०|

(सु. उ. तं. अ. ४७) |

हृद्गात्रतोदकफसंस्रवकण्ठधूमा मूर्छावमिज्वरशिरोरुजनप्रदाहाः ||२०||

द्वेषः सुरान्नविकृतेष्वपि तेषु तेषु तं पानविभ्रममुशन्त्यखिलेन धीराः |

(सु. उ. तं. अ. ४७) |

Panajirna means indigestion of alcoholic drink. In this condition the symptoms including profound distension of the abdomen, vomiting, burning sensation and the drink not undergoing digestion at all - are seen.

Pana-vibhramaPana Vibhrama – Pricking (throbbing) pain in the region of the heart and of the whole body, excess salivation and running in the nose, feeling as though hot fumes are coming out of the throat, fainting, vomiting, fever, headache, severe burning sensation in the body, hatred even towards different kinds of alcoholic drinks and food are the symptoms of pānavibhrama as described by experts. (20)

Symptoms of incurability

हीनोत्तरौष्ठमतिशीतममन्ददाहं तैलप्रभास्यमपि पानहतं त्यजेत्तु ||२१||

जिह्वौष्ठदन्तमसितं त्वथवाऽपि नीलं पीते च यस्य नयने रुधिरप्रभे वा |

(सु. उ. तं. अ. ४७) |

Hanging down of upper lip, feeling of excessive cold externally (outside of the body) and excessive heat or burning sensation internally (inside the body) i.e., the body is cold to touch but is very hot inside (burns from within), face of the person appears as if smeared with oil, blackish or bluish discolouration of the tongue, lips and teeth, and eyes very red, seen in a patient intoxicated by alcohol should be refused treatment. (21)

Upadrava – complications of madatyaya

हिक्काज्वरौ वमथुवेपथुपार्श्वशूलाः कासभ्रमावपि च पानहतं भजन्ते ||२२||

(सु. उ. तं. अ. ४७)

The complications of alcoholic intoxication are – hiccough, fever, vomiting, rigors, pain in the flanks, cough and giddiness. (22)

इति श्रीमाधवकरविरचिते माधवनिदाने पानात्ययपरमदपानाजीर्णपानविभ्रमनिदानं समाप्तम् ||१८||

Thus ends the chapter on Panatyaya Paramada Panajirna Panavibhrama Nidanam in Madhava Nidana text written by Acharya Madhavakara.

19

Madhava Nidana Chapter 19 Daha Nidanam

Daha Nidanam

त्वचं प्राप्तः स पानोष्मा पित्तरक्ताभिमूर्छितः |
दाहं प्रकुरुते घोरं पित्तवत्तत्र भेषजम् ||१||

The heat produced by indiscriminate (violating the ideal procedure of alcoholic consumption as mentioned in the texts) consumption of alcoholic drinks gets associated with pitta and rakta (blood), reaches the skin and gets localized therein and produces a severe burning sensation. The treatment for burning sensation is similar to that of aggravated pitta (pitta mitigating treatments). (1)

Raktaja Daha

कृत्स्नदेहानुगं रक्तमुद्रिक्तं दहति ध्रुवम् |
स उष्यते तृष्यते च ताम्राभस्ताम्रलोचनः ||२||
लोहगन्धाङ्गवदनो वह्निनेवावकीर्यते |
(सु. उ. तं. अ. ४७) |

Burning sensation caused by blood tissue (rakta Dhatu)

The rakta which has aggravated to severe proportions would spread all over the body and cause burning sensation. In this condition the person feels as if his body is being burnt by fire. Apart from this there would be severe thirst, coppery red coloration of the skin and eyes, smell of iron from the body and face (mouth). These are the symptoms of raktaja daha. (2)

Pittaja Daha

पित्तज्वरसमः पित्तात्स चाप्यस्य विधिः स्मृतः ||३||

(सु. उ. तं. अ. ४७) |

Burning sensation caused by pitta

In dāha caused due to pitta aggravation, the symptoms and treatment are similar to those of pitta jwara (fever caused by aggravated pitta). (3)

Trishna Nirodhaja Daha

तृष्णानिरोधादब्धातौ क्षीणे तेजः समुद्धतम् |
सबाह्याभ्यन्तरं देहं प्रदहेन्मन्दचेतसः ||४||
संशुष्कगलताल्वोष्ठो जिह्वां निष्कृष्य वेपते |

(सु. उ. तं. अ. ४७) |

Burning Sensation caused by suppressing the thirst

By suppressing thirst (not drinking water even when thirsty) the water component (body fluids) of the body gets depleted. This increases teja (pitta, heat of the body). This heat produces burning sensation internally as well as externally (inside the body and on the surface of the body). The activity of the mind of the person gets reduced (causes unconsciousness or semi-conscious state) and he suffers from dryness of the throat, palate and lips. The person puts his tongue out of his mouth and experiences shaking of body parts (tremors, convulsions). These are the symptoms of trsna nirodhaja daha. (4-5)

Raktapurna Koshtaja Daha

असृजः पूर्णकोष्ठस्य दाहोऽन्यः स्यात् सुदुःसहः ||५||

(सु. उ. तं. अ. ४७) |

Burning Sensation caused due to 'blood filled visceral organs

Another kind of dāha occurs due to accumulation of blood in the various visceral organs caused by injury. This type of burning sensation is called as raktapurna koshtaja daha. This condition is dreadful. (5)

Dhatu Kshayaja Daha

धातुक्षयोत्थो यो दाहस्तेन मूर्छातृडर्दितः |
क्षामस्वरः क्रियाहीनः स सीदेद्भृशपीडितः ||६||

(सु. उ. तं. अ. ४७) |

Burning sensation caused due to depletion of tissues
Dhatu Kshayaja Daha is the burning sensation which is caused as an effect of depletion of the body tissues. This produces fainting (unconsciousness), thirst and feeble (tired) voice (loss of voice). The person becomes inactive (or unfit to undergo any kind of treatment – no treatment would give him relief) and might also face death. This type of daha is called as dhatu kshayaja daha. (6)

Kshataja Daha
क्षतजोऽनश्नतश्चान्नं शोचतो वाऽप्यनेकधा |
तेनान्तर्दह्यतेऽत्यर्थं तृष्णामूर्छाप्रलापवान् ||७||
This type of burning sensation is caused in a person who becomes incapable of eating food due to injury and also gets afflicted with many types of grief / worries. The symptoms of Kshataja Daha include burning sensation experienced in the interior of the body, excessive thirst, unconsciousness and delirium. (7)

Marmabhighataja Daha
मर्माभिघातजोऽप्यस्ति सोऽसाध्यः सप्तमो मतः |
सर्व एव च वर्ज्याः स्युः शीतगात्रस्य देहिनः ||८||
(सु. उ. तं. अ. ४७) |
Burning Sensation caused by injury to vital organs
Marmabhighataja Daha is the seventh type of burning sensation. This is caused due to the injury to the vital organs including heart, urinary bladder and head. This type of burning sensation is incurable. All types of daha – burning sensation should be refused treatment (should not be treated and rejected because they are incurable) if the body of the patient has become cold (in spite of severe burning sensation inside the body). (8)

इति श्रीमाधवकरविरचिते माधवनिदाने दाहनिदानं समाप्तम् ||१९||
Thus ends the chapter on Daha Nidanam in Madhava Nidana text written by Acharya Madhavakara.

20

Madhava Nidana Chapter 20 Unmada Nidanam

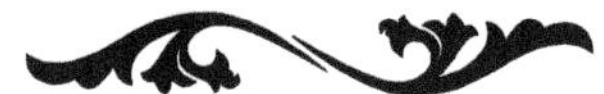

Unmada Nirukti

मदयन्त्युद्गता दोषा यस्मादुन्मार्गमागताः |
मानसोऽयमतो व्याधिरुन्माद इति कीर्तितः ||१||
(सु. उ. तं. अ. ६२) |

Meaning and definition of unmada

Unmada is a disease in which the doshas which have undergone abnormal increase and traversing upwards (through the channels of the mind) get localized in the mind and cause its abnormality. (1)

Types of Unmada

एकैकशः सर्वशश्च दोषैरत्यर्थमूर्छितैः |
मानसेन च दुःखेन स च पञ्चविधो मतः ||२||
विषाद्भवति षष्ठश्च यथास्वं तत्र भेषजम् |
स चाप्रवृद्धस्तरुणो मदसञ्ज्ञां बिभर्ति च ||३||
(सु. उ. तं. अ. ६२) |

Unmada is basically of 6 types. They are, one from each dosha, the fourth type is from the combination of all the three doshas, fifth from grief etc mind factors and the sixth type is caused by poisons.

The treatment of these shall be done in accordance and as appropriate to the cause. When unmada is not completely developed and is of recent onset it will be called as mada. (2-3)

Unmada Nidana

विरुद्धदुष्टाशुचिभोजननि प्रधर्षणं देवगुरुद्विजानाम् |
उन्मादहेतुर्भयहर्षपूर्वो मनोऽभिघातो विषमाश्च चेष्टाः ||४||
(च. चि. अ. ९) |

Unmada Causes (samanya hetu) – common etiological factors of unmada excessive indulgence in foods which are incompatible, spoilt (contaminated) and unclean;
showing disrespect to gods, preceptors (elders) and the twice born (Brahmans) affection of the mind due to sudden emotions like fear, joy, etc. and violent physical activities (4)

Unmada Samprapti

तैरल्पसत्त्वस्य मलाः प्रदुष्टा बुद्धेर्निवासं हृदयं प्रदूष्य |
स्रोतांस्यधिष्ठाय मनोवहानि प्रमोहयन्त्याशु नरस्य चेतः ||५||
(च. चि. अ. १) |

Pathogenesis of Unmada

In persons who are mentally weak (the sattvika quality of the mind has been immensely decreased), the doṣhas having undergone abnormal increase invade and contaminate the hrdaya which is the seat of mind, get spread (lodged) in all the channels of the mind and bring about the derangement of the mind in quick time. This state of derangement of the mind is called as Unmada. (5)

Note – Hrdaya generally means heart. This word has also been mentioned to explain the brain. So, it has to be understood contextually. Therefore, it is good to consider hrdaya as the brain in this context of Unmada.

Unmada Samanya Lakshana

धीविभ्रमःसत्त्वपरिप्लवश्चपर्याकुलादृष्टिरधीरताच।
अबद्धवाक्त्वंहृदयंचशून्यंसामान्यमुन्मादगदस्यलिङ्गम्।।६।।
(च.चि.अ.९)

General symptoms of Unmada

The generalized symptoms of Unmada are - improper understanding and unsteadiness of the mind, in-coordination of sight (seeing here and there or not making eye to eye coordination without any reason), lack of courage (feeling of fear), irrelevant talk, and feeling of emptiness of heart (mind).

(6)

Vataja Unmada

रूक्षाल्पशीतान्नविरेकधातुक्षयोपवासैरनिलोऽतिवृद्धः |
चिन्तादिदुष्टं हृदयं प्रदूष्य बुद्धिं स्मृतिं चाप्युपहन्ति शीघ्रम् ||७||
अस्थानहासस्मितनृत्यगीतवागङ्गविक्षेपणरोदनानि |
पारुष्यकार्श्यारुणवर्णताश्च जीर्णे बलं चानिलजस्य रूपम् ||८|||
(च. चि. अ. ९) |

Causes - Vata gets abnormally increased in the body due to indulgence in foods which are dry, scanty (foods less in quantity) or cold, (frequent) purgation (inclusive of vomiting), depletion of tissues, fasting (starvation) and other factors.

Pathogenesis - This Vāta, in turn invades and further contaminates the hrdaya (brain) which has already been weakened (contaminated) by emotions like worry etc and further brings about derangement of intellect and memory, leading to manifestation of vataja unmada.

Symptoms – The signs and symptoms of unmada caused by abnormal increase of vata are –

laughing, smiling, dancing, singing, speaking, making movement of body parts and weeping at improper time and place (unnecessarily and without any reason);

hardness / roughness, emaciation, blackish red discolouration of the body and exacerbation of symptoms after digestion of food (7-8)

Pittaja Unmada

अजीर्णकट्वम्लविदाह्यशीतैर्भोज्यैश्चितं पित्तमुदीर्णवेगम् |
उन्मादमत्युग्रमनात्मकस्य हृदि स्थितं पूर्ववदाशु कुर्यात् ||९||
अमर्षसंरम्भविनग्नभावाः सन्तर्जनातिद्रवणौष्ण्यरोषाः |
प्रच्छायशीतान्नजलाभिलाषः पीता च भाः पित्तकृतस्य लिङ्गम् ||१०||
(च. चि. अ. ९) |

Causes – Pitta gets abnormally increased in the body due to indulgence in foods which are not properly cooked, very pungent or sour, corrosive (cause heartburn), or those which are hot etc.

Pathogenesis – This aggravated pitta reaches the hrdaya – brain (which has already been weakened / contaminated by emotions like worry, anger etc) and affects the mind quickly as described earlier, in people who are not self controlled and further brings about derangement of intellect and memory,

leading to the manifestation of pittaja unmada.
Symptoms - The signs and symptoms of unmada caused by abnormal increase of pitta are –intolerance,
uncontrollability,
casting away the clothes and remaining naked,
threatening others,
running away (to beat / harm others)
feeling of excessive heat in the body (burning sensation),
desiring shade, cold water and cold foods,
yellowish discolouration of the body (9-10)

Kaphaja Unmada

सम्पूरणैर्मन्दविचेष्टितस्य सोष्मा कफो मर्मणि सम्प्रदुष्टः |
बुद्धिं स्मृतिं चाप्युपहत्य चित्तं प्रमोहयन् सञ्जनयेद्विकारम् ||११||
वाक्चेष्टितं मन्दमरोचकश्च नारीविविक्तप्रियताऽतिनिद्रा |
छर्दिश्च लाला च बलं च [१] भुक्ते नखादिशौक्ल्यं च कफात्मके स्यात् |
(च. चि. अ. ९) ||१२||

Causes – Kapha along with pitta gets abnormally increased in the body due to excessive indulgence in over-eating, lack of physical exercise etc.
Pathogenesis - This Kapha (with pitta), in turn invades and further contaminates the hrdaya (brain) which has already been weakened (contaminated) by emotions like worry etc and further brings about derangement of intellect and memory, leading to manifestation of kaphaja unmada. This occurs on the backdrop of derangement of mind caused by kapha and pitta.
Symptoms - The signs and symptoms of unmada caused by abnormal increase of kapha are –
slow / weak / sluggish voice (or talk) and body movements,
anorexia,
desire for women (or sex) and
solitude,
excessive sleep,
vomiting,
saliva dribbling out,
symptoms pronounced immediately after taking food,
whitish discoloration of nails, etc. (11-12)

Sannipataja Unmada

यः सन्निपातप्रभवोऽतिघोरः सर्वैः समस्तैः स च हेतुभिः स्यात् |
सर्वाणि रूपाणि बिभर्ति तादृग्विरुद्धभैषज्यविधिर्विवर्ज्यः ||१३||
(च. चि. अ. ९) |

Causes and pathogenesis - Sannipataja unmäda is produced by increase of all the three došhas together by their respective causes.

Symptoms – This condition is said to be very dreadful. The symptoms of all the doshas are seen in the patient. Since the treatment of this condition is mutually antagonistic (treatment to balance one dosha aggravates the other) it is regarded as incurable and hence treatment of this type of unmada shall be denied (refused). (13)

Shokadi Janya Unmada

चौरैर्नरेन्द्रपुरुषैररिभिस्तथाऽन्यैर्वित्रासितस्य धनबान्धवसङ्क्षयाद्वा |
गाढं क्षते मनसि च प्रियया रिरंसोर्जायेत चोत्कटतमो मनसो विकारः ||१४||
चित्रं ब्रवीति च मनोऽनुगतं विसञ्ज्ञो गायत्यथो हसति रोदिति चापि मूढः |
(सु. उ. तं. अ. ६२) |

Causes and pathogenesis - Getting frightened by (sudden appearance or presence) of robbers, government officials (like police, etc.) enemies and others (wild animals, weapons and anything causing fear), loss of money, death of relatives (next of kin such as wife, lover, sons, daughters, parents etc.) excessive desire for sex with beloved partner and not being able to obtain that and such other factors cause great injury to the mind and produce dreadful mental disorder - unmada.

Symptoms - Person so affected talks indifferently, which he likes most and sometimes reveals even the secrets hidden in his mind, sings, laughs or weeps on his own accord and behaves senselessly. (14-15)

Visha janya unmada

रक्तेक्षणो हतबलेन्द्रियभाः सुदीनः श्यावाननो विषकृतेऽथ भवेद्विसञ्ज्ञः ||१५||
(सु. उ. तं. अ. ६२) |

Symptoms of Visha janya unmada

In unmada produced by poisons, the person will have red shot eyes, loss of strength of body, senses and complexion. He will have a sense of helplessness, black / bluish-black discolouration of the mouth or face and loss of consciousness. (15)

Symptoms of incurability of Unmada

अवाञ्ची वाऽप्युदञ्ची वा क्षीणमांसबलो नरः |
जागरूको ह्यसन्देहमुन्मादेन विनश्यति ||१६||
(सु. उ. तं. अ. ६२) |

Patient of unmāda who is found always keeping his head bent down or bent up, whose muscles have decreased (is emaciated), whose strength has been decreased (weak) and always awake (without sleep) is sure to die. (16)

General symptoms of Bhutonmada

अमर्त्यवाग्विक्रमवीर्यचेष्टो ज्ञानादिविज्ञानबलादिभिर्यः |
उन्मादकालोऽनियतश्च [१] तस्य भूतोत्थमुन्मादमुदाहरेत्तम् ||१७||
(च. चि. अ. ९) |

Bhütonmāda (unmāda caused due to possession by "spirits") is described as the disease in which the speech, valour, strength, activities, intellect and knowledge of the affected person are super-human and the time of onset of the symptoms is unspecific (not in accordance with that of the doshas). (17)

Devajushta Unmada

सन्तुष्टः शुचिरतिदिव्यमाल्यगन्धो निस्तन्द्रीरवितथसंस्कृतप्रभाषी |
तेजस्वी स्थिरनयनो वरप्रदाता ब्रह्मण्यो भवति नरः स देवजुष्टः ||१८||
(सु. उ. तं. अ. ६०) |

The symptoms of a person possessed by Deva Graha (Gods, Goddesses) are - contentment (not expressing any desires), cleanliness, desire for very pleasant garlands and scents etc. (excessive smell of divine perfumed flowers or flower garlands emitted from his body without the person applying any such perfumes), not getting stupor or sleep (always alert and / or awake), always speaking refined (cultured) language and truth, possessing bright complexion (on the face), unruffled (un-winking) eyes, bestowing favours and blessings and such other acts as seen (done by) in brāhmaṇas or respecting and worshipping Brahmanas. (18)

Devashatru jushta Unmada

संस्वेदी द्विजगुरुदेवदोषवक्ता जिह्माक्षो विगतभयो विमार्गदृष्टिः |
सन्तुष्टो न भवति चान्नपानजातैर्दुष्टात्मा भवति स देवशत्रुजुष्टः ||१९||
(सु. उ. तं. अ. ६०) |

Symptoms of Devashatru (Danava / Asura) jushta Unmada (possessed by demons)

The symptoms of a person possessed by Devashatru / Danava / Asura Graha (Demons) are – heavily sweating, always abusing brahmanas, teachers, gods, etc. having distorted look (crooked eyes / squint), absence of any fear, always taking wrong paths to achieve anything (critical of everything), never getting satisfied with foods and drinks and indulging in sinful acts. (19)

Gandharvajushta Unmada

हृष्टात्मा पुलिनवनान्तरोपसेवी स्वाचारः प्रियपरिगीतगन्धमाल्यः |
नृत्यन् वै प्रहसति चारु चाल्पशब्दं गन्धर्वग्रहपरिपीडितो मनुष्यः ||२०||
(सु. उ. तं. अ. ६०) |

Symptoms of Gandharvajushta Unmada (possessed by Gandharva)

The symptoms of a person possessed by Gandharva are – always in contentment, loves to roam around river banks, gardens etc, indulging in good deeds (pure character), fond of good company, songs (music), scents, garlands, dancing with passion, laughing and speaking less (man of less words). (20)

Yaksha jushta Unmada

ताम्राक्षः प्रियतनुरक्तवस्त्रधारी गम्भीरो द्रुतगतिरल्पवाक्सहिष्णुः |
तेजस्वी वदति च किं ददामि कस्मै यो यक्षग्रहपरिपीडितो मनुष्यः ||२१||
(सु. उ. तं. अ. ६०) |

Symptoms of Yaksha jushta Unmada (possessed by Yaksha)

The symptoms of a person possessed by Yaksha are – red shot eyes, desire for beautiful, thin and red coloured dress, steadiness in all activities and quick pace (walking fast), very less speech, enduring any trouble (has good tolerance), bright complexion of the face (attractive), and enquiring others what they want from him (ready to help). (21)

Pitr jushta Unmada

प्रेतानां स दिशति संस्तरेषु पिण्डान् शान्तात्मा जलमपि चापसव्यवस्त्रः |
मांसेप्सुस्तिलगुडपायसाभिकामस्तद्भक्तो भवति पितृग्रहाभिजुष्टः ||२२||
(सु. उ. तं. अ. ६०) |

Symptoms of Pitr jushta Unmada (possessed by Pitr - ancestor)

The symptoms of a person possessed by Pitr are – The person is engaged in the act of offering pinda (balls of cooked rice offered to the departed souls of ancestors / forefathers during ceremonial procedures) and water, on the seat prepared with kusha grass etc, by being calm and composed, and putting clothes etc on his right shoulder. He has developed desires towards foods prepared with mutton (meat), sesame, jaggery and milk puddings (sweets prepared in milk base) and is also a devotee of pitr (respects them immensely). (22)

Sarpa / Bhujanga Graha Jushta Unmada

यस्तूर्व्यां प्रसरति सर्पवत् कदाचित् सृक्कण्यौ विलिहति जिह्वया तथैव |
क्रोधालुर्गुडमधुदुग्धपायसेप्सुर्ज्ञातव्यो भवति भुजङ्गमेन जुष्टः ||२३||
(सु. उ. तं. अ. ६०) |

Symptoms of Sarpa / Bhujanga Graha Jushta Unmada (possessed by snakes)

The symptoms of a person possessed by Sarpa / Bhujanga Graha are – The person afflicted by this graha is seen moving on the ground lying on his chest, just like a snake does, keeps licking his lips with his tongue, is extremely angry, and develops desire for jaggery, honey, milk and sweet dish prepared on milk base. (23)

Rakshasa Graha Jushta Unmada

मांसासृग्विविधसुराविकारलिप्सुर्निर्लज्जो भृशमतिनिष्ठुरोऽतिशूरः |
क्रोधालुर्विपुलबलो निशाविहारी शौचद्विड् भवति स राक्षसैर्गृहीतः ||२४||
(सु. उ. तं. अ. ६०) |

Symptoms of Rakshasa Graha Jushta Unmada

The symptoms of a person possessed by Rakshasa Graha are – This person possessed with Rakshasa Graha will show immense desire for foods prepared with meat (mutton) and blood, and various types of alcohols / intoxicating drinks. He is devoid of shyness; very cruel and very courageous (brave). He gets very angry and also has great strength. He roams around at night time and hates cleanliness. (24)

Pishaca Graha Jushta Unmada

उद्धस्तः कृशपरुषो अचिरप्रलापी दुर्गन्धो भृशमशुचिस्तथाऽतिलोलः |
बह्वाशी विजनवनान्तरोपसेवी व्याचेष्टन् भ्रमति रुदन् पिशाचजुष्टः ||२५||
(सु. उ. तं. अ. ६०) |

The symptoms of a person possessed by Pishaca Graha are – the person is always seen keeping his shoulders elevated or keeping himself naked, is emaciated, speaks irrelevantly with intermittent gaps, emits bad smell from his body, unclean, greedy, eats large quantities of food, roams around in deserted forests and uninhabited places, who does untoward (weird, opposite) activities, and roams around weeping loudly all alone. (25)

Symptoms of incurability in unmada

स्थूलाक्षो द्रुतमटनः स फेनलेही निद्रालुः पतति च कम्पते च यो हि |
यश्चाद्रिद्विरदनगादिविच्युतः स्यात् सोऽसाध्यो भवति तथा त्रयोदशाब्दे ||२६||
(सु. उ. तं. अ. ६०) |

Bulging out of the eyes
running / walking fast,
licking the froth (saliva) coming out of his mouth,
sleeping in excess,
falling off suddenly,
has tremors,
unmada caused due to fall from a mountain, back of an elephant or tree,
unmada persisting for 13 long years (any type of unmada which is 13 years old) (26)

Periodicity of attack of different grahas

देवग्रहाः पौर्णमास्यामसुराः सन्ध्ययोरपि |
गन्धर्वाः प्रायशोऽष्टम्यां, यक्षाश्च प्रतिपद्यथ ||२७||
पित्र्याः कृष्णक्षये हिंस्युः, पञ्चम्यामपि चोरगाः |
रक्षांसि रात्रौ, पैशाचाश्चतुर्दश्यां विशन्ति हि ||२८||
(सु. उ. तं. अ. ६०) |

Deva grahas seize the person on full-moon days,
Asura grahas seize the person in the mornings (junction of night and early morning) or evening (junction of noon and evening)
Gandharva grahas seize the person on the eighth day,
Yaksa grahas seize the person on the first day,
Pitr grahas seize the person during the dark half of the month,
Naga grahas seize the person on the fifth day,
Rakshasa grahas seize the person during nights and
Pisaca grahas seize the person on the fourteenth day. (27-28)

Analogy to describe the attack and presence of grahas

दर्पणादीन् यथा छाया शीतोष्णं प्राणिनो यथा |
स्वमणिं भास्करार्चिश्च यथा देहं च देहधृक् |
विशन्ति च न दृश्यन्ते ग्रहास्तद्वच्छरीरिणः ||२९||
(सु. उ. तं. अ. ६०) |

Just as an image enters into the mirror, the heat and cold which are invisible enter our body, the sunrays enter the suryakanti gem (or the heat enters the fire), the soul which cannot be seen enters the physical body and all these cannot be perceived by our physical eyes. We cannot see these happening. Similarly, the grahas also enter the human body but cannot be seen or perceived by our physical eyes. Though the grahas are present in the body they cannot be felt or seen. (29)

Entry and existence of (attack, seize) grahas as explained by other texts

प्रविश्याशु शरीरं हि पीडां कुर्वन्ति दुःसहाम् ||३०||

Having entered the body (being invisible), the grahas (spirits) create intolerable sufferings. (30)

तपांसि तीव्राणि तथैव दानं व्रतानि धर्मो नियमश्च सत्यम् |
गुणास्तथाऽष्टावपि तेषु नित्या व्यस्ताः समस्ताश्च यथाप्रभावम् ||३१||
न ते मनुष्यैः सह संविशन्ति न वा मनुष्यान् क्वचिदाविशन्ति |
ये त्वाविशन्तीति वदन्ति मोहात्ते भूतविद्याविषयादपोह्याः ||३२||
तेषां ग्रहाणां परिचारका ये कोटीसहस्रायुतपद्मसङ्ख्याः |
असृग्वसामांसभुजः सुभीमा निशाविहाराश्च तथाऽऽविशन्ति ||३३||

Observance of austerities, charity, vows, right conduct, rigid discipline, truth, the eight extraordinary capabilities — are the qualities always found in the grahas, more in deva graha and less in others. Depending on the graha and their impact, the above said qualities are present either partially or in entirety. This means to tell that these qualities are found partially (few) in asura etc grahas and in entirety (full, almost) in deva graha. Being endowed with these good qualities the deva graha etc do not sit along with human beings nor do enter the unclean bodies of the human beings all by themselves. But those who still, due to ignorance, say that these grahas enter the human body, should be considered as having absolutely no knowledge of bhuta vidhya i.e., demonology. It is in fact the thousands and millions of servants or retinue of the grahas, who are fond of blood and flesh, who are very terrific and who roam about at nights, which enter into the human body and take possession of the person. (31-33)

इति श्रीमाधवकरविरचिते माधवनिदान उन्मादनिदानं समाप्तम्||२०||

Thus ends the chapter on Unmāda Nidanam in Madhava Nidana text written by Acharya Madhavakara.

Ashta Siddhis - The eight extraordinary capabilities are

1. Anima - capacity to assume minute size
2. Mahima - capacity to assume very huge size
3. Garima - capacity to become very heavy
4. Laghima - to become very light
5. Prapti - obtaining any desired thing
6. Prakamya - fulfilling all desires
7. Isatwa – over-lordship on anything and
8. Vasitva - subjugating or controlling anything

According to another version, the extraordinary powers are –

1. Capacity to enter into the body of another person
2. Extraordinary sense perception
3. To understand all sounds or meanings of all words / language
4. Capacity to see
5. Hear and
6. Remember things which are impossible by others
7. Unusual bright complexion and
8. Capacity to vanish out of sight-are the extraordinary powers.

21

Madhava Nidana Chapter 21 Apasmara Nidanam

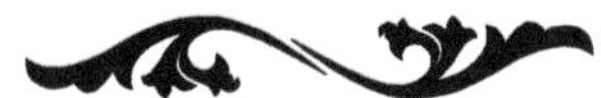

Apasmara Samprapti, Swarupa

(चिन्ताशोकादिभिर्दोषाः क्रुद्धा हृत्स्रोतसि स्थिताः |
कृत्वा स्मृतेरपध्वंसमपस्मारं प्रकुर्वते) |
तमःप्रवेशः संरम्भो दोषोद्रेकहतस्मृतेः |
अपस्मार इति ज्ञेयो गदो घोरश्चतुर्विधः ||१||

(The doshas having become increased (aggravated) by worry, grief, etc. get lodged in the channels of the hrdaya (mind, brain), make for loss of memory (knowledge, consciousness) and produce the disease apasmāra).

In Apasmāra the person experiences a feeling as if entering into a zone of utter darkness (the person experiences darkness in front of his eyes and he experiences entering into a zone of ignorance which is in the form of darkness, loss of consciousness), and does many types of activities including violent movements of the eyes, limbs (convulsions) etc.

All these happen due to the destruction (loss) of memory caused by severely aggravated doshas. This dreaded disease is called Apasmara and is of four kinds. (1)

The four types of apasmara are – vataja, pittaja, kaphaja and tridoshaja.

Aasmara Purvarupa

हृत्कम्पः शून्यता स्वेदो ध्यानं मूर्छा प्रमूढता |

निद्रानाशश्च तस्मिंश्च भविष्यति भवत्यथ ||२||
(सु. उ. तं. अ. ६१) |
Premonitory symptoms of apasmara are – palpitation of the heart, feeling of emptiness (of the mind), perspiration, worry, fainting, destruction of activities of mind and senses (delusion), and loss of sleep. (2)

Symptoms of Vataja Apasmara

कम्पते प्रदशेद्दन्तान् फेनोद्वामी श्वसित्यपि |
परुषारुणकृष्णानि पश्येद्रूपाणि चानिलात् ||३||
(च. चि. अ. १०) |
The **symptoms of vataja apasmara** are – tremors (convulsions), grinding of teeth, frothy vomiting, dyspnoea (increased respiration), and roughness of the body. All things around him appear to be of reddish black colour before the attack (before he falls and goes into unconsciousness). (3)

Symptoms of Pittaja Apasmara

पीतफेनाङ्गवक्त्राक्षः पीतासृग्रूपदर्शकः |
सतृष्णोष्णानलव्याप्तलोकदर्शी च पैत्तिकः ||४||
(च. चि. अ. १०) |
The **symptoms of pittaja** apasmara are - yellow coloured froth around the mouth, yellowish skin, face and eyes. He sees all things around him being yellow or red coloured (before the attack, before going into unconsciousness). He also will have severe thirst, feeling of excessive heat in the body and would see the surroundings as if covered (burning) with fire (that everything around him is being burnt by the fire). (4)

Symptoms of Kaphaja Apasmara

शुक्लफेनाङ्गवक्त्राक्षः शीतहृष्टाङ्गजो गुरुः |
पश्येच्छुक्लानि रूपाणि श्लैष्मिको मुच्यते चिरात् ||५||
(च. चि. अ. १०) |
The **symptoms of kaphaja apasmara** are - whitish froth at the mouth, white colour of the skin, face and eyes, (feeling of) coldness and heaviness of the body, horripilation, and seeing white coloured things (he sees all things around him being white in colour, before the attack). The attacks of this type of apasmara ends very late i.e. the person regains consciousness long time after the attack. (5)

Tridoshaja Apasmara

सर्वैरेतैः समस्तैश्च लिङ्गैर्ज्ञेयस्त्रिदोषजः |
अपस्मारः स चासाध्यो यः क्षीणस्यानवश्च यः ||६||
(च. चि. अ. १०) |

Symptoms of Tridoshaja / Sannipataja Apasmara and symptoms of incurability of apasmara

In tridoshaja / sannipataja apasmara is caused by the aggravation of all the three doshas and the symptoms of all three doshas are seen in this condition.

This type of apasmara (tridoshaja), the apasmara manifested in persons who are emaciated and apasmara which is not of recent onset (chronic apasmara) - are all said to be incurable. (6)

Other symptoms of incurability of apasmara

प्रतिस्फुरन्तं बहुशः क्षीणं प्रचलितभ्रुवम् |
नेत्राभ्यां च विकुर्वाणमपस्मारो विनाशयेत् ||७||

When apasmara occurs with too much of (severe and continuous) tremors (convulsions), emaciation, fierce movement of eyebrows (eyebrows deviated in upward direction) and eyes (deformities in the eyes), it would kill the person (it becomes incurable). (7)

Period of aggravation of apasmara

पक्षाद्वा द्वादशाहाद्वा मासाद्वा कुपिता मलाः |
अपस्माराय कुर्वन्ति वेगं किञ्चिदथान्तरम् ||८||
(च. चि. अ. १०) |
देवे वर्षत्यपि यथा भूमौ बीजानि कानिचित् |
शरदि प्रतिरोहन्ति तथा व्याधिसमुच्छ्रयाः ||९||
(सु. उ. तं. अ. ६१) |

The doshas get aggravated (regularly) on 5, 12 or 30-days intervals and produce episodes of apasmāra (epileptic seizures). Sometimes the episodes (attacks) can take place at any other interval of time, even apart from these intervals (whenever there is aggravation of accumulated and latent doshas). Just as the seeds which lay in the earth even during rainy season sprout only during sarat ritu (autumn season) i.e., when the favourable season for their sprouting appears, the diseases also, (in spite of being latent in the body) develop only after a certain period of time. (8-9)

इति श्रीमाधवकरविरचिते माधवनिदानेऽपस्मारनिदानं समाप्तम् ||२१||

Thus ends the chapter on Apasmara Nidanam in Madhava Nidana text written by Acharya Madhavakara.

22

Madhava Nidana Chapter 22 Vata Vyadhi Nidanam

Vata Vyadhi Nidana, Samprapti

रूक्षशीताल्पलघ्वन्नव्यवायातिप्रजागरैः |
विषमादुपचाराच्च दोषासृक्स्रवणादपि ||१||
लङ्घनप्लवनात्यध्वव्यायामादिविचेष्टितैः |
धातूनां सङ्क्षयाच्चिन्ताशोकरोगातिकर्षणात् ||२||
वेगसन्धारणादामादभिघातादभोजनत् |
मर्माबाधाद्गजोष्ट्राश्वशीघ्रयानापतंसनात् ||३||
देहे स्रोतांसि रिक्तानि पूरयित्वाऽनिलो बली |
करोति विविधान् व्याधीन् सर्वाङ्गैकाङ्गसंश्रयान् ||४||
(च. चि. अ. २८) |

Causes of Vata Vyadhi -

Excessive indulgence in foods which are dry, cold, scanty, light (quickly digestible);

sexual intercourse, keeping awake at nights, improper treatments (administering Panchakarma treatments at wrong times, in wrong conditions or consuming foods and activities which are incompatible as well as opposite to the nature of land and season), excessive discharge (elimination) of doṣhas and blood from the body (during the course of treatments like emesis, purgation, bloodletting, etc.),

jumping, swimming, long distance walking and such other exercises and

untoward activities (opposite to one's nature);
loss or depletion of body tissues, worry, grief, extreme debility due to protracted diseases, habit of suppression of natural urges of the body, production of āma (undigested intermediary metabolites),
trauma, fasting or diseases of vital organs (pain or damage to vital organs), riding fast on elephants, camels and horses (other similar animals or vehicles), or falling during such rides.

Vatavyadhi Samprapti

Pathogenesis – Due to the above said etiological factors aggravation of vata takes place and the channels (of vāta) in the body become empty or dry. This aggravated vata later occupies (fills) these channels and produces different diseases affecting one or more parts of the body. (1-4)

Vata Vyadhi Purvarupa

अव्यक्तं लक्षणं तेषां पूर्वरूपमिति स्मृतम् ।
आत्मरूपं तु यद्व्यक्तमपायो लघुता पुनः ॥५॥
(च. चि. अ. २८) ।

Premonitory stage of Vata Vyadhi is characterised by appearance of the symptoms of the disease which are in milder form. When the same symptoms (found in milder form in the premonitory stage) become well marked and severe, they denote the stage of manifestation of the disease (vata vyadhi).
On the other hand, absence of characteristic symptoms and lightness of the body (during the course of specific diseases to be described further on) are the signs of cure of such diseases.(5)

Vata Vyadhi Lakshanas

सङ्कोचः पर्वणां स्तम्भो भङ्गोऽस्थ्नां पर्वणामपि ।
रोमहर्षः प्रलापश्च पाणिपृष्ठशिरोग्रहः ॥६॥
खाञ्ज्यपाङ्गुल्यकुब्जत्वं शोथोऽङ्गानामनिद्रता ।
गर्भशुक्ररजोनाशः स्पन्दनं गात्रसुप्तता ॥७॥
शिरोनासाक्षिजत्रूणां ग्रीवायाश्चापि हुण्डनम् ।
भेदस्तोदोऽर्तिराक्षेपो मुहुश्चायास एव च ॥८॥
एवंविधानि रूपाणि करोति कुपितोऽनिलः ।
हेतुस्थानविशेषाच्च भवेद्रोगविशेषकृत् ॥९॥
(च. चि. अ. २८) ।

The **general symptoms of vata vyadhi** are - contractures of small joints of hands and feet (body parts), rigidity of joints, fracture & dislocation of joints including small joints of hands and feet, horripilation, delirium, stiffness (gripping pain, rigidity) of hands, back and head, limping and lameness of one or both legs, curvature of the back (hunchback), wasting of the body parts, loss of sleep, loss or destruction of foetus, semen and ovum (menstrual blood); tremors, and loss of sensation pain in the body parts.
This also occurs crookedness (drawing in of) head, nose, eyes, shoulders and neck; cutting or throbbing type of pain in the body parts, frequent convulsions and tiredness. These and other similar symptoms are produced by increased vata. The aggravated vata also produces special and newer diseases corresponding to the specific causes and sites of affection. (6-9)

Koshtashrita Vata

तत्र कोष्ठाश्रिते दुष्टे निग्रहो मूत्रवर्चसोः |
ब्रध्नहृद्रोगगुल्मार्शःपार्श्वशूलं च मारुते ||१०||

If the aggravated vāta is localised in the kostha (alimentary tract) there will be obstruction to passage of urine and faeces, enlargement of the scrotum (swelling in the groin), heart diseases, tumours of the abdomen, haemorrhoids and pain in the flanks. (10)

Sarvanga Vata

सर्वाङ्गकुपिते वाते गात्रस्फुरणभञ्जनम् |
वेदनाभिः परीताश्च स्फुटन्तीवास्य सन्धयः ||११||

If vāta gets increased all over the body, there will be tremors (throbbing, twitching, pulsations, etc.) cutting, crushing and other types of pain, feeling of pain in the joints and the person feels as if there is a blast (bursting) in the joints. (11)

Guda Sthita (Gudagata) Vata

ग्रहो विण्मूत्रवातानां शूलाध्मानाश्मशर्कराः |
जङ्घोरुत्रिकपात्पृष्ठरोगशोषौ गुदे स्थिते ||१२||

When the aggravated vāta gets localized and occupies in the gudā (rectum), it causes stoppage of movement of urine, faeces and flatus; pain (colic) and distension of the abdomen, formation of urinary gravel (calculus), pain in the calves, thighs, pelvis, legs (feet) and back and emaciation. (12)

Amashaya Sthita (Amashaya gata) Vata

रुक् पार्श्वोदरहृन्नाभेस्तृष्णोद्गारविसूचिकाः |
कासः कण्ठास्यशोषश्च श्वासश्चामाशयस्थिते ||१३||
(च. चि. अ. २८) |

If increased vāta resides in the āmāśaya (stomach) it causes pain in the flanks, abdomen, region of the heart and umbilicus, thirst, belching / eructation, vomiting and diarrhoea (occurring together), cough, dryness of throat and mouth and dyspnoea are found. (13)

Pakwasaya Sthita (Pakwasaya Gata) Vata

पक्वाशयस्थोऽन्त्रकूजं शूलाटोपौ करोति च |
कृच्छ्रमूत्रपुरीषत्वमानाहं त्रिकवेदनाम् ||१४||

If the aggravated vata gets lodged in the pakwāśaya (large intestine and rectum) it will cause intestinal gurgling and pain, gurgling sounds in the abdomen, difficulty for defecation and urination, flatulence (distension) of abdomen and pain in the sacral region. (14)

Srotradi Gata Vata

श्रोत्रादिष्विन्द्रियवधं कुर्याद्दुष्टसमीरणः | (सु. नि. अ. १) |

If vāta gets increased and localised in the Indriyas (sense organs) it will produce loss of function of those organs.

Twak Gata Vata

त्वग्रूक्षा स्फुटिता सुप्ता कृशा कृष्णा च तुद्यते |
आतन्यते सरागा च पर्वरुक् त्वग्गतेऽनिले ||१५||
(च. चि. अ. २८) |

If the increased vata is located in the twak (skin), it produces dryness, cracks, loss of sensation, thinning, blackish discolouration, pricking pain, stretching, redness and pain in the small joints of the hands and feet (and other joints of the body). (15)

Raktagata Vata

रुजस्तीव्राः ससन्तापा वैवर्ण्यं कृशताऽरुचिः |
गात्रे चारूंषि भुक्तस्य स्तम्भश्चासृग्गतेऽनिले ||१६||
(च. चि. अ. २८) |

If vata gets located in asrk (blood), it will cause severe pain, increased feeling of heat, discolouration, emaciation, loss of taste, appearance of ulcers or boils on the skin and stiffness of the body after meals. (16)

Mamsa Medogata Vata

गुर्वङ्गं तुद्यतेऽत्यर्थं दण्डमुष्टिहतं यथा |
सरुक् श्रमितमत्यर्थं मांसमेदोगतेऽनिले ||१७||

If vāta gets lodged in māmsa and medas (muscles and fat) it produces a feeling of heaviness of the body parts (body parts would become heavy and inactive) associated with severe throbbing (pricking) pain and pain as though beaten by a stick or fist. The person would also experience severe pain in the entire body and extreme exhaustion. (17)

Majja-Asthigata Vata

भेदोऽस्थिपर्वणां सन्धिशूलं मांसबलक्षयः |
अस्वप्नः सन्तता रुक् च मज्जास्थिकुपितेऽनिले ||१८||
(च. चि. अ. २८) |

When the aggravated vata is located in the majjā (bone marrow) and asthi (bone) it causes splitting pain in the bones and joints of the body including the small joints of the hands and feet, loss of muscles and strength of the body, loss of sleep and constant pain of the body.(18)

Shukragata Vata

क्षिप्रं मुञ्चति बध्नाति शुक्रं गर्भमथापि वा |
विकृतिं जनयेच्चापि शुक्रस्थः कुपितोऽनिलः ||१९||
(च. चि. अ. २८) |

If the aggravated vata gets localized in the shukra (semen, reproductive tissue) it would cause premature ejaculation. Similarly, the foetus created by such shukra (sperm) would either be delivered too soon (aborted / miscarriage) or would be delivered too late. This vata would also cause abnormalities of sperm (semen) and embryo. (19)

Siragata, Snayugata, Sandhigata Vata

कुर्यात् सिरागतः शूलं सिराकुञ्चनपूरणम् |
स बाह्याभ्यन्तरायामं खल्लीं कौब्ज्यमथापि वा ||२०||
सर्वाङ्गैकाङ्गरोगांश्च कुर्यात् स्नायुगतोऽनिलः | (च. चि. अ. २८) |
हन्ति सन्धिगतः सन्धीन् शूलाटोपौ करोति च ||२१|| (सु. नि. अ. १७) |

Siragata Vata - Vata (aggravated) located in the siras (veins and arteries) would cause pain, contractures or shortening and engorgement (with accumulation of blood).

Snayugata Vata – When the aggravated vata gets located in the snayus (ligaments, tendons, nerves) it would cause bow-like bending of the body either inwards or outwards, contractures of the fingers, shortening of the body due to the abnormal curvature of the back, and other diseases of either the whole body or any particular part or parts of the body.

Sandhigata Vata - If the aggravated vata is localized in the joints, it causes destruction of joints and their functions. Along with this, there also occurs pain and cracking sound (swelling) in the joints. (20-21)

Avarana of Vata subtypes by Pitta and Kapha

प्राणोदानौ समानश्च व्यानश्चापान एव च |
स्थानस्था मारुताः पञ्च यापयन्ति शरीरिणम्) | (सु. नि. अ. १) |
प्राणे पित्तावृते छर्दिर्दाहश्चैवोपजायते |
दौर्बल्यं सदनं तन्द्रा वैरस्यं च कफावृते ||२२|| (सु. नि. अ. १) |
उदाने पित्तयुक्ते तु दाहो मूर्छा भ्रमः क्लमः |
अस्वेदहर्षौ मन्दोऽग्निः शीतता च कफावृते ||२३||
स्वेददाहौष्ण्यमूर्छाः स्युः समाने पित्तसंवृते |
कफेन सक्ते विण्मूत्रे गात्रहर्षश्च जायते ||२४||
अपाने पित्तयुक्ते तु दाहौष्ण्यं रक्तमूत्रता |
अधःकाये गुरुत्वं च शीतता च कफावृते ||२५||
व्याने पित्तावृते दाहो गात्रविक्षेपणं क्लमः |
स्तम्भनो दण्डकश्चापि शूलशोथौ कफावृते ||२६|| (सु. नि. अ. १) |२७|

Prana, Udana, Samana, Vyana and Apana are the five types of vata. In their normal state, these vata subtypes residing in their own seats would nourish and sustain the body and good health of the body.

Avarana is a condition wherein vata and its normal functioning and movements are clouded (encompassed, masked, surrounded, blocked, obstructed or interfered) by pitta, kapha, tissues, food or excreta. One subtype of vata can cause avarana of another subtype of vata also.

Pittavrita Prana - If prana vata gets obstructed by pitta the person would have vomited and burning sensation.

Kaphavrita Prana – If prana vata is encompassed by kapha, the person would suffer from debility, tiredness (loss of strength), stupor and bad taste (manifestation of opposite tastes) in the mouth.

Pittavrita Udana – When udana vata is encompassed or enveloped by pitta it produces burning sensation, fainting (unconsciousness), dizziness and exhaustion.
Kaphavrita Udana – If Udana Vata is encompassed or enveloped by kapha it causes loss of perspiration, loss of enthusiasm, poor digestive ability and feeling of coldness.
Pittavrita Samana – When Samana Vata is encompassed by pitta it gives rise to perspiration, burning sensation, increased temperature and fainting (unconsciousness).
Kaphavrita Samana – When Samana Vata is enveloped by Kapha, it causes obstruction to the elimination of urine and faeces and horripilations in the body.
Pittavrita Apana – When Apana Vata is encompassed by pitta it causes burning sensation, increase of heat / temperature and elimination of blood mixed urine.
Kaphavruta Apana – When Apana Vata is obstructed by kapha, it causes heaviness of the lower portion of the body (limbs) and feeling of coldness.
Pittavruta Vyana – When Vyana Vata is encompassed by pitta it gives rise to burning sensation, abnormal movements of the parts of the body and exhaustion.
Kaphavruta Vyana – If Vyana Vata is clouded by Kapha the body becomes stiff like a log. Along with this there is pain and swelling.

Akshepaka

यदा तु धमनीः सर्वाः कुपितोऽभ्येति मारुतः |
तदाऽऽक्षिपत्याशु मुहुर्मुहुर्देहं मुहुश्चरः ||२७||
मुहुर्मुहुश्चाक्षेपणादाक्षेपक इति स्मृतः |
(सु. नि. अ. १) |

When the increased vata gets localized in all the dhamanis (blood vessels) of the body, it produces quick, frequent and jerky movements of the body. Since there are repeated convulsions, this condition is called Aksepaka (convulsions). (22-27)

Apatantraka, Apatanaka, Dandapatanaka

क्रुद्धः स्वैः कोपनैर्वायुः स्थानादूर्ध्वं [१] प्रवर्तते ||२८||
पीडयन् हृदयं गत्वा शिरःशङ्खौ च पीडयन् |
धनुर्वन्नमयेद्गात्राण्याक्षिपेन्मोहयेत्तदा ||२९||

स कृच्छ्रादुच्छ्वसेच्चापि स्तब्धाक्षोऽथ निमीलकः |
कपोत इव कूजेच्च निःसञ्ज्ञः सोऽपतन्त्रकः ||३०||
दृष्टिं संस्तभ्य सञ्ज्ञां च हत्वा कण्ठेन कूजति |
हृदि मुक्ते नरः स्वास्थ्यं याति मोहं वृते पुनः ||३१||
वायुना दारुणं प्राहुरेके तदपतानकम् |
(च. सि. अ. १) |
कफान्वितो भृशं वायुस्तास्वेव यदि तिष्ठति ||३२||
दण्डवत् स्तम्भयेद्देहं स तु दण्डापतानकः |
(सु. नि. अ. १) |

Apatantraka and Apatanaka are the variants of Aksepaka.

Apatantraka - Vata undergoing increase by its own moves in an upward direction towards the head (leaving its seats of predominance like colon etc). While doing so, it causes pain in the heart, head and temples. It further makes the body bend like a bow and produces convulsions and loss of consciousness.

The patient will find difficulty in breathing, the eyes are kept wide open at times (without the movement of lids) and at other times they remain half closed (or lids completely closed). The person remains in a state of unconsciousness and makes sounds from within the throat like a pigeon. This condition which is a variant of aksepaka is called apatantraka.

Apatanaka – Apatanaka is yet another variant of apatanaka (described by other scholars) in which the patient will have completely fixed gaze (incapable of perceiving any visual objects), complete loss of consciousness, produces cooing sounds in the throat, and will have intermittent relief of symptoms when the heart (brain) becomes free from the affliction of aggravated vata but once again enters into a state of unconsciousness when there is another attack. This dreadful disease caused by severely aggravated vata is called apatanaka.

Dandapatanaka – This is a variant of apatanaka. If in apatānaka, vāta gets associated with kapha, the body of the patient will become stiff like a log of wood. This condition is called as Dandāpatānaka. (28-32)

Dhanustambha, Abhyantarayama, Bahyayama

धनुस्तुल्यं नमेद्यस्तु स धनुःस्तम्भसञ्ज्ञकः ||३३|| (सु. नि. अ. १)
अङ्गुलीगुल्फजठरहृद्वक्षोगलसंश्रितः |
स्नायुप्रतानमनिलो यदाऽऽक्षिपति वेगवान् ||३४||

विष्टब्धाक्षः स्तब्धहनुर्भग्नपार्श्वः कफं वमन् |
अभ्यन्तरं धनुरिव यदा नमति मानवम् ||३५||
तदाऽस्याभ्यन्तरायामं कुरुते मारुतो बली |
बाह्यस्नायुप्रतानस्थो बाह्यायामं करोति च ||३६||
तमसाध्यं बुधाः प्राहुर्वक्षःकट्यूरुभञ्जनम् | (सु. नि. अ. १) |

Dhanustambha – It is a condition wherein the aggravated vata makes the body bent like a bow.

Abhyantarayama (dhanustambha) – It is a variant of dhanustambha. Here the powerful (aggravated) vata affects the network of snayus (ligaments, tendons, nerves) located in the toes (and fingers), ankle joints, abdomen, and region of the heart, chest and throat. By doing so, it causes severe convulsive movements. The patient develops fixed gaze, stiffness of the jaw (lower) fracture (collapse or in-drawing) of the flanks, ribs), and vomiting of phlegm (mucus). Here the bending of the body will be inwards and is bent like a bow. This condition caused by severely aggravated vata is called as Abhyantharayama dhanustambha.

Bahyayama (dhanustambha) – It is also a variant of dhanustambha. When severely aggravated vata affects the tendons (nerves) of the external part of the body, the body of the person gets bent outwards like a bow. In this condition there is a threat of fracture (damage) to the chest, waist and thighs and hence is incurable. This condition is known as Bahyayama dhanustambha and in the opinion of scholars is an incurable condition. (33-36)

Abhighataja Aksepaka

कफपित्तान्वितो वायुर्वायुरेव च केवलः ||३७||
कुर्यादाक्षेपकं त्वन्यं चतुर्थमभिघातजम् |
गर्भपातनिमित्तश्च शोणितातिस्रवाच्च यः ||३८||
अभिघातनिमित्तश्च न सिध्यत्यपतानकः | (सु. नि. अ. १) |

Dosha association in Aksepaka and symptoms of incurability of Apatanaka

Vata associated with kapha and pitta or even alone produces aksepaka. A fourth kind of aksepaka is caused due to trauma to the body parts and is called abhighataja aksepaka.

Apatanaka caused by abortions, excessive haemorrhage and trauma are incurable. (37-38)

Paksavadha

गृहीत्वाऽर्धं तनोर्वायुः सिराः स्नायूर्विशोष्य च ||३९||
पक्षमन्यतरं हन्ति सन्धिबन्धान् विमोक्षयन् |
कृत्स्नोऽर्धकायस्तस्य स्यादकर्मण्यो विचेतनः ||४०||
एकाङ्गरोगं तं केचिदन्ये पक्षवधं विदुः |
सर्वाङ्गरोगस्तद्वच्च सर्वकायाश्रितेऽनिले ||४१||
(वा. नि. अ. १५) |

Pathogenesis and symptoms

The aggravated vata gets lodged in and affects any half side of the body (right or left side of the body), causes dryness (destruction) of the siras and snayus (blood vessels and ligaments / tendons / nerves), causes looseness of the joints and destroys the functions and sensation of half side of the body. This condition is called as Ekanga Roga by some people and Paksavadha by some others. When the entire body i.e., both halves of the body are affected in a similar way by the aggravated vata, it is called Sarvanga Vata. (39-41)

Dosha association and symptoms of incurability in Paksavadha

दाहसन्तापमूर्छाः स्युर्वायौ पित्तसमन्विते |
शैत्यशोथगुरुत्वानि तस्मिन्नेव कफान्विते ||४२||
शुद्धवातहतं पक्षं कृच्छ्रसाध्यतमं विदुः |
साध्यमन्येन संयुक्तमसाध्यं क्षयहेतुकम् ||४३||
(सु. नि. अ. १) |

In the above disease (paksavadha), if vāta is associated with pitta, there will be burning sensation, increase of temperature of the affected parts and fainting (unconsciousness).

In paksavadha if vata is associated with kapha, there will be coldness, swelling and heaviness of the affected parts.

Pakşavadha caused by vāta alone is difficult to cure. Paksavadha caused by vata associated with other doshas (pitta and kapha) is easily curable. Pakdavadha caused by destruction of tissues (emaciation, wasting) is incurable. (42-43)

Other symptoms of incurability of Paksavadha

(गर्भिणीसूतिकाबालवृद्धक्षीणेष्वसृक्स्रुते | पक्षाघातं परिहरेत् वेदनारहितो यदि) |

(Paksāghāta seen in pregnant women, in women who has recently delivered, children, old people, emaciated persons and that caused by heavy bleeding and that in which the patient has no pain (sensation) at all in the affected limbs (and affected parts) should be refused treatment because this condition is incurable.)

Ardita

उच्चैर्व्याहरतोऽत्यर्थं खादतः कठिनानि वा |
हसतो जृम्भतो वाऽपि भाराद्विषमशायिनः ||४४||
शिरोनासौष्ठचिबुकललाटेक्षणसन्धिगः |
अर्दयत्यनिलो वक्त्रमर्दितं जनयत्यतः |
वक्रीभवति वक्त्रार्धं ग्रीवा चाप्यपवर्तते ||४५||
शिरश्चलति वाक्सङ्गो नेत्रादीनां च वैकृतम् |
ग्रीवाचिबुकदन्तानां तस्मिन् पार्श्वे च वेदना ||४६||

Speaking in loud voice (high pitch) for long periods, eating (biting) hard food substances, excessive laughing (by opening the mouth), excessive yawning, carrying heavy loads on the head, and sleeping in uneven or irregular posture.

Pathogenesis - The vata getting aggravated by the above said etiological factors spreads to and occupies the head, nose, lips, chin, forehead and joints of the eye affects the face and causes a disease called as Ardita.

Symptoms - In this condition one half of the face gets crooked (deviated to the other side) and the neck also becomes crooked (turned outwards). There is also shaking of the head, obstruction of voice / speech (inability to speak), and deformities of eyes, nose, neck, jaw and teeth. The person also experiences pain (in the mentioned parts) on the afflicted side. (44-46)

Premonitory symptoms and symptoms of incurability of ardita

(यस्याग्रजो रोमहर्षो वेपथुर्नेत्रमाविलम् |
वायुरूर्ध्वं त्वचि स्वापस्तोदो मन्याहन्ग्रहः) |
तमर्दितमिति प्राहुर्व्याधिं व्याधिविचक्षणाः |
क्षीणस्यानिमिषक्षस्य प्रसक्ताव्यक्तभाषिणः ||४७||
न सिध्यत्यर्दितं गाढं त्रिवर्षं वेपनस्य च |
(सु. नि. अ. १) |

(The premonitory symptoms of ardita include horripilations, tremors, accumulation of dirt in the eyes (dirty looking eyes), belching (eructation), loss of sensation in the skin (of the face), pricking pain, stiffness of the neck and lower jaw.)

Expert clinicians call this disease Ardita.

Symptoms of incurability of ardita

Ardita is said to be incurable in emaciated persons, in those who do not wink their eyes, whose speech is slurred and incoherent and in whom ardita is persisting for more than three years. (47)

Attacks and episodes of Aksepaka and other disorders

गते वेगे भवेत् स्वास्थ्यं सर्वेष्वाक्षेपकादिषु ||४८|| (वा. नि. अ. १५) |

In all types of aksepakas (convulsive disorders) the patient gets periods of health (normalcy) when the episodes of attack pass off. (48)

Hanugraha

जिह्वानिर्लेखनाच्छुष्कभक्षणादभिघाततः |
कुपितो हनुमूलस्थः स्रंसयित्वाऽनिलो हनुम् ||४९||
करोति विवृतास्यत्वमथवा संवृतास्यताम् |
हनुग्रहः स तेन स्यात् कृच्छ्राच्चर्वणभाषणम् ||५०|| (वा. नि. अ. १५) |

Causes

Opening the mouth in excess and for long periods (and also putting out the tongue) for the purpose of cleaning the teeth (brushing) and tongue with the help of brushes and tongue cleaners, eating foods which are dry, and injury are the etiological factors of hanugraha.

Pathogenesis

Due to the above said causes, the vata located at the root of the jaw causes loosening and dislocation of the joints of the jaw.

Symptoms

The mouth of the person will either remain open or closed tight all the time. This would cause difficulty in chewing the food as well as speaking. This disease is known as Hanugraha. (49-50)

Manyastambha

दिवास्वप्नासनस्थानविवृतोर्ध्वनिरीक्षणैः |
मन्यास्तम्भं प्रकुरुते स एव श्लेष्माणऽऽवृतः ||५१|| (सु. नि. अ. १) |

Causes

Excessive sleeping during daytime, sleeping at irregular places and in irregular postures and looking in upward direction for long periods are the causes of manyastambha.

Pathogenesis and symptoms

Vata aggravated due to the above said etiological factors either singly or in association with kapha will afflict the sides of the neck and cause manyastambha.

Symptoms

Stiffness of the neck is the main symptom of this disease, which is also the name of the disease. (51)

Jihvastambha

वाग्वाहिनीसिरासंस्थो जिह्वां स्तम्भयतेऽनिलः |
जिह्वास्तम्भः स तेनान्नपानवाक्येष्वनीशता ||५२||
(वा. नि. अ. १५) |

Jihva stambha (stiffness or loss of movement of the tongue) is caused when the aggravated vata affects the tendons / nerves near the voice box (responsible for the production of voice) and causes inability for chewing the food, drinking or talking. (52)

Siragraha

रक्तमाश्रित्य पवनः कुर्यान्मूर्धधराः सिराः |
रूक्षाः सवेदनाः कृष्णाः सोऽसाध्यः स्यात् सिराग्रहः ||५३||
(वा. नि. अ. १५) |

Vata increases, getting localised in the blood makes the blood vessels of the neck dry, painful and black coloured. This condition is known as Siragraha (or sirograha) and is incurable. (53)

Gridhrasi

स्फिक्पूर्वा कटिपृष्ठोरुजानुजङ्घापदं क्रमात् |
गृध्रसी स्तम्भरुक्तोदैर्गृह्णाति स्पन्दते मुहुः ||५४||
वाताद्वातकफात्तन्द्रागौरवारोचकान्विता | (च. चि. अ. २८) |
वातजायां भवेत्तोदो देहस्यापि प्रवक्रता |
जानुकट्यूरुसन्धीनां स्फुरणं स्तब्धता भृशम् ||५५||
वातश्लेष्मोद्भवायां तु निमित्तं वह्निमार्दवम् |
तन्द्रा मुखप्रसेकश्च भक्तद्वेषस्तथैव च ||५६||

Pathogenesis of Gridhrasi

Vata either alone or associated with kapha produces (a disease called) Grdhrasi. This condition is characterised by a peculiar type of pain. The pain typically starts from the buttock and descends downwards encroaching (spreading in, radiating) the back portions of pelvis (lumbar region), thigh, knee joint, calf muscles (back of the leg – the portion of the lower limb between knee and ankle joints) and foot.

Vataja Gridhrasi

Due to this there is also (apart from pain) stiffness (inability to move), severe pain and throbbing (pricking pain) in the regions mentioned above along with repeated (and intermittent) pulsations. These symptoms are characteristic of Vataja (vata predominant) Grdhrasi.

Vata-Kaphaja Gridhrasi

In Grdhrasi if there is association of kapha with vata the person will experience stupor, heaviness and anorexia.

(Vataja Grdhrasi presents with pricking pain, crookedness of the body parts (irregular shape of the body parts), throbbing and severe stiffness in the joints of the knee, pelvis and thigh (hip). In Vata-Kaphaja Grdhrasi sluggishness of digestive fire / capacity (poor digestive capacity), stupor, excessive salivation and aversion towards food are predominantly seen as symptoms.) (54-60)

Vishvachi

तलं प्रत्यङ्गुलीनां याः कण्डरा बाहुपृष्ठतः ||५७||
बाह्वोः कर्मक्षयकरी विश्वाची चेति सोच्यते |
(सु. नि. अ. १) |

Visvahci is an affection of the tendons / nerves of the fingers, the arms and the shoulders, leading to loss of function of the arm as caused by the aggravated vata.

The aggravated vata afflicts the tendons / nerves of the upper limb beginning from the back of the arm and reaching up to the back of the fingers and also involving the upper portions of the forearm and hands ultimately leading to the loss of functions in these regions. (57)

Krostuka Sirsa

वातशोणितजः शोथो जानुमध्ये महारुजः ||५८||
ज्ञेयः क्रोष्टुकशीर्षस्तु स्थूलः क्रोष्टुकशीर्षवत् | (सु. नि. अ. १) |

Vata and rakta getting affected together produces a very painful swelling of the knee joint (in the centre of the knee joint). The swelling is big and resembles the head of a fox and hence is known by the name Krostuka-Sirsa. (58)

Khanja and Pangu

वायुः कट्याश्रितः सक्थ्नः कण्डरामाक्षिपेद्यदा ||५९||
खञ्जस्तदा भवेज्जन्तुः पङ्गुः सक्थ्नोर्द्वयोर्वधात् |
(सु. नि. अ. १) |

Khanja – The aggravated vata gets lodged in the waist of the person, affects the tendons of one lower limb and causes loss of functions therein. This condition is called Khanja. Here the person cannot walk properly and experiences limping.

Pangu – When the aggravated vata, instead of one lower limb, affects the tendons and nerves of both the lower limbs and causes loss of functions therein the person would become lame. This condition is called as Pangu. (59)

Kalayakhanja

प्रक्रामन् वेपते यस्तु खञ्जन्निव च गच्छति ||६०||
कलायखञ्जं तं विद्यान्मुक्तसन्धिप्रबन्धनम् |
(सु. नि. अ. १) |

A condition in which there are tremors (in the legs, lower limbs) when the person begins to walk and later walks with a limp (limping gait, just like a person who has limp) is called Kalayakhanja. In this condition there is also looseness of the joints of the lower limb. This condition is caused due to excessive consumption of Kalaya (pea, lentil, masura dala) and hence the name Kalayakhanja. (60)

Vatakantaka

रुक् पादे विषमेन्यस्ते श्रमाद्वा जायते यदा ||६१||
वातेन गुल्फमाश्रित्य तमाहुर्वातकण्टकम् |
(वा. नि. अ. १५) |

Due to improper placing of the feet on the ground (walking on an irregular surface) while walking or exhaustion due to exertion of walking, the vata gets aggravated and gets localized in the ankle joints and causes severe pain therein. This condition is called as Vatakantaka. (61)

Padadaha

पादयोः कुरुते दाहं पित्तासृक्सहितोऽनिलः ||६२||
विशेषतश्चङ्क्रमतः पाददाहं तमादिशेत् |

(सु. नि. अ. १) |

The vitiated Vata gets associated with pitta and rakta (blood) and causes burning sensation in the feet. The burning sensation is experienced more when the person walks. This condition is called as Padadaha. (62)

Padaharsa

हृष्येते चरणौ यस्य भवेतां चापि सुप्तकौ ||६३||
पादहर्षः स विज्ञेयः कफवातप्रकोपतः |
(सु. नि. अ. १) |

Vitiated vata along with kapha produces a feeling of pins and needles or feeling of loss of sensation in the feet. This condition is called as padaharsa. (63)

Amsa Sosa and Apabahuka

अंसदेशस्थितो वायुः शोषयेदंसबन्धनम् ||६४|| (सु. नि. अ. १) |
सिराश्चाकुञ्च्य तत्रस्थो जनयेदवबाहुकम् |६५| (सु. नि. अ. १) |

Amsa Sosa - Vāta located in the region of the shoulder (shoulder blade) causes emaciation (of muscles) of the shoulder joint. (This is known as Amsa sosa.)

Avabahuka / Apabahuka – The aggravated vata located in the region of the shoulder (blades) causes constriction / dryness of the tendons / nerves located therein and causes another condition called as Apabahuka. (64)

Mukadi

आवृत्य वायुः सकफो धमनीः शब्दवाहिनीः ||६५||
नरान् करोत्यक्रियकान्मूकमिन्मिनगद्गदान् |
(सु. नि. अ. १) |

The aggravated vata along with kapha invades and obstructs the shabda vahini dhamanis (vessels / nerves which are responsible for the production of voice, vessels and nerves around the voice box) and cause inability to speak in the person. The person would become mute or would develop nasal speech or stammer. (65)

Tuni and Pratituni

अधो या वेदना याति वर्चोमूत्राशयोत्थिता ||६६||
भिन्दतीव गुदोपस्थं सा तूनी नाम नामतः | (सु. नि. अ. १) |

गुदोपस्थोत्थिता या तु प्रतिलोमं प्रधाविता ||६७||
वेगैः पक्वाशयं याति प्रतितूनीति सोच्यते |(सु. नि. अ. १) |

Tuni - The disease in which severe cutting pain begins in the colon (rectum?) and urinary bladder and moves downwards towards anus and penis is called Tuni.

Pratituni – In this condition the movement of the pain is in reverse direction as compared to that of tuni. Here the cutting type of pain first starts in the anus and penis and moves upwards towards the colon (large intestine). Here the pain quickly moves up in bouts, as if thrown in an upward direction (colic). (66-67)

Adhmana and Pratyadhmana

साटोपमत्युग्ररुजमाध्मातमुदरं भृशम् ||६८||
आध्मानमिति तं विद्याद् घोरं वातनिरोधजम् |
विमुक्तपार्श्वहृदयं तदेवामाशयोत्थितम् ||६९||
प्रत्याध्मानं विजानीयात् कफव्याकुलितानिलम् |
(सु. नि. अ. १) |

Adhmana - Adhmana is a condition caused due to the obstruction to the movements of vata. It is characterised by gurgling noise in the abdomen (intestines), severe pain and distension of the abdomen. This is considered to be a dreadful condition (life threatening).

Pratyadhmana – When the same symptoms of adhmana manifest in the stomach excluding (not manifesting) the regions of flanks and heart and is caused by vata associated with kapha, it is known as Pratyadhmana. (68-69)

Vatasthila and Pratyasthila

नाभेरधस्तात् सञ्जातः सञ्चारी यदि वाऽचलः ||७०||
अष्ठीलावद्घनो ग्रन्थिरूर्ध्वमायत उन्नतः |
वाताष्ठीलां विजानीयाद्बहिर्मार्गावरोधिनीम् ||७१||
एतामेव रुजोपेतां वातविण्मूत्ररोधिनीम् |
प्रत्यष्ठीलामिति वदेज्जठरे तिर्यगुत्थिताम् ||७२||
(सु. नि. अ. १) |

Ashthila / Vatashthila – A tumour / cyst (like outgrowth / protuberance) occurring below the umbilicus, which is either mobile or immobile, hard like a stone, which projects upwards and causes obstruction to the passage of faeces and urine is called as Vatashthila or Ashthila.

Pratyashthila – If the same stony projection (as that found in ashthila) is found lying obliquely in the abdomen, produces pain and obstruction to flatus, faeces and urine it is called as pratyashthila. (70-72)

Mutravarodha

मारुतेऽनुगुणे बस्तौ मूत्रं सम्यक् प्रवर्तते |
विकारा विविधाश्चात्र प्रतिलोमे भवन्ति च ||७३||
(सु. नि. अ. ३) |

When the vata (present in the urinary bladder) has its normal downward movement (anuloma), it causes proper elimination of urine from teh urinary bladder. But when the same vata moves in an upward direction (pratiloma), it causes many disorders (like mutrakrchchra, mutraghata, ashmari etc). (73)

Kampavata / Vepathu and Khalli

सर्वाङ्गकम्पः शिरसो वायुर्वेपथुसञ्ज्ञकः |७४|
खल्ली तु पादजङ्घोरुकरमूलावमोटनी ||७४||
(च. चि. अ. २८) |

Vepathu is that condition caused by vata in which there will be tremors in the entire body or all the parts of the body including the head. (Vepathu may occur with or without shaking or tremors in the head).
Khalli is that condition in which there will be cramps (distortions) of the foot (legs), calves, thighs, chest and wrist joints (arms). (74)

Urdhvavata

अधः प्रतिहतो वायुः श्लेष्मणा मारुतेन वा |
करोत्युद्गारबाहुल्यमूर्ध्ववातः स उच्यते ||७५||

Vata, getting obstructed in its downward movement either by kapha or by itself (another subtype of vata), begins to move upwards and produces too many belchings (eructation). This condition is known as Urdhvavata. (75)

Anukta Vataroga

स्थाननामानुरूपैश्च लिङ्गैः शेषान् विनिर्दिशेत् |
सर्वेष्वेतेषु संसर्गं पित्ताद्यैरुपलक्षयेत् ||७६||
(च. चि. अ. २८) |

Other vatavyadhi which are not explained
Symptoms of the remaining kinds of vata vyadhis are to be diagnosed with

respect to their site of affection and names. Similarly, the association of pitta, kapha and ama with vata shall be inferred based on the existing symptoms (of the associated dosha in the disease). (76)

Incurability of Vata Vyadhi

हनुस्तम्भार्दिताक्षेपपक्षाघातापतानकाः |
कालेन महता वाता यत्नात् सिध्यन्ति वा न वा ||७७||
नरान् बलवतस्त्वेतान् साधयेन्निरुपद्रवान् |
(च. चि. अ. २८) |

Hanustambha, ardita, akshepa, pakshaghata, apatanaka, become severe and difficult to cure or even incurable with lapse of time. These diseases, in the availability of all equipments and facilities of treatment and with proper treatment being administered will sometimes get cured and sometimes not. Treatment of these conditions shall be attempted in patients who are physically strong and when they are not associated with complications. (77-78)

Upadravas

विसर्पदाहरुक्सङ्गमूर्छारुच्यग्निमार्दवैः ||७८||
क्षीणमांसबलं वाता घ्नन्ति पक्षवधादयः |

Complications of Vata

Visarpa (erysipelas), burning sensation, severe pain, stiffness of body parts (ankylosis) or non-elimination of flatus, faeces, urine, etc. fainting (unconsciousness), anorexia, poor digestive capacity, wasting of muscles, and loss of strength are the complications of vata vyadhi. In the presence of these diseases / conditions, the vata disorders such as paksawadha become fatal. (78)

शूनं सुप्तत्वचं भग्नं कम्पाध्माननिपीडितम् |
रुजार्तिमन्तं च नरं वातव्याधिर्विनाशयेत् ||७९||
(सु. सू. अ. ३३) |

Swelling of the body (or its parts), loss of tactile sensation, fractures of bones, tremors, distension of the abdomen (flatulence) or severe pain found in vata vyadhis are also to be considered as fatal signs. (79)

Symptoms of Prakrutastha Vata

अव्याहतगतिर्यस्य स्थानस्थः प्रकृतिस्थितः |

वायुः स्यात् सोऽधिकं जीवेद्वीतरोगः समाः शतम् ||८०||
(च. चि. अ. २८) |

The person in whom the movements (functions) of vata are not obstructed anywhere in the body, the subtypes of vata (Prana, Udana, Vyana, Samana and Apana Vata) remaining in their normal locations render normal functions, will live for hundred years without suffering from any disease. (80)

इति श्रीमाधवकरविरचिते माधवनिदाने वातव्याधिनिदानं समाप्तम् ||२२||

Thus ends the chapter on Vatavyadhi Nidanam in Madhava Nidana text written by Acharya Madhavakara.

23

Madhava Nidana Chapter 23 Vata Raktha Nidanam

Vatarakta Nidana Samprapti

लवणाम्लकटुक्षारस्निग्धोष्णाजीर्णभोजनः |
क्लिन्नशुष्काम्बुजानूपमांसपिण्याकमूलकैः ||१||
कुलत्थमाषनिष्पावशाकादिपललेक्षुभिः |
दध्यारनालसौवीरशुक्ततक्रसुरासवैः ||२||
विरुद्धाध्यशनक्रोधदिवास्वप्नप्रजागरैः |
प्रायशः सुकुमाराणां मिथ्याहारविहारिणाम् |(च. चि. अ. २९) |
स्थूलानां सुखिनां चापि कुप्यते वातशोणितम् ||३|| (सु. चि. अ. १) |
हस्त्यश्वोष्ट्रैर्गच्छतश्चाश्नतश्च विदाह्यन्नं सविदाहोऽशनस्य |
कृत्स्नं रक्तं विदहत्याशु तच्च स्रस्तं दुष्टं पादयोश्चीयते तु |
तत् सम्पृक्तं वायुना दूषितेन तत्प्राबल्यादुच्यते वातरक्तम् ||४|| (सु. नि. अ. १) |

Excessive indulgence in foods which are salty, sour, pungent, alkaline, unctuous (fatty), hot or uncooked (unprocessed),

Excessive consumption of flesh of animals or birds belonging to marshy or desert like regions – which are either wet (soaked in water for long time) or dry (devoid of moisture)

Excessive consumption of eatables having sesame paste, radish, horse gram, black gram, cow pea, green leafy vegetables, meat (mutton), sugarcane (juice),

Excessive consumption of curds, fermented drinks like aranala, sauviraka,

sukta, takra (fermented buttermilk), sura, asava etc
Excessive consumption of incompatible (foods having opposite qualities),
Eating food in excess
Anger
Habit of sleeping during day time and keeping awake at night (and many such other unhealthy foods and activities)
The above-mentioned etiological factors produce a disease called Vatarakta especially in those who are very tender (those people who are not accustomed to hardships of life, those having soft and tender organs or body parts), who are obese and people who are always happy and content (have not experienced hardships or misery of any kind.

Vatarakta Samprapti

Pathogenesis of Vatarakta - Excessive riding on elephants, horses, camels etc (animal back) for long durations of time or regularly (as a habit or part of profession) and excessive indulgence (consumption of) in foods which cause burning sensation (inside the body) during or after digestion etc. will burn the food which in turn would quickly burn (vitiate or contaminate) the blood.
This burnt and improperly processed blood will flow downwards and accumulate in the foot. Here this blood gets associated with vata which has been aggravated due to its etiological factors (like riding on the elephants etc. mentioned above) and causes the disease therein. Since vata is predominant in this disease it is called as Vatarakta. (1-4)

Vatarakta Purvarupa

स्वेदोऽत्यर्थं न वा कार्ष्ण्यं स्पर्शाज्ञत्वं क्षतेऽतिरुक् |
सन्धिशैथिल्यमालस्यं सदनं पिडकोद्गमः ||५||
जानुजङ्घोरुकट्यंसहस्तपादाङ्गसन्धिषु |
निस्तोदः स्फुरणं भेदो गुरुत्वं सुप्तिरेव च ||६||
कण्डूः सन्धिषु रुग्भूत्वा भूत्वा नश्यति चासकृत् |
वैवर्ण्यं मण्डलोत्पत्तिर्वातासृक्पूर्वलक्षणम् ||७||
(च. चि. अ. २९) |

Premonitory Symptoms of Vatarakta
Excessive or absence of perspiration, black discolouration, loss of tactile sensation,
severe pain even on slight injury (pain in the seat of injury), looseness of joints,

laziness (lethargy), debility, appearance of boils (eruptions, blisters) in joints of knee, leg, thigh (hip), pelvis (waist), shoulder (blade, axillary region), hands (fingers), feet (toes) and the entire body.
There will also be severe pain which present in different ways, like throbbing (gnawing), pulsating and cutting (in the above-mentioned joints and body) along with heaviness and loss of sensation. Apart from these, there is itching, the pain keeps coming and going in the joints (intermittent pain), discolouration and appearance of circular rashes. (5-7)

Vatadhika Vatarakta

वातेऽधिकेऽधिकं तत्र शूलस्फुरणभञ्जनम् |
शोथस्य रौक्ष्यं कृष्णत्वं श्यावता वृद्धिहानयः ||८||
धमन्यङ्गुलिसन्धीनां सङ्कोचोऽङ्गग्रहोऽतिरुक् |
शीतद्वेषानुपशयौ स्तम्भवेपथुसुप्तयः ||९||

If vāta is very predominant in vatarakta, there will be excessive (severe) pain, like pulsating or tearing (cutting) pain. The swelling over the joints will appear dry, black or blue (bluish black). The symptoms increase or decrease often. There will be contractures of arteries (blood vessels) and joints of the fingers, stiffness of the body parts and severe pain. The person will have dislike (aversion) towards cold things and the symptoms would increase by consumption of or exposure to cold things, stiffness, tremors and loss of sensation etc (in other parts of the body). (8-9)

Raktadhika Vatarakta

रक्ते शोथोऽतिरुक्तोदस्ताम्रश्चिमिचिमायते |
स्निग्धरूक्षैः शमं नैति कण्डूक्लेदसमन्वितः ||१०||

If in vatarakta, rakta is affected profoundly; the swelling will be having severe pain, pricking or a feeling of pins and needles, coppery red in colour, and tingling sensation. There will be no relief with unctuous (oily) or dry comforts (like massage etc). The person will also have itching and exudation from the joints. (10)

Pittadhika Vatarakta

पित्ते विदाहः सम्मोहः स्वेदो मूर्छा मदस्तृषा |
स्पर्शासहत्वं रुग्रागः शोथः पाको भृशोष्मता ||११||

If pitta is predominant (in vatarakta) the person would experience burning sensation in the body, delusion, perspiration, unconsciousness (fainting), intoxication and thirst. There will also be tenderness, pain, redness, swelling, suppuration (formation of pus) and increased heat (temperature). (11)

Kaphadhika Vataraka

कफे स्तैमित्यगुरुतासुप्तिस्निग्धत्वशीतताः |
कण्डूर्मन्दा च रुग्द्वन्द्वं सर्वलिङ्गं च सङ्करात् ||१२|| (वा. नि. अ. १६) |

If kapha is predominant (in vatarakta), the person would feel as if his body has been wrapped with wet cloth and would experience heaviness of the body, loss of sensation, unctuousness (greasy feel), coldness, itching and mild pain (in the joints).

Dwandwa and Sannipataja Vatarakta

When there is predominance of two doshas in vatarakta, the symptoms of both doshas will be present mixed together.

When there is predominance of three doshas in vatarakta, the symptoms of all the three doshas will be present mixed together. (12)

Mode of spread of vatarakta

पादयोर्मूलमास्थाय कदाचिद्धस्तयोरपि |
आखोर्विषमिव क्रुद्धं तद्देहमुपसर्पति ||१३|| (सु. नि. अ. १) |

The (pain of) vatarakta usually starts from the root of the legs (toes or ankle joint) or from the root of the hands (fingers or wrist joint) and spreads to the other parts of the body, slowly, just like a rat poison. (13)

Symptoms of incurability

आजानु स्फुटितं यच्च प्रभिन्नं प्रस्रुतं च यत् |
उपद्रवैश्च यज्जुष्टं प्राणमांसक्षयादिभिः ||१४||
वातरक्तमसाध्यं स्याद्याप्यं संवत्सरोत्थितम् | (सु. नि. अ. १) |
अस्वप्नारोचकश्वासमांसकोथशिरोग्रहाः ||१५||
सम्मूर्छामदरुक्तृष्णाज्वरमोहप्रवेपकाः |
हिक्कापाङ्गुल्यवीसर्पपाकतोदभ्रमक्लमाः ||१६||
अङ्गुलीवक्रतास्फोटदाहमर्मग्रहार्बुदाः |
एतैरुपद्रवैर्वर्ज्यं मोहेनैकेन वाऽपि यत् ||१७||
अकृत्स्नोपद्रवं याप्यं, साध्यं स्यान्निरुपद्रवम् |
एकदोषानुगं साध्यं नवं, याप्यं द्विदोषजम् |
त्रिदोषजमसाध्यं स्याद्यस्य च स्युरुपद्रवाः ||१८|| (च. चि. अ. २९) |

Vatarakta is said to be incurable if –
It has started in the toe and has spread to the knee joint (all the joints from foot to knee are affected)
The skin over the joints has peeled off or has cracked and if there is exudation from the cracked skin
It is associated with many complications (like loss of sleep etc enumerated below) which bring about
Destruction of muscles (muscular wasting) and loss of vital functions of the body (prana)
Vatarakta is said to be manageable (persists for the rest of the life but would require regular treatment to keep it under control – yapya) if it has not existed for more than one year.
Vatarakta associated with complications is also incurable.
The complications of vatarakta are –
loss of sleep, anorexia, dyspnoea (increased / difficult respiration),
putrefaction of muscles, headache, unconsciousness (fainting), intoxication,
pain (colic), thirst, fever, delusion, rigors (tremors), hiccough,
lameness (inability to walk), herpes / erysipelas (or other skin diseases),
suppuration, pricking sensation (pain), giddiness, exhaustion (tiredness),
crookedness / contractures of fingers (or toes), blisters, burning sensation,
diseases / pain in the vital organs and appearance of tumours (nodules).
The patient of vatarakta having these complications shall be refused treatment. Vatarakta is incurable even if unconsciousness is the only complication associated with it.
When vatarakta is not associated with all the above-mentioned complications (only few complications exist), the condition is said to be manageable (disease would persist for life but would require regular treatment).
When vatarakta is devoid of any of the above-mentioned complications it is said to be curable.
Vatarakta is caused by only one dosha and that which is of recent onset is curable.
Vatarakta caused by two doshas is manageable (persists for life but needs regular treatment).
Vatarakta caused by all three aggravated doshas is incurable. Similarly, vatarakta associated with complications is also incurable. (14-18)

इति श्रीमाधवकरविरचिते माधवनिदाने वातरक्तनिदानं समाप्तम् ||२३||

Thus ends the chapter on Vātarakta Nidanam in Madhava Nidana text written by Acharya Madhavakara.

24

Madhava Nidana Chapter 24 Urustambha Nidanam

Nidana of Urustambha

शीतोष्णद्रवसंशुष्कगुरुस्निग्धैर्निषेवितैः ।
जीर्णाजीर्णे तथाऽऽयाससङ्क्षोभस्वप्नजागरैः ॥१॥
सश्लेष्ममेदःपवनः साममत्यर्थसञ्चितम् ।
अभिभूयेतरं दोषमूरू चेत् प्रतिपद्यते ॥२॥
सक्थ्यस्थिनी प्रपूर्यान्तः श्लेष्मणा स्तिमितेन च ।
तदा स्तभ्नाति तेनोरू स्तब्धौ शीतावचेतनौ ॥३॥
परकीयाविव गुरू स्यातामतिभृशव्यथौ ।
ध्यानाङ्गमर्दस्तैमित्यतन्द्राच्छर्द्यरुचिज्वरैः ॥४॥
संयुक्तौ पादसदनकृच्छ्रोद्धरणसुप्तिभिः ।
तमूरुस्तम्भमित्याहुराढ्यवातमथापरे ॥५॥
(वा. नि. अ. १५) ।

Causes of Urustambha - stiffness of the thigh - Excessive indulgence in foods and other activities which are mixture of opposites such as cold and hot, watery and dry, heavy and light, fatty (unctuous) and non-fatty (non-unctuous), cooked and uncooked (eating food when the previously taken food is not digested or partially digested), etc.

Severe exertion, mental strain, over-sleeping or keeping awake and such other factors

Samprapti

Pathogenesis - Due to the above said factors – the aggravated vata getting associated with excessively accumulated ama (intermediate products of digestion or products formed due to sluggish digestion in the stomach), kapha and meda (adipose tissue) taking the pitta together with them, moves downwards and accumulate in the thigh. The thick consolidated kapha fills up the bones of the thighs and causes stiffness of the thighs.

Lakshanas of Urusthambha

Symptoms of Urustambha – This condition causes stiffness of lower limbs (thighs), coldness and loss of sensation (loss of control).

The patient feels heaviness in his lower limbs, as if his legs are not his own and his legs have been replaced by someone else's legs (he feels as though his legs belong to somebody else and that is why they are heavy to him).

He will also experience severe pain in the lower limbs.

The patient also experiences grief or anxiety, pain in the body parts, immobility of lower limbs (as if his limbs are covered by wet clothes), stupor, vomiting, anorexia, fever, weakness in the legs (lower limbs), difficulty in lifting the legs and loss of sensation in the lower limbs.

This disease is known as Urustambha. Others call the same condition as Adhyavata. (1-5)

Purvarupa

प्राग्रूपं तस्य निद्राऽतिध्यानं स्तिमितता ज्वरः |
रोमहर्षोऽरुचिश्छर्दिर्जङ्घोर्वोः सदनं तथा ||६||

Premonitory symptoms of urustambha

The premonitory symptoms of urustambha are – excessive sleep, too much worry, loss of movements, (feeling as if the body or affected parts have been covered by a wet leather or cloth), fever, horripilation, anorexia, vomiting, and weakness in the legs and thighs. (6)

Anupashaya, Sadhyasadhyata

वातशङ्किभिरज्ञानात्तस्य स्यात् स्नेहनात् पुनः |
पादयोः सदनं सुप्तिः कृच्छ्रादुद्धरणं तथा ||७||
जङ्घोरुग्लानिरत्यर्थं शश्वच्चादाहवेदने |
पादं च व्यथते न्यस्तं शीतस्पर्शं न वेत्ति च ||८||
संस्थाने पीडने गत्यां चालने चाप्यनीश्वरः |
अन्यस्येव हि सम्भग्नावूरू पादौ च मन्यते ||९||

Conditions in which the symptoms of urustambha get aggravated, symptoms of curability and incurability (prognosis)

Without knowing the specific features of this disease (urustambha) and suspecting it to be a disease of vata (on observing vata predominant symptoms like numbness, contracture, tremor etc), if unctuous remedies like oil massage etc. are done (considering that oil remedies are the best in treating vata disorders and vata symptoms), the symptoms will exacerbate (increase) quickly, causing severe debility in the legs, and loss of sensation, difficulty in lifting the lower limbs, severe exhaustion (tiredness) of the legs and thighs, constant mild burning sensation (heat) and pain. The patient gets pain on placing the foot on the ground, and he (his feet) will not be able to appreciate cold touch.

The patient suffering from urustambha will be unable to stand (keep the leg in any one posture), press something from his foot, move the foot, walk around or do any type of activity. The patient will feel that his thigh and feet has been replaced by someone else's thighs or that his thighs have been fractured. (7-9)

यदा दाहार्तितोदार्तो वेपनः पुरुषो भवेत् |
ऊरुस्तम्भस्तदा हन्यात्, साधयेदन्यथा नवम् ||१०||(च. चि. अ. २७) |

If urustambha is associated with complications like burning sensation, severe pain, pricking pain and tremors in the legs it is considered as incurable. At the same time if urustambha is not associated with these symptoms (complications) and if it has developed very recently, it is curable. (10)

इति श्रीमाधवकरविरचिते माधवनिदाने ऊरुस्तम्भनिदानं समाप्तम् ||२४||

Thus ends the chapter on Urustambha Nidanam in Madhava Nidana text written by Acharya Madhavakara.

25

Madhava Nidana Chapter 25 Amavata Nidanam

Amavata Nidana

विरुद्धाहारचेष्टस्य मन्दाग्नेर्निश्चलस्य च |
स्निग्धं भुक्तवतो ह्यन्नं व्यायामं कुर्वतस्तथा ||१||
वायुना प्रेरितो ह्यामः श्लेष्मस्थानं प्रधावति |
तेनात्यर्थं विदग्धोऽसौ धमनीः प्रतिपद्यते ||२||
वातपित्तकफैर्भूयो दूषितः सोऽन्नजो रसः |
स्रोतांस्यभिष्यन्दयति नानावर्णोऽतिपिच्छिलः ||३||
जनयत्याशु दौर्बल्यं गौरवं हृदयस्य च |
व्याधीनामाश्रयो ह्येष आमसञ्ज्ञोऽतिदारुणः ||४||
युगपत्कुपितावन्तस्त्रिकसन्धिप्रवेशकौ |
स्तब्धं च कुरुतो गात्रमामवातः स उच्यते ||५||

Etiological factors - indulgence in incompatible (mutually opposite, incompatible and antagonistic) foods and habits,
having low digestion fire (capacity),
lack of physical activity, or
doing exercise (indulgence in physical activities) immediately after taking unctuous (fatty) foods

Samprapti

Pathogenesis - The above said etiological factors produce plenty of ama (improperly digested food, intermediate products of digestion produced due to the action of weak digestive fire in the stomach on the food consequently leading to sluggish and incomplete digestion). The vata too is aggravated.

This ama being stimulated and pushed by aggravated vata moves towards different seats of kapha and gets lodged therein.

Being excessively contaminated (further) and pushed further by the aggravated vata, this ama reaches the dhamanis (blood vessels).

This ama is further contaminated by all the three doshas i.e., vata, pitta and kapha located in the dhamanis.

Due to the contamination by all the three doshas, ama acquires different colours and becomes excessively sticky (slimy), produces excessive fluidity in all the channels of the body and causes obstruction therein.

All these events produce quick weakness (debility) and heaviness in the region of the heart.

This ama becomes the root source and causative factors of many diseases and hence is considered dreadful and dangerous.

These vata and ama aggravated simultaneously would enter and lodge in the trika sandhi – pelvis and other joints of the body.

This dreadful disease which produces stiffness of the entire body in due course of time is called as amavata. (1-5)

(**Note** - Trika Sandhi shall be considered as the joints in the pelvis or the meeting of three bones in the region of shoulder blade / shoulder girdle. This also includes sacro-iliac and sacro-coccygeal joints including lower lumbar vertebrae. Some have considered the words trika and sandhi separately. In this condition trika sandhi should be understood as the pelvis and other joints of the body.)

Amavata Lakshanas

अङ्गमर्दोऽरुचिस्तृष्णा आलस्यं गौरवं ज्वरः |
अपाकः शूनताऽङ्गानामामवातस्य लक्षणम् ||६||

General symptoms of amavata - The general symptoms of amavata include – pain all over the body (in all parts of the body and joints), tastelessness, thirst, laziness (loss of enthusiasm), heaviness of the body, fever, indigestion and swelling of the body parts (and joints). (6)

Pravruddha Amavata Lakshanas

स कष्टः सर्वरोगाणां यदा प्रकुपितो भवेत् |

हस्तपादशिरोगुल्फत्रिकजानूरुसन्धिषु ||७||
करोति सरुजं शोथं यत्र दोषः प्रपद्यते |
स देशो रुज्यतेऽत्यर्थं व्याविद्ध इव वृश्चिकैः ||८||
जनयेत् सोऽग्निदौर्बल्यं प्रसेकारुचिगौरवम् |
उत्साहहानिं वैरस्यं दाहं च बहुमूत्रताम् ||९||
कुक्षौ कठिनतां शूलं तथा निद्राविपर्ययम् |
तृट्छर्दिभ्रममूर्छाश्च हृद्ग्रहं विड्विबद्धताम् |
जाड्यान्त्रकूजमानाहं कष्टांश्चान्यानुपद्रवान् ||१०||

Symptoms of advanced stage of amavata

The severely aggravated and advanced stage of amavata (when it has become chronic due to long standing symptoms) is considered to be the most difficult one to treat in comparison to many other diseases i.e., it becomes incurable.

In this condition there is painful swelling of the joints of hands, feet, head, ankle, pelvis / waist, knee and thigh (hip), wherever the doshas tend to reach and get lodged. Apart from this, the person would experience severe pain resembling the pain of a scorpion sting in any place or joints of the body where the doshas reach (doshas here mean vata along with ama and other doshas as explained in the pathogenesis of amavata).

The other symptoms of amavata include – weakness of digestive fire (poor digestion), excessive salivation, anorexia, heaviness of the body, lack of enthusiasm and drive, manifestation of bad / odd tastes in the mouth, burning sensation, profuse (excessive) urination – polyuria, hardness of the abdomen, pain in the abdomen (colic), and erratic sleep patterns (excessive sleepiness in the morning and loss of sleep at night).

Along with these there is also excessive thirst, vomiting, giddiness, loss of consciousness, stiffness in the region of the heart, constipation, inability to do any work (loss of movements of the body parts – severe stiffness), gurgling sounds in the abdomen, flatulence (distension) and many other difficult complications. (7-10)

Symptoms of associated doshas in amavata

पित्तात् सदाहरागं च, सशूलं पवनानुगम् |
स्तिमितं गुरुकण्डूं च कफदुष्टं तमादिशेत् ||११||

In amavata associated with pitta there will be burning sensation and redness of the affected joint (part).

If vata is predominant in amavata the patient would experience severe pain.

In case of kapha predominance in amavata there will be feeling as if his joints (and other parts of the body) are covered by a wet leather or cloth, heaviness and itching. (11)

Prognosis

एकदोषानुगः साध्यो, द्विदोषो याप्य उच्यते |
सर्वदेहचरः शोथः स कृच्छ्रः सान्निपातिकः ||१२||

Symptoms of incurability of amavata

Amavata caused by predominant involvement of any one dosha is curable.

If amavata is caused by two doshas it will be manageable (persists for the rest of the life but needs regular and prompt treatment).

Amavata, wherein all the three doshas are involved and presents with swelling which has spread all over the body (including all the joints) is said to be incurable. (12)

इति श्रीमाधवकरविरचिते माधवनिदाने आमवातनिदानं समाप्तम् ||२५||

Thus ends the chapter on Amavāta Nidanam in Madhava Nidana text written by Acharya Madhavakara.

26

Madhava Nidana Chapter 26 Shula Parinama shoola Annadrava shula Nidanam

Types of Sula

दोषैः पृथक् समस्तामद्वन्द्वैः शूलोऽष्टधा भवेत् ।
सर्वेष्वेतेषु शूलेषु प्रायेण पवनः प्रभुः ॥१॥

Shula (colic, pain in the abdomen) is of eight types; one from each doṣha, one from the combination of all three doshas, one each from the combination of two doṣhas and the eighth from āma. In all types, vāta is the predominant causative dosha. (1)

To sum up, sula is of 8 types and are named as mentioned below –

1. Vataja Shoola
2. Pittaja Shula
3. Kaphaja Sula
4. Tridoshaja / Sannipataja Shoola
5. Vata-Pittaja Sula
6. Kapha-Pittaja Sula

7. Kapha-Vataja Sula
8. Amaja Sula

Vataja Sula

व्यायामयानादतिमैथुनाच्च प्रजागराच्छीतजलातिपानात् |
कलायमुद्गाढकिकोरदूषादत्यर्थरूक्षाध्यशनाभिघातात् ||२||
कषायतिक्तातिविरूढजान्नविरुद्धवल्लूरकशुष्कशाकात् |
विट्शुक्रमूत्रानिलवेगरोधाच्छोकोपवासादतिहास्यभाष्यात् ||३||
वायुः प्रवृद्धो जनयेद्धि शूलं हृत्पार्श्वपृष्ठत्रिकबस्तिदेशे |
जीर्णे प्रदोषे च घनागमे च शीते च कोपं समुपैति गाढम् ||४||
मुहुर्मुहुश्चोपशमप्रकोपी विड्वातसंस्तम्भनतोदभेदैः |
संस्वेदनाभ्यञ्जनमर्दनाद्यैः स्निग्धोष्णभोज्यैश्च शमं प्रयाति ||५||

Nidana

Etiological factors of Vataja Sula - Excessive indulgence in physical exercises, riding, sexual intercourse, keeping awake at nights, and excessive drinking of very cold water

Excessive ingestion of food articles like peas, green gram, tuvar dāl, kora dūsa and other foods which cause dryness inside the body,

Excessive consumption of foods (over-eating)

Injury / trauma,

Consumption in excess of foods which are predominant in astringent and bitter taste; germinated grains and foods which have mutually opposite qualities (mutually incompatible foods), dried up flesh and dried leafy vegetables

Suppression of urges of faeces, semen, urine and flatus;

Excessive grief

Starvation or fasting

Excessive laughing and speaking

Samprapti (Pathogenesis) – The vata gets abnormally increased due to the above said etiological factors and causes colic. This condition is called Vataja Sula.

Lakshanas (Symptoms) - pain is manifested in the region of the heart, flanks, back, waist and urinary bladder,

pain gets exacerbated after the digestion of food, in the evenings, during cloudy (rainy season) and cold weather;

pain frequently keeps increasing or decreasing on its own accord,

there is obstruction to the movement (expulsion) of faeces and flatus,
pain is of pricking or tearing nature
the pain subsides on administration of sudation (hot fomentation), massage with oils, rubbing or tapping, and foods and drinks which are unctuous (fatty) and hot (2-5)

Pittaja Sula

क्षारातितीक्ष्णोष्णविदाहितैलनिष्पावपिण्याककुलत्थयूषैः |
कट्वम्लसौवीरसुराविकारैः क्रोधानलायासरविप्रतापैः ||६||
ग्राम्यातियोगादशनैर्विदग्धैः पित्तं प्रकुप्याशु करोति शूलम् |
तृण्मोहदाहार्तिकरं हि नाभ्यां संस्वेदमूर्छाभ्रमचोषयुक्तम् ||७||
मध्यन्दिने कुप्यति चार्धरात्रे विदाहकाले जलदात्यये च |
शीते च शीतैः समुपैति शान्तिं सुस्वादुशीतैरपि भोजनश्च ||८||

Nidana

Etiological factors - Excessive consumption of foods which are alkaline, deep penetrating, excessive hot, which produces burning sensation (or heat),
Excessive consumption of oils, cow-pea, and cake made from paste of sesame, horse gram soup
Excessive consumption of foods which are predominant in pungent and sour taste
Excessive consumption of fermented beverages like sauvira, sura etc
Excessive anger
Exposure to fire
Fatigue
Prolonged exposure to heat of the sun
Excessive indulgence in sexual intercourse

Samprapti

Pathogenesis - The consumption of the above-mentioned etiological factors will cause improper digestion of food (burning of food). This in turn causes aggravation of pitta and this aggravated pitta causes colic. This colic is called Pittaja Sula.

Lakshanas - Symptoms

Severe thirst
Delusion
Severe burning sensation around the umbilicus
Perspiration (excessive sweating)

Unconsciousness
Giddiness
Localised burning sensation
The pain increases during afternoon, midnight, during the digestion of food and in Sharad Ritu (autumn season)
The pain subsides in cold season, by cold comforts, and by consumption of sweet and cold foods (6-8)

Kaphaja Sula

आनूपवारिजकिलाटपयोविकारैर्मांसेक्षुपिष्टकृशरातिलशष्कुलीभिः |
अन्यैर्बलासजनकैरपि हेतुभिश्च श्लेष्मा प्रकोपमुपगम्य करोति शूलम् ||९||
हृल्लासकाससदनारुचिसम्प्रसेकैरामाशये स्तिमितकोष्ठशिरोगुरुत्वैः |
भुक्ते सदैव हि रुजं कुरुतेऽतिमात्रं सूर्योदयेऽथ शिशिरे कुसुमागमे च ||१०||

Nidana

Etiological factors - Excessive consumption of foods prepared from the flesh of animals and birds living in the marshy lands and also that prepared from the flesh of aquatic animals (animals living in water)
Excessive consumption of Kilata (a buttermilk preparation) and milk products
Excessive consumption of meat (mutton), sugarcane (and sugarcane juice), flour (made of black gram), krshara (gruel prepared using sesame, rice and black gram) and large round cake prepared from sesame
Excessive consumption of other etiological factors (foods and activities) which tend to cause aggravation of kapha

Samprapti

Pathogenesis – Kapha gets abnormally increased due to the consumption of the above-mentioned etiological factors and causes colic. This type of colic is called Kaphaja Sula.

Lakshanas (Symptoms)

Nausea (oppression of the chest)
Cough,
Debility,
Tastelessness,
Excessive salivation (excessive production of phlegm in the mouth),
Pain in the stomach,
Loss of movement (hardness) and fullness in the abdomen,
Heaviness in the head

The pain increases immediately after taking the food, early in the morning, late winter (shishira rtu) and spring season (kusumagame – vasanta rtu) (9-10)

Sannipataja Sula

सर्वेषु दोषेषु च सर्वलिङ्गं विद्याद्भिषक् सर्वभवं हि शूलम् |
सुकष्टमेनं विषवज्रकल्पं विवर्जनीयं प्रवदन्ति तज्ज्ञाः ||११||

Symptoms and nature of Sannipataja Sula

The colic produced by the combination of all the three dosas together is called sannipataja shula.

This condition is marked by the presence of the symptoms of all the three doshas. This colic will occur in severe form and is troublesome. According to experts this condition is difficult to treat (incurable) just like poison and diamond and hence should be refused treatment. (11)

Amaja Shula

आटोपहृल्लासवमीगुरुत्वस्तैमित्यकानाहकफप्रसेकैः |
कफस्य लिङ्गेन समानलिङ्गमामोद्भवं शूलमुदाहरन्ति ||१२||

The symptoms of amaja shula (colic caused due to material produced due to indigestion) are - gurgling sounds in the abdomen (intestines), nausea (oppression in the chest), vomiting, feeling of heaviness, feeling as if the body has been wrapped with wet leather or cloth, flatulence (distension of the abdomen), excessive salivation, and manifestation of other symptoms similar to those found in kaphaja type of colic. (12)

Dwidoshaja Sula

बस्तौ हृत्पार्श्वपृष्ठेषु स शूलः कफवातिकः |
कुक्षौ हृन्नाभिमध्येषु स शूलः कफपैत्तिकः ||१३||
दाहज्वरकरो घोरो विज्ञेयो वातपैत्तिकः |१४|

Symptoms of Dwidoshaja Sula (colic caused by predominant aggravation of two doshas)

Kapha-Vataja Sula - If the pain / colic is found in the region of the urinary bladder, heart, flanks and back it is probably due to combined vitiation of kapha and vata.

Kapha-Pittaja Sula – If the pain / colic is found in the centre of abdomen, heart and umbilicus, it is probably due to combined vitiation of kapha and pitta.

Vata-Pittaja Sula – If there is burning sensation and fever accompanied by severe pain in the region of urinary bladder and navel, it is probably caused due to combined vitiation of vata and pitta. (13)

Prognosis of Shoola

एकदोषोत्थितः साध्यः, कृच्छ्रसाध्यो द्विदोषजः ||१४||
सर्वदोषोत्थितो घोरस्त्वसाध्यो भूर्युपद्रवः |१५|

Colic produced by the increase of any one dosha is easily curable. The colic caused by simultaneously vitiating 2 doshas is said to be difficult to cure.
The colic caused by simultaneous vitiation of all three doshas, is severe and dreadful in nature, and associated with many complications is incurable. (14)

Parinama Shoola

Pathogenesis

स्वैर्निदानैः प्रकुपितो वायुः सन्निहितस्तदा ||१५||
कफपित्ते समावृत्य शूलकारी भवेद्बली |
भुक्ते जीर्यति यच्छूलं तदेव परिणामजम् ||१६||
तस्य लक्षणमप्येतत् समासेनाभिधीयते |१७|

The vata gets aggravated due to its own etiological factors (etiological factors responsible for aggravation of vata) on getting lodged in specific seats (in the stomach and intestine) will get powerful (severely aggravated), gets enveloped (blocked, obstructed) by kapha and pitta and produces severe colic during the process of digestion of food. This colic occurs during the digestion of food (transformation of food) and hence called as parinama sula. This itself (colic appearing during the process of digestion of food) is the characteristic symptom of parinama sula. (15-16)

Symptoms

Vataja Parinama Sula Symptoms

आध्मानाटोपविण्मूत्रविबन्धारतिवेपनैः ||१७||
स्निग्धोष्णोपशमप्रायं वातिकं तद्वदेद्भिषक्

The symptoms of parinama sula caused due to vata predominance are – distension of the abdomen, gurgling sounds in the abdomen (intestines), obstruction to the elimination of (excretion of) faeces and urine, restlessness (not able to focus in any work) and tremors. The symptoms pacify by using unctuous and hot comforts (fatty and warm foods). (16-17)

Pittaja Parinama Sula Symptoms

तृष्णादाहारतिस्वेदं कट्वम्ललवणोत्तरम् ||१८||
शूलं शीतशमप्रायं पैत्तिकं लक्षयेद्बुधः |

The symptoms of parinama sula caused due to pitta predominance are – thirst, burning sensation, restlessness and perspiration. The pain increases by use of pungent, sour and salty foods. On the other hand, the pain gets reduced due to use of cold foods and comforts. (18)

Kaphaja Parinama Sula Symptoms

छर्दिहृल्लाससम्मोहं स्वल्परुग्दीर्घसन्तति ||१९||
कटुतिक्तोपशान्तं च तच्च ज्ञेयं कफात्मकम् |

The symptoms of parinama sula caused due to kapha predominance are – vomiting, nausea, and unconsciousness. The pain is mild in nature and persists for a long duration. The pain gets reduced by use of pungent and bitter foods. (19)

Dwidoshaja Parinama Sula and Tridoshaja Parinama Sula Symptoms

संसृष्टलक्षणं बुद्ध्वा द्विदोषं परिकल्पयेत् ||२०||
त्रिदोषजमसाध्यं तु क्षीणमांसबलानलम् |२१|

When in parainama sula there are combined symptoms of two doshas it should be considered as dwidoshaja parinama sula.

Similarly, when there are combined symptoms of three doshas in parinama shula it should be considered as tridoshaja parinama sula.

Tridoshaja Shoola is considered to be incurable. Likewise, any shoola associated with loss of muscles (emaciation), loss of strength and decrease of digestive fire (digestive capacity) is considered to be incurable. (20)

Annadrava Sula Symptoms

जीर्णे जीर्यत्यजीर्णे वा यच्छूलमुपजायते ||२१||
पथ्यापथ्यप्रयोगेण भोजनभोजनन च |
न शमं याति नियमात् सोऽन्नद्रव उदाहृतः ||२२||
(अन्नद्रवाख्यशूलेषु न तावत् स्वास्थ्यमश्नुते |
वान्तमात्रे जरत्पित्तं शूलमाशु व्यपोहति) ||१||

When the colic occurs after the digestion of food, during the process of digestion of food and also before the digestion of food (immediately after consumption of food) i.e., the colic can occur at any time (and doesn't subside at any time) – it is called as annadrava sula. Such type of pain doesn't pacify with use of compatible or incompatible foods, by eating food on not eating it.

(In annadrava sula the pain persists constantly and the patient never feels relieved with anything. The pain subsides when the aggravated pitta is expelled out through vomiting i.e., when the patient vomits or is induced). (21-22)

इति श्रीमाधवकरविरचिते माधवनिदाने शूलपरिणामशूलान्नद्रवशूलनिदानं समाप्तम् ||२६||

Thus ends the chapter on Thus ends the chapter on Shula Parinamashula Annadravashula Nidanam in Madhava Nidana text written by Acharya Madhavakara.Nidanam in Madhava Nidana text written by Acharya Madhavakara.

27

Madhava Nidana Chapter 27 Udavarta Anaha Nidanam

Udavarta Nidana

वातविण्मूत्रजृम्भाश्रुक्षवोद्गारवमीन्द्रियैः |
क्षुत्तृष्णोच्छ्वासनिद्राणां धृत्योदावर्तसम्भवः ||१||

Etiological Factors of Udavarta - Suppression of the urges of flatus, faeces, urine, yawning, tears, sneezing, belching, vomiting, semen, hunger, thirst, respiration and sleep, is the cause for the disease Udāvarta. (1)

Vata Nigrahaja Udavarta

वातमूत्रपुरीषाणां सङ्गो ध्मानं क्लमो रुजा |
जठरे वातजाश्चान्ये रोगाः स्युर्वातनिग्रहात् ||२||
(च. सू. अ. ७) |

The symptoms of 'suppression of urge of flatus' are –
obstruction (difficulty in) to expulsion of flatus, faeces and urine
distension of abdomen,
weakness
pain (in the abdomen or body parts)
manifestation of other symptoms of abnormal increase of vata (in the abdomen) (2)

Purishaja Udavarta

आटोपशूलौ परिकर्तिका च सङ्गः पुरीषस्य तथोर्ध्ववातः |
पुरीषमास्यादथवा निरेति पुरीषवेगेऽभिहते नरस्य ||३||
(सु. उ. तं. अ. ५५) |
The symptoms of suppression of 'urge for defecation (excretion of faeces)' are –
gurgling sounds in the abdomen (intestines),
pain in the abdomen (colic)
cutting pain in the rectum (anus and also in the penis and urinary bladder)
constipation (obstruction to excretion of faeces),
excessive belching
upward movement of flatus and faeces through the mouth (3)

Mutra Udavarta
बस्तिमेहनयोः शूलं मूत्रकृच्छ्रं शिरोरुजा |
विनामो वङ्क्षणानाहः स्याल्लिङ्गं मूत्रनिग्रहे ||४||
(च. सू. अ. ७) |
The symptoms of suppression of 'urge for urination (expulsion or excretion of urine)' are –
pain in the urinary bladder and penis,
difficulty in urination (dysuria)
headache
bending of the body forwards
distension / obstruction / tension / swelling in the groins (4)

Jrimbha Nirodhaja Udavarta
मन्यागलस्तम्भशिरोविकारा जृम्भोपघातात् पवनात्मकाः स्युः |
तथाऽक्षिनासावदनामयाश्च भवन्ति तीव्राः सह कर्णरोगैः ||५||
The symptoms of suppression of 'urge for yawning' are –
stiffness of the nape of the neck and neck (throat)
diseases of the head (headache)
other symptoms / diseases of vata increase
diseases of the eyes, nose, face (mouth)
severe diseases of the ears (5)

Ashruja (ashru nirodhaja) Udavarta
आनन्दजं वाऽप्यथ शोकजं वा नेत्रोदकं प्राप्तममुञ्चतो हि |
शिरोगुरुत्वं नयनामयाश्च भवन्ति तीव्राः सह पीनसेन ||६||

(सु. उ. तं. अ. ५५) |

The symptoms of suppression of 'urge for tearing (weeping, shedding tears)' of pleasure or grief origin are –
heaviness of the head
disorders of the eyes
severe nasal catarrh (6)

Kshavathu Nirodhaja Udavarta

मन्यास्तम्भः शिरःशूलमर्दितार्धावभेदकौ |
इन्द्रियाणां च दौर्बल्यं क्षवथोः स्याद्विधारणात् ||७||
(च. सू. अ. ७) |

The symptoms of suppression of 'urge for sneezing' are –
stiffness of the neck (nape of the neck),
headache
facial paralysis
headache on one side (hemicrania, migraine)
weakness of the sense organs (inability or decreased ability of sense organs to perceive their respective objects) (7)

Udgara Nirodhaja Udavarta

कण्ठास्यपूर्णत्वमतीव तोदः कूजश्च वायोरथवाऽप्रवृत्तिः |
उद्गारवेगेऽभिहते भवन्ति घोरा विकाराः पवनप्रसूताः ||८||
(सु. उ. तं. अ. ५५) |

The symptoms of suppression of 'urge for belching' are –
feeling of fullness (obstruction) in the throat and mouth
severe pricking pain in the throat
gurgling sounds in the abdomen
obstruction to breathing
other diseases or symptoms of vata increase (8)

Chardi Nigrahajanya Udavarta

कण्डूकोठारुचिव्यङ्गशोथपाण्ड्वामयज्वराः |
कुष्ठवीसर्पहृल्लासाश्छर्दिनिग्रहजा गदाः ||९||
(च. सू. अ. ७) |

The symptoms of suppression of 'urge for vomiting' are –
itching
appearance of rashes

tastelessness / anorexia
black spots / patches on the face
oedema
anaemia
fever
leprosy / skin diseases
erysipelas / herpes
nausea (9)

Shukra Nirodhaja Udavarta

मूत्राशये वै गुदमुष्कयोश्च शोथो रुजा मूत्रविनिग्रहश्च |
शुक्राश्मरी तत्स्रवणं भवेच्च ते ते विकारा विहते च शुक्रे ||१०||

The symptoms of suppression of 'urge for ejaculation of semen' are –
oedema / swelling and pain in the urinary bladder, rectum (anus) and scrotum
obstruction to the elimination of urine
formation and discharge (expulsion) of stones / gravel in the seminal passages (seminal calculi) (10)

Kshuda Nirodhaja Udavarta

तन्द्राङ्गमर्दावरुचिः श्रमश्च क्षुधाभिघातात् कृशता च दृष्टेः |

The symptoms of suppression of 'urge for eating food (hunger)' are –
stupor
body aches,
tastelessness (anorexia),
exhaustion,
darkness in front of the eyes / loss of vision

Trsna Nirodhaja Udavarta

कण्ठास्यशोषः श्रवणावरोधस्तृष्णाविघातादधृदये व्यथा च ||११||

The symptoms of suppression of 'urge for thirst' are –
dryness of the throat and mouth,
difficulty in hearing (deafness),
pain in the region of heart (11)

Svasa Nigrahajanya Udavarta

श्रान्तस्य निःश्वासविनिग्रहेण हृद्रोगमोहावथवाऽपि गुल्मः |

The symptoms of suppression of 'exertion induced dyspnoea' are –
Exertion causes difficulty in breathing for a short duration. If one suppresses this, it would cause –
diseases of the heart,
unconsciousness
abdominal tumours

Nidra Nirodhaja Udavarta

जृम्भाऽङ्गमर्दोऽक्षिशिरोऽतिजाड्यं निद्राभिघातादथवाऽपि तन्द्रा ||१२||
(सु. उ. तं. अ. ५५) |

The symptoms of suppression of 'urge for sleep' are –
yawning,
body aches
heaviness in the eyes and head
stupor (12)

Vatajanya Udavarta

वायुः कोष्ठानुगो रूक्षैः कषायकटुतिक्तकैः |
भोजनः कुपितः सद्य उदावर्तं करोति हि ||१३||
वातमूत्रपुरीषासृक्कफमेदोवहानि वै |
स्रोतांस्युदावर्तयति पुरीषं चातिवर्तयेत् ||१४||
ततो हृद्बस्तिशूलार्तो हृल्लासारतिपीडितः |
वातमूत्रपुरीषाणि कृच्छ्रेण लभते नरः ||१५||
श्वासकासप्रतिश्यायदाहमोहतृषाज्वरान् |
वमिहिक्काशिरोरोगमनःश्रवणविभ्रमान् |
बहूनन्यांश्च लभते विकारान् वातकोपजान् ||१६||
(सु. उ. तं. अ. ५५) |

Vata located in the abdomen gets suddenly aggravated due to excessive consumption of foods which are dry and predominant in astringent, pungent and bitter tastes and produce a disease called udavarta instantly.
The normal direction of movement in the passages of flatus, urine, faeces, blood, kapha and medas (adipose tissue) gets reversed (or obstructed). The faeces would get dried up.
The person would experience severe pain in the region of the heart and urinary bladder, nausea and restlessness.
The flatus, urine and faeces get eliminated with difficulty.
The other symptoms include – dyspnoea (increased respiration), cough,

running in the nose, burning sensation, unconsciousness / confusion, thirst, fever, vomiting, hiccough, headaches (diseases of the head), confusion (deviations in the mind), disorders of hearing (manifestation of abnormal sounds in the ears) and many other symptoms / diseases of vata increase. (13-16)

Anaha

आमं शकृद्वा निचितं क्रमेण भूयो विबद्धं विगुणानिलेन |
प्रवर्तमानं न यथास्वमेनं विकारमानाहमुदाहरन्ति ||१७||
तस्मिन् भवन्त्यामसमुद्भवे तु तृष्णाप्रतिश्यायशिरोविदाहाः |
आमाशये शूलमथो गुरुत्वं हृत्स्तम्भ उद्गारविघातनं च ||१८||
स्तम्भः कटीपृष्ठपुरीषमूत्रे शूलोऽथ मूर्छा शकृतश्च छर्दिः |
शोथश्च पक्वाशयजे भवन्ति तथाऽलसोक्तानि च लक्षणानि ||१९||
(सु. उ. तं. अ. ५६) |

Anaha Definition, Types

Anaha is a disease wherein gradually accumulated ama (undigested food, intermediated products of digestion caused by sluggishness of the digestive fire) in the stomach or faeces in the colon get obstructed in a more severe way as caused by aggravated vata and do not get eliminated through their normal routes.

Amaja Anaha – If anaha is caused by accumulation of ama in the stomach it produces – thirst, running in the nose, burning sensation in the head, pain and heaviness in the stomach, stiffness in the region of the heart, and absence of (obstruction of) belching.

Purishaja Anaha – If anaha is caused by accumulation of faeces in the large intestine (colon) it causes – stiffness of the waist and back, obstruction of faeces and urine, pain (colic), unconsciousness, vomiting of faecal material (vomited material appearing and smelling like faeces), dyspnoea, and other symptoms mentioned in the context of Alasaka disease. (17-19)

Symptoms of incurability of udavarta

तृष्णार्दितं परिक्लिष्टं क्षीणं शूलैरभिद्रुतम् |
शकृद्वमन्तं मतिमानुदावर्तिनमुत्सृजेत् ||२०||
(सु. उ. तं. अ. ५५) |

A patient of udavarta suffering from severe thirst, restlessness or severe distress, emaciation, continuous obstinate abdominal pain and faecal vomiting should be refused treatment because this condition is incurable.

(20)

इति श्रीमाधवकरविरचिते माधवनिदाने उदावर्तानाहनिदानं समाप्तम् ||२७||
Thus ends the chapter on Udavarta Anaha Nidanam in Madhava Nidana text written by Acharya Madhavakara.

28

Madhava Nidana Chapter 28 Gulma Nidanam

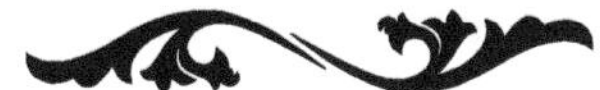

Gulma Samprapti

दुष्टा वातादयोऽत्यर्थं मिथ्याहारविहारतः |
कुर्वन्ति पञ्चधा गुल्मं कोष्ठान्तर्ग्रन्थिरूपिणम् |
तस्य पञ्चविधं स्थानं पार्श्वहृन्नाभिबस्तयः ||१||

Pathogenesis of Gulma - Due to excessive indulgence in incompatible / erroneous foods and activities (habits and daily activities) Vata and other doshas undergo severe vitiation. These doshas cause five types of gulma which are of the form and shape of a cyst / tumour inside the abdomen (abdominal cavity).

Seats of Gulma – Gulma manifests in five seats. The five common sites of gulma are – two parsva (flanks, sides of the abdomen), hrdaya (heart, cardiac region, epigastrium), nabhi (umbilicus, umbilical region) and vasti (region of urinary bladder). (1)

Definition of Gulma

हृन्नाभ्योरन्तरे ग्रन्थिः सञ्चारी यदि वाऽचलः |
वृत्तश्चयापचयवान् स 'गुल्म' इति कीर्तितः ||२||
(सु. उ. तं. अ. ४२) |

Gulma is defined as a mass in between the region of the heart and the umbilicus, which is either moving (from one place to the other) or stationary, round in shape and undergoing increase or decrease in size. (2)

Bheda – Types of gulma

स व्यस्तैर्जायते दोषैः समस्तैरपि चोच्छ्रितैः |
पुरुषाणां तथा स्त्रीणां ज्ञेयो रक्तेन चापरः ||३||
(सु. उ. तं. अ. ४२) |

There are five types of gulma. Among these four types of gulma are caused in both men and women (common in men and women). These four types of gulma are caused due to vitiation of individual doshas i.e., vata, pitta, kapha, combined vitiation of all three doshas together. The fifth type of gulma is caused by an increase of rakta (blood) and is manifested only in women. (3) In short, the five types of gulma are –

उद्गारबाहुल्यपुरीषबन्धतृप्त्यक्षमत्वान्त्रविकूजनानि |
आटोप आध्मानमपक्तिशक्तिरासन्नगुल्मस्य वदन्ति चिह्नम् ||४||
(वा. नि. अ. ११) |

1. Vataja Gulma
2. Pittaja Gulma
3. Kaphaja Gulma
4. Sannipataja Gulma
5. Raktaja Gulma (manifested only in women)

Purvarupa

Premonitory symptoms of Gulma - The premonitory symptoms of gulma are excessive belching, constipation, disinterest towards food (a morbid feeling of contentment), lack of endurance, gurgling sounds in the abdomen (intestines), painful irritation in the abdomen, distension of abdomen and poor digestion capacity. (4)

Gulma Samanya Lakshana

अरुचिः कृच्छ्रविण्मूत्रवातताऽन्त्रविकूजनम् |
आनाहश्चोर्ध्ववातत्वं सर्वगुल्मेषु लक्षयेत् ||५||

General symptoms / presentation of gulma - The symptoms commonly seen in all types of gulma are – loss of taste, difficulty in elimination of faeces, urine and flatus, gurgling sounds in the abdomen (intestines), flatulence, & upward movement of vata. (5)

Vataja Gulma

रूक्षान्नपानं विषमातिमात्रं विचेष्टनं वेगविनिग्रहश्च |
शोकोऽभिघातोऽतिमलक्षयश्च निरन्नता चानिलगुल्महेतुः ||६||
यः स्थानसंस्थानरुजां विकल्पं विड्वातसङ्गं गलवक्त्रशोषम् |
श्यावारुणत्वं शिशिरज्वरं च हृत्कुक्षिपार्श्वांसशिरोरुजं च ||७||
करोति जीर्णे त्वधिकं प्रकोपं भुक्ते मृदुत्वं समुपैति यश्च |
वातात् स गुल्मो नच तत्र रूक्षं कषायतिक्तं कटु चोपशेते ||८||
(च. चि. अ. ५) |

Etiological factors – Excessive indulgence in dry foods and drinks (foods devoid of fats), imbalanced and incompatible foods, and excessive consumption of foods (in large quantities), unsuitable physical activities, suppression of natural urges, excessive grief, trauma, excessive depletion of faeces and starvation (not consuming food) are the etiological factors of vataja gulma.

Symptoms – In vataja gulma the seat, shape and nature of pain keeps changing constantly (they are not fixed or well defined, fluctuant in nature). The other symptoms include – obstruction to (non elimination) the elimination of faeces and flatus, dryness of throat and mouth, blackish or reddish discolouration, fever accompanied by cold, pain in the region of heart, abdomen, flanks, shoulder blades (shoulders) and head. The pain increases after the digestion of food and subsides immediately after consuming food. The pain and discomfort are not relieved (worsened, increased) by consumption of foods which are dry, astringent, bitter and pungent. (6-8)

Pittaja Gulma

कट्वम्लतीक्ष्णोष्णविदाहिरूक्षक्रोधातिमद्यार्कहुताशसेवा |
आमाभिघातो रुधिरं च दुष्टं पैत्तस्य गुल्मस्य निमित्तमुक्तम् ||९||
ज्वरः पिपासा वदनाङ्गरागः शूलं महज्जीर्यति भोजन च |
स्वेदो विदाहो व्रणवच्च गुल्मः स्पर्शासहः पैत्तिकगुल्मरूपम् ||१०||
(च. चि. अ. ५) |

Etiological factors – Excessive indulgence in foods which are pungent, sour, penetrating, causing burning sensation (corrosive) and dry (devoid of fats and unctuous substances), anger, excessive use of alcohol, excessive exposure to sunlight and fire, excessive accumulation of ama in the body, injury, and vitiation (contamination) of blood are the causative factors for pittaja gulma.

Symptoms – The symptoms of pittaja gulma are – fever, thirst, redness of the face and body, severe pain (colic) in the abdomen experienced during the digestion of food, excessive sweating, burning sensation, and tenderness as found in (resembling) ulcers. (9-10)

Kaphaja Gulma

शीतं गुरु स्निग्धमचेष्टनं च सम्पूरणं प्रस्वपनं दिवा च |
गुल्मस्य हेतुः कफसम्भवस्य सर्वस्तु दुष्टो निचयात्मकस्य ||११||
स्तैमित्यशीतज्वरगात्रसादहृल्लासकासारुचिगौरवाणि |
शैत्यं रुगल्पा कठिनोन्नतत्वं गुल्मस्य रूपाणि कफात्मकस्य ||१२||
(च. चि. अ. ५) |

Etiological factors – Excessive indulgence in foods which are too cold, heavy to digest, and excessively unctuous (fatty), sedentary life devoid of any physical activities or exercise, eating foods till satiation (eating in excess) & excessive sleep during day time are the causative factors of kaphaja gulma.

Etiological factors of sannipataja Gulma – Sannipataja or Tridoshaja Gulma are caused by a combination of etiological factors mentioned for individual doshaja gulma.

Symptoms of kaphaja gulma – The symptoms of kaphaja gulma are – feeling as if the body (abdomen) has been covered by wet cloth, fever with cold, weakness, nausea, cough, tastelessness, and heaviness of the body. The gulma is cold in touch (person feels cold), has mild pain, hard and elevated (bulged out). (11-12)

Dwandwaja Gulma

निमित्तरूपाण्युपलभ्य गुल्मे द्विदोषजे दोषबलाबलं च |
व्यामिश्रलिङ्गानपरांश्च गुल्मांस्त्रीनादिशेदौषधकल्पनार्थम् ||१३||
(च. चि. अ. ५) |

Tumors of abdomen caused by two doshas

The combination of any two doshas will also cause three other types of gulma. This should be identified and diagnosed based on the availability of etiological factors, symptoms and strength of two doshas together. They are recognised for the purpose of providing suitable treatment. (13)

Sannipataja Gulma Symptoms

महारुजं दाहपरीतमश्मवद्घनोन्नतं शीघ्रविदाहि दारुणम् |
मनःशरीराग्निबलापहारिणं त्रिदोषजं गुल्ममसाध्यमादिशेत् ||१४||
(च. चि. अ. ५) |

Sannipataja or Tridoshaja Gulma is marked by the presence of severe pain and burning sensation, the mass is bulged out and has stone-like feel and consistency (on touch). The mass will undergo suppuration very quickly and is considered to be very dreadful. This condition would produce weakness of the mind, body, digestive fire and strength. This gulma is incurable in nature. (14)

Rakta Gulma

नवप्रसूताऽहितभोजन या या चामगर्भं विसृजेद्दतौ वा |
वायुर्हि तस्याः परिगृह्य रक्तं करोति गुल्मं सरुजं सदाहम् |
पैत्तस्य लिङ्गेन समानलिङ्गं विशेषणं चाप्यपरं निबोध ||१५||
(सु. उ. तं. अ. ४२) |
यः स्पन्दते पिण्डित एव नाङ्गैश्चिरात् सशूलः समगर्भलिङ्गः |
स रौधिरः स्त्रीभव एव गुल्मो मासे व्यतीते दशमे चिकित्स्यः ||१६||
(च. चि. अ. ५) |

Causes of Rakta Gulma – Consumption of unsuitable / incompatible foods and indulgence in incompatible activities by women who have recently delivered a child, have undergone miscarriage or abortion or during menstruation.

Pathogenesis – In women consuming the above-mentioned etiological factors, vata gets aggravated in the uterus (reproductive system of the women). This vata causes obstruction of rakta (menstrual blood) and causes gulma (tumour) along with pain and burning sensation. This condition is called rakta gulma.

Symptoms – Rakta Gulma is associated with pain and burning sensation. The symptoms are similar to those of pittaja gulma. In addition, this condition will also have some special symptoms. Due to the mass, the woman experiences all the signs of pregnancy but on palpation (by the doctor) the gulma pulsates in a single mass and not by organs i.e., the palpating hands of the physician can appreciate a pulsating mass (single) but will not be able to detect different parts of the fetus (since the foetus is not there in the womb). The pulsating pain occurs at long intervals along with signs of pregnancy. This condition occurs only in women. It shall be treated only after the completion of ten months. (This is to rule out pregnancy in case of chance of wrong diagnosis. If it is pregnancy, the foetus will be naturally delivered at the end of 9 months. If it is rakta gulma it doesn't get delivered. This will confirm the diagnosis and hence shall be treated after 10 months.) (15-16)

Symptoms of incurability

सञ्चितः क्रमशो गुल्मो महावास्तुपरिग्रहः |
कृतमूलः सिरानद्धो यदा कूर्म इवोत्थितः ||१७||
दौर्बल्यारुचिहृल्लासकासच्छर्द्यरतिज्वरैः |
तृष्णातन्द्राप्रतिश्यायैर्युज्यते स न सिध्यति ||१८||
गृहीत्वा सज्वरं श्वासच्छर्द्यतीसारपीडितम् |
हृन्नाभिहस्तपादेषु शोथः कर्षति गुल्मिनम् ||१९|| (च. चि. अ. ५) |

Gulma is incurable when the mass -
grows steadily,
has assumed very big size,
occupies the entire abdomen
is deeply rooted,
has visible networks of veins on the abdomen (mass), i.e. accompanied with venous engorgement,
is elevated like the shell of a tortoise,
It is also incurable when associated with the below mentioned symptoms –
weakness / debility
tastelessness
nausea
cough
vomiting
restlessness
fever
thirst
drowsiness / stupor
running in the nose,

Other symptoms of incurability are –
continuous fever
dyspnoea
vomiting
diarrhoea

swelling / oedema in the region of the heart, umbilicus, hands and feet (17-19)

Other symptoms of incurability of gulma

श्वासः शूलं पिपासाऽन्नविद्वेषो ग्रन्थिमूढता |
जायते दुर्बलत्वं च गुल्मिनो मरणाय वै ||२०||
(सु. सू. अ. ३३) |

Dyspnoea (difficulty in breathing), colic, thirst, aversion towards food, sudden disappearance of the mass (of gulma), and severe tiredness are the fatal signs of gulma. (20)

इति श्रीमाधवकरविरचिते माधवनिदाने गुल्मनिदानं समाप्तम् ||२८||

Thus ends the chapter on Gulma Nidanam in Madhava Nidana text written by Acharya Madhavakara.

29

Madhava Nidana Chapter 29 Hridroga Nidanam

Hridroga Nidana

अत्युष्णगुर्वन्नकषायतिक्तश्रमाभिघाताध्यशनप्रसङ्गैः |
सञ्चिन्तनैर्वेगविधारणैश्च हृदामयः पञ्चविधः प्रदिष्टः ||१||

Etiological factors of heart diseases

Regular and excessive consumption of foods which are very hot, heavy (hard to digest), predominantly astringent and bitter in taste, excess fatigue, injury, eating before the previous food has been digested, excessive worry, and suppression of the urges of the body are the causative factors of five kinds of heart diseases. (1)

Hrudroga Samprapti

दूषयित्वा रसं दोषा विगुणा हृदयं गताः |
हृदि बाधां प्रकुर्वन्ति हृद्रोगं तं प्रचक्षते ||२||
(सु. उ. तं. अ. ४३) |

Pathogenesis of heart diseases

The doshas having undergone morbid increase by their etiological factors, vitiate the rasa dhaatu, and get localised in the heart which is the seat of rasa dhatu and causes disease (pain) in the heart. This condition is called as Hridroga. (2)

Vataja Hridroga

आयम्यते मारुतजे हृदयं तुद्यते तथा |
निर्मथ्यते दीर्यते च स्फोट्यते पाट्यतेऽपि च ||३||
(सु. उ. तं. अ. ४३) |

Symptoms

In Vātaja hridroga – the pain in the heart is pulling (constricting), piercing / pricking, churning, bursting or tearing in nature. (3)

Pittaja Hrudroga Symptoms

तृष्णोष्मादाहचोषाः स्युः पैत्तिके हृदयक्लमः |
धूमायनं च मूर्छा च स्वेदः शोषो मुखस्य च ||४||
(सु. उ. तं. अ. ४३) |

In Pittaja Hridroga – the person would have thirst, increased heat (temperature) in the body, burning sensation, localized heat, tiredness / weakness of the heart, feeling of movement of hot smoke (of hot air) inside the chest, unconsciousness (loss of consciousness), increased sweating and dryness of the mouth. (4)

Kaphaja Hrudrog Symptoms

गौरवं कफसंस्रावोऽरुचिः स्तम्भोऽग्निमार्दवम् |
माधुर्यमपि चास्यस्य बलासावतते हृदि ||५||
(सु. उ. तं. अ. ४३) |

In Kaphaja Hridroga – there will be feeling of heaviness of the body, excessive salivation (watery secretions from the mouth, nose, eyes), loss of taste, stiffness of the body parts, weak digestive fire (poor digestion capacity), and manifestation of sweet taste in the mouth. (5)

Tridoshaja and Krimija Hrdroga Symptoms

विद्यात्त्रिदोषं त्वपि सर्वलिङ्गं तीव्रार्तितोदं क्रिमिजं सकण्डूम् | (च. चि. अ. २६) |
उत्क्लेदः ष्ठीवनं तोदः शूलं हृल्लासकस्तमः |
अरुचिः श्यावनेत्रत्वं शोथश्च क्रिमिजे भवेत् ||६|| (सु. उ. तं. अ. ४३) |

Tridoshaja Hridroga – In this condition the symptoms of all the three doshas will be present in mixed proportions.

Krimija Hridroga

Krimija Hridroga – There will be severe pain, pricking sensation and itching (in the chest or in the region of the heart). (Master Charaka)

According to Master Sushruta Krimija Hridroga will manifest with nausea, severe and repeated spitting, pricking pain, severe pain, nausea (oppression in the chest), experiencing darkness in front of the eyes, tastelessness (loss of taste of food), blackish appearance of the eyes (around the eyes) and oedema (swelling). (6)

Hridroga Upadrava

क्लमः सादो भ्रमः शोषो ज्ञेयास्तेषामुपद्रवाः |
क्रिमिजे क्रिमिजातीनां श्लैष्मिकाणां च ये मताः ||८||

Complications of Heart diseases

Debility, exhaustion, giddiness and emaciation are the complications of Hridroga . The complications explained in Kaphaja Krimi Roga (worm or parasitic infestation caused by excessive kapha) are found in Krimija Hridroga also. (7)

इति श्रीमाधवकरविरचिते माधवनिदाने हृद्रोगनिदानं समाप्तम् ||२९||

Thus ends the chapter on Hridroga Nidanam in Madhava Nidana text written by Acharya Madhavakar

30

Madhava Nidana Chapter 30 Mutrakrichra Nidanam

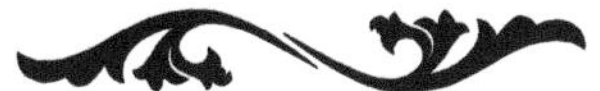

Mutrakrichra Nidana, Samprapti

व्यायामतीक्ष्णौषधरूक्षमद्यप्रसङ्गनित्यद्रुतपृष्ठयानात् |
आनूपमांसाध्यशनादजीर्णात्स्युर्मूत्रकृच्छ्राणि नृणां तथाऽष्टौ ||१||
पृथङ्मलाः स्वैः कुपिता निदानैः सर्वेऽथवा कोपमुपेत्य बस्तौ |
मूत्रस्य मार्गं परिपीडयन्ति यदा तदा मूत्रयतीह कृच्छ्रात् ||२|| (च. चि. अ. २६) |

Nidana

Etiological Factors - Excessive indulgence in exercise, medicines which are penetrating in nature (heat producing), dry foods and alcoholic drinks, riding regularly on the backs of animals like horses which basically run fast (or riding any other vehicles with fast pace regularly), regular and excessive consumption of flesh of animals and birds living in the marshy places, eating food in excess and indigestion of foods are the etiological factors of mutra krchra.

Mutrakrichra Samprapti

Pathogenesis – The above-mentioned etiological factors aggravate one or all doshas and cause 8 kinds of mutrakrchra. The vata and other doshas aggravated by their respective etiological factors reach the urinary bladder (urinary tract) either singly or collectively and get lodged therein. These doshas cause constriction, pressure or irritation of the urinary passages. As an effect, the person will find difficulty in voiding the urine. This condition marked by 'difficulty in urination' is called Mutrakrchra. This is of 8 types. (1-2)

Types

8 types of Mutrakrchra are –

1. Vataja Mutrakrchra
2. Pittaja Mutrakrchra
3. Kaphaja Mutrakrchra
4. Sannipataja Mutrakrchra
5. Shalyabhighataja Mutrakrchra (caused due to injury caused by foreign object)
6. Purishaja / Shakrdvighataja Mutrakrchra (caused by forcibly holding the urge for defecation)
7. Shukraja Mutrakrchra (dysuria caused by impaction of urinary passages by semen)
8. Ashmarijanya Mutrakrchra (dysuria caused by urinary stones)

Vataja Mutrakruchra

तीव्रार्तिरुग्वङ्क्षणबस्तिमेढ्रे स्वल्पं मुहुर्मूत्रयतीह वातात् |
पीतं सरक्तं सरुजं सदाहं कृच्छ्रं मुहुर्मूत्रयतीह पित्तात् ||३||
बस्तेः सलिङ्गस्य गुरुत्वशोथौ मूत्रं सपिच्छं कफमूत्रकृच्छ्रे |
सर्वाणि रूपाणि तु सन्निपाताद्भवन्ति तत्कृच्छ्रतमं हि कृच्छ्रम् ||४||
(च. चि. अ. २६) |

In this type, severe pain in the groins, urinary bladder and penis, scanty and frequent urination are the symptoms.

Pittaja Mutrakrichra

In this type of dysuria the patient will pass urine which is yellow in colour and mixed with blood. The patient will experience pain and burning sensation along with difficulty in passing the urine.

Kaphaja Mutrakrichra

In this condition the patient will have heaviness and swelling in the region of the urinary bladder and penis. The urine will be thick and viscid (sticky, slimy).

Tridoshaja Mutrakrichra

Sannipataja Mutrakrchra – In this condition all the above-mentioned symptoms in the individual doshaja types of mutrakrchra (vataja, pittaja, kaphaja) are found together and in severe form. (3-4)

Shalya abhighataja Mutrakrichra

मूत्रवाहिषु शल्येन क्षतेष्वभिहतेषु वा |
मूत्रकृच्छ्रं तदाघाताज्जायते भृशदारुणम् ||५||
वातकृच्छ्रेण तुल्यानि तस्य लिङ्गानि निर्दिशेत् |

This condition occurs due to the injury caused by the foreign bodies inside the urinary tract or due to external injury. The difficulty in urination is of a severe form and will have symptoms similar to those of vataja type of mutrakrchra. (5)

Shakrd Vighataja Mutrakruchra

शकृतस्तु प्रतीघातादवायुर्विगुणतां गतः ||६||
आध्मानं वातशूलं च मूत्रसङ्गं करोति च |

Due to the obstruction to the movement of the faeces as caused by habitual suppression of the urge for defecation will cause vata aggravation. This vata will move in an abnormal route (upward direction against its normal downward course) and produces distension of abdomen, colic of vataja type and difficulty in urination. (6)

Ashmarijanya & Shukraja Mutrakrchra

अश्मरीहेतु तत्पूर्वं मूत्रकृच्छ्रमुदाहरेत् ||७||
(सु. उ. तं. अ. ५९) |
शुक्रे दोषैरुपहते मूत्रमार्गे विधाविते
सशुक्रं मूत्रयेत् कृच्छ्राद्बस्तिमेहनशूलवान् ||८||

Ashmarijanya Mutrakrichra

If mutrakrchra (dysuria) is caused due to asmari (urinary calculi) it is called Ashmarijanya Mutrakrchra. Here calculus is the cause and difficulty in urination is the effect.

Shukraja Mutrakruchra

When the semen which has been displaced from its place (and has not been ejaculated) gets vitiated and obstructed by the aggravated doshas in the urinary passages it leads to difficulty in micturation. Since this condition is caused by the obstruction of semen it is called shukraja (shukra = semen) mutrakrchra. In this condition the urine mixed with semen is eliminated with great difficulty. It is also associated with pain in the region of the urinary bladder and penis. (7-8)

Difference between Asmari and Sarkara

अश्मरी शर्करा चैव तुल्यसम्भवलक्षणे |
विशेषणं शर्करायाः शृणु कीर्तयतो मम ||९||
पच्यमानाऽश्मरी पित्ताच्छोष्यमाणा च वायुना |
विमुक्तकफसन्धाना क्षरन्ती शर्करा मता ||१०||
हृत्पीडा वेपथुः शूलं कुक्षावग्निश्च दुर्बलः |
तया भवति मूर्छा च मूत्रकृच्छ्रं च दारुणम् ||११||
मूत्रवेगनिरस्ताभिः प्रशमं याति वेदना |
यावदस्याः पुनर्नैति गुडिका स्रोतसो मुखम् ||१२||
(सु. उ. तं. अ. ५९) |

Asmari (calculii) and sarkara (gravel) are similar in their causes and symptoms. But there is a difference in both these conditions.
Sarkara – The asmari (calculus) undergoing processing by pitta, dried by vata (dehydration of asmari by vāta) and losing the property of cohesion (or sticking together) of kapha, broken into tiny particles and passed out is called as sharkara (gravel).
Symptoms of dysuria (mutrakrchra) caused by ashmari or sarkara - pain in the region of the heart, shivering (tremors), pain in the abdomen (epigastrium), weakness of the digestive fire (poor digestive capacity), loss of consciousness (fainting) and great difficulty in urination are the symptoms caused by calculi or gravel.
Pain of the urinary tract subsides after the gravel gets eliminated along with the force of urination. The relief will be only until the urinary passage is impacted / obstructed by yet another gravel or stone. This means to tell that the symptoms recur (dysuria) when a new gravel or stone passes into the urinary tract and causes obstruction therein. (9-12)

इति श्रीमाधवकरविरचिते माधवनिदाने मूत्रकृच्छ्रनिदानं समाप्तम् ||३०||
Thus ends the chapter on Asmarī Nidanam in Madhava Nidana text written by Acharya Madhavakara.

31

Madhava Nidana Chapter 31 Mutraghata Nidana

Mutraghata Nidana, Samkhya

जायन्ते कुपितैर्दोषैर्मूत्राघातास्त्रयोदश |
प्रायो मूत्रविघाताद्यैर्वातकुण्डलिकादयः ||१||

Etiological factors and number of mutraghata

Causes – Suppression of natural urge for urination and other urges (like that of defecation, ejaculation etc.) and consumption of dry foods (and other etiological factors which cause predominant vitiation of vata) are the chief causes of mutraghata – suppression of urine.

Pathogenesis and number of mutraghata – The doshas (one or more of the doshas), predominantly vata, aggravated by the above mentioned etiological factors cause thirteen types of mutraghata commencing with Vatakundalika. (1)

Vatakundalika

रौक्ष्याद्वेगविघाताद्वा वायुर्बस्तौ सवेदनः |
मूत्रमाविश्य चरति विगुणः कुण्डलीकृतः ||२||
मूत्रमल्पाल्पमथवा सरुजं सम्प्रवर्तते |
वातकुण्डलिकां तां तु व्याधिं विद्यात् सुदारुणम् ||३||
(सु. उ. तं. अ. ५८) |

Excessive indulgence in dry foods, suppression of natural urges of the body etc. are the etiological factors of Vatakundalika. These causes lead to aggravation of vata located in the urinary bladder. This vata moves all around in a circular way obstructing the urine and also causes pain in the urinary bladder.

There is either scanty urination (frequent passage of small quantities of urine) or painful urination. This dreadful condition is known as Vatakundalika. (2-3)

Asthila

आध्मापयन् बस्तिगुदं रुद्ध्वा वायुश्चलोन्नताम् |
कुर्यात्तीव्रार्तिमष्ठीलां मूत्रविण्मार्गरोधिनीम् ||४||

The vata which has abnormally increased in the urinary bladder causes distension of the urinary bladder and rectum and would cause an enlargement (cyst like structure) which resembles an asthila (round pebble or stone ball) and hence the name asthila. This is elevated and mobile. It will produce severe pain and obstruction in the passages of urine and faeces. (4)

Vatavasti / Vatabasti

वेगं विधारयेद्यस्तु मूत्रस्याकुशलो नरः |
निरुणद्धि मुखं तस्य बस्तेर्बस्तिगतोऽनिलः ||५||
मूत्रसङ्गो भवेत्तेन बस्तिकुक्षिनिपीडितः |
वातबस्तिः स विज्ञेयो व्याधिः कृच्छ्रप्रसाधनः ||६||
(सु. उ. तं. अ. ५८) |

Vatavasti or Vatabasti is a condition caused in unwise persons who suppress their urge for urination and make the habit of the same (suppress urge for urination of long durations and long time). In these people the vata located in the urinary bladder gets aggravated and blocks the opening of the urinary bladder (urinary passages) and abdomen. This causes total retention of urine and also pain in the region of the urinary bladder. This disease is known as Vatavasti and is difficult to cure. (5-6)

Mutratita

चिरं धारयतो मूत्रं त्वरया न प्रवर्तते |
मेहमानस्य मन्दं वा मूत्रातीतः स उच्यते ||७||

When a person is habituated to suppress the urge of urination for a long time (and also has suppressed it for a long time) he fails to void the urine with normal force (and speed). Even if he voids the urine, it will be in a very slow stream. This condition is called as Mootraatita. (7)

Mutrajathara

मूत्रस्य वेगेऽभिहते तदुदावर्तहेतुकः |
अपानः कुपितो वायुरुदरं पूरयेद्भृशम् ||८||
नाभेरधस्तादाध्मानं जनयेत्तीव्रवेदनम् |
तन्मूत्रजठरं विद्यादधोबस्तिनिरोधनम् ||९||
(सु. उ. तं. अ. ५८) |

Suppression of the urge of urination is the cause for udavarta (reverse / upward movement of vata). Apaanavata getting increased begins to move upwards and accumulates in the abdomen, causing distension of the abdomen below the umbilicus, along with severe pain and obstruction in the lower part (opening) of the urinary bladder. This condition is known as Mootrajathara. (8-9)

Mutrotsanga

बस्तौ वाऽप्यथवा नाले मणौ वा यस्य देहिनः |
मूत्रं प्रवृत्तं सज्जेत सरक्तं वा प्रवाहतः ||१०||
स्रवेच्छनैरल्पमल्पं सरुजं वाऽथ नीरुजम् |
विगुणानिलजो व्याधिः स मूत्रोत्सङ्गसञ्ज्ञितः ||११||
(सु. उ. तं. अ. ५८) |

Mutrotsanga is a disease in which the urine which has left its seat (to get voided) gets obstructed in the urinary bladder, urethra or glans penis. If the person forcibly tries to void the urine in this condition (strains), the urine flows out mixed with blood or gets voided slowly and in small quantities, with or without pain. This condition is caused by aggravated vata. (10-11)

Mutraksaya

रूक्षस्य क्लान्तदेहस्य बस्तिस्थौ पित्तमारुतौ |
मूत्रक्षयं सरुग्दाहं जनयेतां तदाह्वयम् ||१२||
(सु. उ. तं. अ. ५८) |

In a person whose body is excessively dry and has fatigue, pitta and vata would undergo aggravation in the urinary bladder. They would cause reduction in the quantity of urine (mutraksaya) associated with pain and burning sensation. This condition is called as mutraksaya. (12)

Mutra Granthi

अन्तर्बस्तिमुखे वृत्तः स्थिरोऽल्पः सहसा भवेत् |
अश्मरीतुल्यरुग्ग्रन्थिर्मूत्रग्रन्थिः स उच्यते ||१३||
(वा. नि. अ. ९) |

A round, small and stationary cyst like mass developing quickly inside the urinary bladder, which resembles a stone and also presents pain (and other symptoms) similar to those of urinary calculi is called as Mutragranthi. (13)

Mutrasukra

मूत्रितस्य स्त्रियं यातो वायुना शुक्रमुद्धतम् |
स्थानाच्च्युतं मूत्रयतः प्राक् पश्चाद्वा प्रवर्तते ||१४||
भस्मोदकप्रतीकाशं मूत्रशुक्रं तदुच्यते |
(वा. नि. अ. ९) |

In a person who indulges in sexual intercourse suppressing the urge of urination, vata gets aggravated. By this, the semen which is dislodged from its seat gets obstructed and flows out of the body either before or after the urination. This disease in which the void urine resembles a solution of ash is called as Mutraksaya. (14)

Ushnavata

व्यायामाध्वातपैः पित्तं बस्तिं प्राप्यानिलान्वितम् ||१५||
बस्तिं मेढ्रं गुदं चैव प्रदहेत् स्रावयेदधः |
मूत्रं हारिद्रमथवा सरक्तं रक्तमेव वा ||१६||
कृच्छ्रात् पुनः पुनर्जन्तोरुष्णवातं ब्रुवन्ति तम् |
(सु. उ. तं. अ. ५८) |

When a person is indulged in excessive physical exercises, long distance walking and exposure to the heat of the sun, the pitta gets aggravated and reaches the urinary bladder. Here it gets associated with vata and causes burning sensation in the urinary bladder, penis (urethra) and rectum (anus). The urine voided is deep yellow in colour (resembling the colour of turmeric) or mixed with blood or only the blood flows out. The urine frequently comes out in small quantities. This disease is known as Usnavata. (15-16)

Mutrasadam

पित्तं कफो द्वावपि वा संहन्येतेऽनिलेन चेत् ||१७||

कृच्छ्रान्मूत्रं तदा पीतं श्वेतं रक्तं घनं सृजेत् |
सदाहं रोचनाशङ्खचूर्णवर्णं भवेत्तु तत् ||१८||
शुष्कं समस्तवर्णं वा मूत्रसादं वदन्ति तम् |
(वा. नि. अ. ९) |

Pitta and kapha either alone or in combination will get condensed (solidified) by the aggravated vata. When this happens there is difficulty in urination. The urine is yellow, white or red in colour, is dense, associated with burning sensation, resembles the colour of the colour of ox bile or conch shell, is dry (the watery portion of the urine is less, non-viscid) and has different colours of all the doshas (due to the aggravation of tridoshas). This condition is called as Mutrasada. (17-18)

Vidvighata

रूक्षदुर्बलयोर्वातेनोदावृत्तं शकृद्यदा ||१९||
मूत्रस्रोतोऽनुपद्येत विट्संसृष्टं तदा नरः |
विड्गन्धं मूत्रयेत् कृच्छ्राद्विड्विघातं विनिर्दिशेत् ||२०||
(वा. नि. अ. ९) |

In a person who has excessive dryness in the body and is also physically weak, the faeces are pushed in its opposite direction (upward direction) by the aggravated vata. The faeces enter the urinary bladder (urinary passages) and cause difficulty in urination. The urine which is void is either mixed with faeces or obtains the smell of faeces. This condition is called as Vidvighata. (19-20)

Vastikundala

द्रुताध्वलङ्घनायासैरभिघातात् प्रपीडनात् |
स्वस्थानाद्बस्तिरुद्वृत्तः स्थूलस्तिष्ठति गर्भवत् ||२१||
शूलस्पन्दनदाहार्तो बिन्दुं बिन्दुं स्रवत्यपि |
पीडितस्तु सृजेद्धारां संस्तम्भोद्वेष्टनार्तिमान् ||२२||
बस्तिकुण्डलमाहुस्तं घोरं शस्त्रविषोपमम् |
पवनप्रबलं प्रायो दुर्निवारमबुद्धिभिः |२४|
तस्मिन् पित्तान्विते दाहः शूलं मूत्रविवर्णता ||२३||
श्लेष्मणा गौरवं शोथः स्निग्धं मूत्रं घनं सितम् |२४|
श्लेष्मरुद्धबिलो बस्तिः पित्तोदीर्णो न सिध्यति ||२४||
अविभ्रान्तबिलः साध्यो, न तु यः कुण्डलीकृतः |२५|
स्याद्बस्तौ कुण्डलीभूते तृण्मोहः श्वास एव च ||२५||

By indulgence in fast walking, jumping and other exercises causing fatigue, injury (by blunt weapons) etc. or due to the pressure (on the urinary bladder, the urinary bladder gets displaced upwards (due to the increased vata) towards the centre of the abdomen and also becomes upside down resembling a pregnant uterus.

In this condition there is pain in the urinary bladder, fluctuations in the region of bladder and burning sensation and the urine is voided with difficulty, drop by drop. The urine flows out in the stream when pressure is applied on the abdomen (the region of the urinary bladder is pressed with hands) but stops when the pressure is released. There is rigidity and cramps. Such a disease is called Vastikundala. It is very dreadful, just like a sharp weapon or poison or a sharp weapon (like an arrow) dipped in poison. Vata is predominantly aggravated in this condition, and should not be treated by a physician with less knowledge.

If pitta gets associated (involved) in Vastikundala it causes burning sensation, pain, and discolouration of urine.

If kapha is involved in Bastikundala it causes heaviness and swelling. The urine is oily, thick and white.

If the orifice of the urinary bladder is blocked by thick kapha or if the urinary bladder (inside) gets afflicted by pitta (inflamed or ulcerated) the disease becomes incurable.

On the other hand, if the orifice of the bladder is not obstructed or if the bladder doesn't get rolled up into a ball like structure Vastikundala becomes curable.

If the urinary bladder becomes rolled up like a ball, it causes thirst, loss of consciousness (delusion) and dyspnoea. (21-26)

इति श्रीमाधवकरविरचिते माधवनिदाने मूत्राघातनिदानं समाप्तम् ||३१||

Thus ends the chapter on Mutraghata Nidanam in Madhava Nidana text written by Acharya Madhavakara.

32

Madhava Nidana Chapter 32 Ashmari Nidanam

Ashmari Bheda

वातपित्तकफैस्तिस्रश्चतुर्थी शुक्रजाऽपरा |
प्रायः श्लेष्माश्रयाः सर्वा अश्मर्यः स्युर्यमोपमाः ||१||

Types of calculi

Asmari is of four types, one from each dosha i.e., vataja, pittaja and kaphaja and the fourth one is that formed from sukra (semen). All types of asmari have predominance of kapha (kapha as the basic dosha involved in the formation of all kinds of asmari). This disease is considered to be dreadful, like the God of Death. (1)

Asmari Samprapti

विशोषयेद्बस्तिगतं सशुक्रं मूत्रं सपित्तं पवनः कफं वा |
यदा तदाऽश्मर्युपजायते तु क्रमेण पित्तेष्विव रोचना गोः ||२||
नैकदोषाश्रयाः सर्वाः... |
(च. चि. अ. २६) |

Pathogenesis of Ashmari

Asmari (stone, calculi) gets formed when vata dries up the semen, urine, pitta or kapha located in the urinary bladder. These stones are formed in the same way as the bile gets dried up and solidified inside the gallbladder of the cow. All types of asmaris are caused by the combined vitiation of all

the three doshas (no asmari is formed by predominance of only one dosha). Therefore, basically all types of asmaris are tridoshaja. (2)
Though all the asmaris are caused by all three doshas, they are named as vataja, pittaja etc. due to the predominance of that particular dosha in the combined vitiation. But for the formation of a stone or calculus kapha is the basic dosha which is required as a base substance or matrix. So, all kinds of asmaris are formed by tridoshas, any dosha may dominate the picture (and hence different types of asmari based on dosha predominance) and kapha is the basic dosha required for the formation of structure of calculi of any type.

Ashmari Purvarupa

... अथासां पूर्वलक्षणम् |
बस्त्याध्मानं तदासन्नदेशेषु परितोऽतिरुक् ||३||
मूत्रे बस्तसगन्धत्वं मूत्रकृच्छ्रं ज्वरोऽरुचिः |
(वा. नि. अ. ९) |

Premonitory symptoms of asmari
The premonitory symptoms of Ashmaris are distension of the urinary bladder, severe pain in and around the urinary bladder, the smell of urine resembling that of a goat, difficulty in urination, fever and loss of taste in food. (3-4)

Asmari Samanya Lakshana

सामान्यलिङ्गं रुङ्नाभिसेवनीबस्तिमूर्धसु ||४||
विशीर्णधारं मूत्रं स्यात्तया मार्गे निरोधिते |
तद्व्यपायात् सुखं मेहेदच्छं गोमेदकोपमम् ||५||
तत्सङ्क्षोभात् क्षते सास्रमायासाच्चातिरुग्भवेत् |
(वा. नि. अ. ९) |

General Symptoms of Ashmari
General signs and symptoms of asmari (calculi) include - pain in the region of the umbilicus, perineum and dome of the bladder. In this condition, since the urinary passage (flow) is interrupted or blocked by the stone, the flow of urine comes out in many streams. When the stone gets dislodged, the person easily voids urine which is clear, having the colour of gomedaka gem (yellowish red in colour), of blood coloured or mixed with blood (due to bleeding in the urinary tract). If the interior of the urinary bladder (and urinary passages) get injured due to the friction by stone, bleeding also

occurs along with urine. When the person tries to void the urine forcibly in spite of the stone being present in the urinary passage, the pressure causes severe pain. (4-5)

Vataja Ashmari

तत्र वाताद्भृशं चार्तो दन्तान् खादति वेपते ||६||
गृह्णाति मेहनं नाभिं पीडयत्यनिशं क्वणन् |
सानिलं मुञ्चति शकृन्मुहुर्मेहति बिन्दुशः ||७||
श्यावारुणाऽश्मरी चास्य स्याच्चिता कण्टकैरिव |
(वा. नि. अ. ९) |

Symptoms of Vataja Asmari – The pain is so severe that the person bites his lips with his teeth and he will have tremors. He would repeatedly squeeze his penis and would press his umbilicus constantly while crying. The faeces of the person are expelled along with flatus. Urine gets voided drop by drop frequently. The colour of the stone will be black or reddish black in colour and is surrounded by thorn like sprouts or projections. (6-7)

Pittaja Asmari

पित्तेन दह्यते बस्तिः पच्यमान इवोष्मवान् ||८||
भल्लातकास्थिसंस्थाना रक्तपीताऽसिताऽश्मरी |
(वा. नि. अ. ९) |

Symptoms of Pittaja Asmari – The person would experience burning sensation inside the urinary bladder and heat similar to the ulcer which is in the process of being ripened (as though smeared by alkali). The region of the bladder is hot to touch. The stone resembles the seed of Bhallataka (Semecarpus anacardium). It is red, yellow or black in colour. (8)

Kaphaja Asmari

बस्तिर्निस्तुद्यत इव श्लेष्मणा शीतलो गुरुः ||९||
अश्मरी महती श्लक्ष्णा मधुवर्णाऽथवा सिता |
(वा. नि. अ. ९) |

Symptoms of Kaphaja Asmari - In this type there is pricking pain, coldness and heaviness in the urinary bladder. The stone will be big in size, smooth, resembles honey (slightly brownish) in colour or is white in colour. (9)

Asmari in children

एता भवन्ति बालानां तेषामेव च भूयसा ||१०||

आश्रयोपचयाल्पत्वाद्ग्रहणाहरणे सुखाः |
(वा. नि. अ. ९) |
The above three types of asmari are common in young boys and girls. These stones can be easily removed through surgical process in children because of the small size of both the urinary bladder and the stone. (10)

Shukrasmari

शुक्राश्मरी तु महतां जायते शुक्रधारणात् ||११||
स्थानाच्च्युतममुक्तं हि मुष्कयोरन्तरेऽनिलः |
शोषयत्युपसङ्गृह्य शुक्रं तच्छुक्रमश्मरी ||१२||
बस्तिरुङ्मूत्रकृच्छ्रत्वमुष्कश्वयथुकारिणी |
तस्यामुत्पन्नमात्रायां शुक्रमेति विलीयते ||१३||
पीडिते त्ववकाशेऽस्मिन्... |
(वा. नि. अ. ९) |
Shukrashmari occurs in adults who withhold (suppress the urge) the ejaculation of the semen. Due to immense sexual excitation or during sex, the semen gets displaced from its seat (of production). In this condition if the person tries to withhold the urge for ejaculation the semen gets blocked (impacted) between the two testicles (in the urethra). The aggravated vata dries up this semen. Being dried by vata the semen becomes hard and assumes the shape and structure of a stone. This further leads to pain in the region of the urinary bladder, dysuria and swelling in the scrotum (testicles). On rubbing over the point of obstruction, the semen gets dissolved and released through the urethral passage. (11-13)

Sarkara – gravel

...अश्मर्येव च शर्करा |१४|
अणुशो वायुना भिन्ना सा तस्मिन्ननुलोमगे ||१४||
निरेति सह मूत्रेण प्रतिलोमे निरुध्यते | (वा. नि. अ. ९) |
मूत्रस्रोतःप्रवृत्ता सा सक्ता कुर्यादुपद्रवान् ||१५||
दौर्बल्यं सदनं कार्श्यं कुक्षिशूलमथारुचिम् |
पाण्डुत्वमुष्णवातं च तृष्णां हृत्पीडनं वमिम् ||१६|| (सु. नि. अ. ३) |
Sarkara (gravel) is the same as ashmari. The aggravated vata breaks the ashmari into minute pieces. Due to the downward course (movement) of vata, the stone particles are expelled out mixed with urine. If the vata has an opposite course i.e., moves in the upward direction they remain inside (and

are not expelled out).
The sarkara having got impacted inside the urinary passages due to the reverse movement of vata causes many complications including debility, exhaustion, emaciation, pain in the lower part of the abdomen, loss of taste, anaemia, burning urination, thirst, pain in the region of the heart and vomiting. (14-16)

Symptoms of incurability of asmari
प्रशूननाभिवृषणं बद्धमूत्रं रुजातुरम् |
अश्मरी क्षपयत्याशु सिकता शर्करान्विता ||१७||
Asmari is going to kill the patient quickly if it is associated with severe swelling in the scrotum (testes) and umbilicus, total obstruction of urine, severe pain and presence of gravel in it (because such asmari is incurable). (17)

इति श्रीमाधवकरविरचिते माधवनिदानेऽश्मरीनिदानं समाप्तम् ||३२||
Thus ends the chapter on Ashmari Nidanam in Madhava Nidana text written by Acharya Madhavakara.

33

Madhava Nidana Chapter 33 Prameha, Prameha Pidaka Nidanam

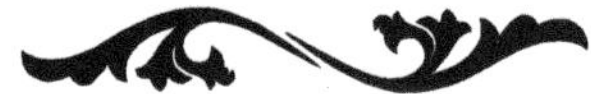

Prameha Nidana

आस्यासुखं स्वप्नसुखं दधीनि ग्राम्यौदकानूपरसाः पयांसि |
नवान्नपानं गुडवैकृतं च प्रमेहहेतुः कफकृच्च सर्वम् ||१||
(च. चि. अ. ७) |

Etiological Factors of Prameha -

- sitting on soft cushions and comfortable beddings for long periods (thus avoiding physical activity)
- sleeping for long hours
- excessive use of curds
- excessive consumption of flesh of domestic animals (and birds) or of those living in aquatic or of marshy places
- excessive consumption of milk and its products / preparations
- excessive use of fresh grains and fresh water (rain water)
- excessive use of puddings made of jaggery / sugar (and other edibles made of jaggery or sugar)
- all other similar factors which bring about increase of kapha in the body (kapha aggravating foods and activities) (1)

Prameha Samprapti

मेदश्च मांसं च शरीरजं च क्लेदं कफो बस्तिगतः प्रदूष्य |
करोति मेहान् समुदीर्णमुष्णैस्तानेव पित्तं परिदूष्य चापि ||२||
क्षीणेषु दोषेष्ववकृष्य धातून् सन्दूष्य मेहान् कुरुतेऽनिलश्च |

Pathogenesis of Kaphaja Prameha - Kapha which has undergone increase due to its own etiological factors and located in the urinary bladder, vitiates the medas (fat), māṁsa (muscle) and kleda (body fluids), and causes kaphaja prameha.

Pathogenesis of Pittaja Prameha – Pitta which has been aggravated due to excessive consumption of foods which are hot in nature (and other pitta aggravating foods and activities) and located in the urinary bladder vitiates the fat, muscle and body fluids (as described in kaphaja prameha) and causes pittaja prameha.

Pathogenesis of Vataja Prameha – The vata aggravated due to decrease of kapha and pitta would vitiate muscle-fat, bone marrow, ojus (essence of all the tissues) and serum (plasma), pulls them into the urinary bladder and causes vataja prameha.

Prognosis of doshaja types of prameha

साध्याः कफोत्था दश, पित्तजाः षड् याप्या, न साध्यः पवनाच्चतुष्कः ||३||
समक्रियत्वाद्विषमक्रियत्वान्महात्ययत्वाच्च यथाक्रमं ते |
(च. चि. अ. ६) |

The ten kinds produced by kapha are easily curable. This is due to the similarity in properties of the causative doshas and vitiated tissues. Due to this similarity the treatment for doshas and tissues will be similar and hence makes these conditions curable.

The six kinds of pittaja prameha are manageable (controllable). This is due to the dissimilarity in the properties of the causative doshas and vitiated tissues. Due to this dissimilarity the treatment for the involved doshas and tissues will be opposite in nature. Therefore, this condition becomes manageable (persists throughout the life but would be under control if timely and prompt treatment is given i.e., requires frequent treatment to manage the disease and have it under control).

The four kinds of vataja prameha are said to be incurable. This is due to the grave consequences and severe complications caused due to severe and quick destruction of tissues due to aggravation of vata and also due to the opposite nature of the treatment for the involved doshas and tissues. (2-3)

Doshas and Dushyas (tissues and other components of the body) involved in the pathogenesis of Prameha

कफः सपित्तः पवनश्च दोषा मेदोऽस्रशुक्राम्बुवसालसीकाः |
मज्जा रसौजः पिशितं च दूष्याः प्रमेहिणां विंशतिरेव मेहाः ||४|| (च. चि. अ. ६) |

Involved doshas - In all the twenty varieties of prameha, vaata, pitta and kapha together form the causative doshas.

Involved dushyas – medas (fat), asrk (blood), sukra (semen), ambu (body fluids), vasa (muscle fat), lasika (tissue fluid), majja (marrow), rasa (lymph), oja (essence of all the dhātus) and pishita (muscle tissue) are the dushyas involved in the causation of prameha. (4)

Premonitory symptoms of Prameha

दन्तादीनां मलाढ्यत्वं प्राग्रूपं पाणिपादयोः |
दाहश्चिक्कणता देहे तृट् स्वाद्वास्यं च जायते ||५||

Premonitory symptoms of prameha are accumulation of dirt on the teeth (mouth, palate, throat, tongue, eyes, nose, and ears), feeling of burning sensation in the palms and soles, stickiness of the skin all over the body, thirst and manifestation of sweet taste in the mouth. (5)

Prameha Samanya Lakshana

सामान्यं लक्षणं तेषां प्रभूताविलमूत्रता |
दोषदूष्याविशेषेऽपि तत्संयोगविशेषतः ||६||
मूत्रवर्णादिभेदेन भेदो मेहेषु कल्प्यते |
(वा. नि. अ. १०) |

General symptoms of Prameha

Increased quantity and turbidity of urine are the characteristic features of prameha. Due to the specificity of doshas and tissues and combination of doşhas and dūşyas, different colours are seen in the urine and the prameha (diabetes) are classified depending upon the colour of the urine, etc. (6-7)

Kaphaja Prameha

अच्छं बहु सितं शीतं निर्गन्धमुदकोपमम् ||७||
मेहत्युदकमेहेन किञ्चिदाविलपिच्छिलम् |
इक्षो रसमिवात्यर्थं मधुरं चेक्षुमेहतः ||८||

सान्द्रीभवेत् पर्युषितं सान्द्रमेहेन मेहति |
सुरामेही सुरातुल्यमुपर्यच्छमधो घनम् ||९||
संहृष्टरोमा पिष्टेन पिष्टवद्बहलं सितम् |
शुक्राभं शुक्रमिश्रं वा शुक्रमेही प्रमेहति ||१०||
मूर्ताणून् सिकतामेही सिकतारूपिणो मलान् |
शीतमेही सुबहुशो मधुरं भृशशीतलम् ||११||
शनैः शनैः शनैर्मेही मन्दं मन्दं प्रमेहति |
लालातन्तुयुतं मूत्रं लालामेहेन पिच्छिलम् ||१२||
(वा. नि. अ. १०) |

Types and symptoms

Udakameha Symptoms – The urine is clear, more in quantity (copious), white, cold, odourless, resembles water, with little turbidity and stickiness.

Iksumeha Symptoms – The urine is sweet – like the juice of sugarcane.

Sandrameha Symptoms – In this condition, the urine kept undisturbed for a while in a vessel becomes thick and dense.

Surameha Symptoms – Here, the urine resembles sura i.e., alcoholic beverages prepared with flour, clear at the top and thick sediments at the bottom.

Pistameha Symptoms – In this condition the urine appears thick like flour (as if mixed with flour) and is white in colour. The patient will experience horripilation.

Sukrameha Symptoms – Here, the urine either resembles (appears like) semen or is mixed with semen.

Sikatameha Symptoms – In this condition the urine contains small particles which resemble sand.

Shitameha Symptoms – In this condition the urine is large in quantity (copious), sweet in taste and very cold.

Sanairmeha Symptoms – In this condition the urine is voided frequently and very slowly.

Lalameha Symptoms – Here the urine resembles saliva along with the appearance of thread like structures and is sticky in nature.

(These ten varieties are predominantly kaphaja). (7-12)

Pittaja Prameha

गन्धवर्णरसस्पर्शैः क्षारेण क्षारतोयवत् |
नीलमेहेन नीलाभं कालमेही मसीनिभम् ||१३||
हारिद्रमेही कटुकं हरिद्रासन्निभं दहत् |

विस्रं माञ्जिष्ठमेहेन मञ्जिष्ठासलिलोपमम् ||१४||
विस्रमुष्णं सलवणं रक्ताभं रक्तमेहतः |१५|
(वा. नि. अ. १०) |

Types and symptoms

Ksarameha Symptoms – In this condition the urine resembles the solution of alkali in smell, colour, taste and touch.

Nilameha Symptoms – The urine is blue in colour in nilameha.

Kalameha Symptoms – In this type the urine resembles the colour of ink.

Haridrameha Symptoms – In this condition the colour of the urine resembles that of turmeric (deep yellow). The urine is pungent in taste and the patient experiences a burning sensation during urination.

Manjisthameha Symptoms – The urine in this type of pittaja prameha resembles the decoction of Manjistha (Rubia cordifolia) and smells foul.

Raktameha Symptoms – The urine in this condition has a foul smell, hot, has salty taste and resembles blood in colour (is blood red in colour). (13-14)

(The above six varieties are predominantly pittaja.)

Vataja Prameha

वसामेही वसामिश्रं वसाभं मूत्रयेन्मुहुः ||१५||
मज्जाभं मज्जमिश्रं वा मज्जमेही मुहुर्मुहुः |
कषायं मधुरं रूक्षं क्षौद्रमेहं वदेद्बुधः ||१६||
हस्ती मत्त इवाजस्रं मूत्रं वेगविवर्जितम् |
सलसीकं विबद्धं च हस्तिमेही प्रमेहति ||१७||
(वा. नि. अ. १०) |

Types and symptoms

Vasameha Symptoms – In this condition the urine voided is either mixed with muscle fat and resembles muscle fat in colour, smell etc and is voided frequently.

Majjameha Symptoms – In this condition the person frequently voids urine mixed with marrow and also appears like marrow in colour, smell etc.

Ksaudrameha Symptoms – It is a condition in which the urine is astringent and sweet in taste and is dry (non-sticky, non-unctuous).

Hastimeha Symptoms – The person suffering from this condition continuously passes urine like an intoxicated elephant. The urine is mixed with laskia i.e., tissue fluid and is composed of matted (small nodular) material.

(The above four varieties are predominantly vātaja.) (15-17)

Prameha Upadrava

अविपाकोऽरुचिश्छर्दिर्निद्रा कासः सपीनसः |
उपद्रवाः प्रजायन्ते मेहानां कफजन्मनाम् ||१८||

Complications of Kaphaja Prameha are - indigestion, loss of taste, vomiting, excessive sleep, cough, and running nose. (18)

बस्तिमेहनयोस्तोदो मुष्कावदरणं ज्वरः |
दाहस्तृष्णाऽम्लिका मूर्छा विड्भेदः पित्तजन्मनाम् ||१९||

Complications of Pittaja Prameha are – pricking pain in the urinary bladder and penis, cracking pain in the scrotum, fever, burning sensation, thirst, sour belching, loss of consciousness and diarrhoea. (19)

वातजानामुदावर्तः कम्पहृद्ग्रहलोलताः |
शूलमुन्निद्रता शोषः कासः श्वासश्च जायते ||२०||
(वा. नि. अ. १०) |

Complications of Vataja Prameha are – movement of vata in upward direction in the abdomen (retrograde peristalsis), tremors, stiffness or gripping pain in the heart (region of the heart), immense desire to eat foods having all tastes, pain in the abdomen (bladder and penis), loss of sleep, emaciation, cough and dyspnoea. (20)

Symptoms of incurability

यथोक्तोपद्रवाविष्टमतिप्रस्रुतमेव च |
पिडकापीडितं गाढः प्रमेहो हन्ति मानवम् ||२१||
(सु. सू. अ. ३३) |

Prameha of long duration (which has become chronic), associated with the above-mentioned complications, in which there is elimination of very large quantities of urine and appearance of carbuncles / tubercles (or ulcers) on the body is going to kill the patient (is incurable). (21)

जातः प्रमेही मधुमेहिनो वा न साध्य उक्तः स हि बीजदोषात् |
ये चापि केचित् कुलजा विकारा भवन्ति तांस्तान् प्रवदन्त्यसाध्यान् ||२२||
(च. चि. अ. ६) |

A person who is born with prameha (hereditary diabetes) or a person who is suffering from madhumeha are said to be incurable because of defect in genes. Likewise, many other hereditary diseases also are said to be incurable. (22)

Transformation of all kinds of prameha into madhumeha

सर्व एव प्रमेहास्तु कालेनाप्रतिकारिणः ।
मधुमेहत्वमायान्ति तदाऽसाध्या भवन्ति हि ॥२३॥ (सु. नि. अ. ६) ।
मधुमेहे मधुसमं जायते स किल द्विधा ।
क्रुद्धे धातुक्षयाद्वायौ दोषावृतपथेऽथवा ॥२४॥

All varieties of prameha, if not treated at appropriate time, will ultimately get transformed into madhumeha. In this condition they will become incurable. Madhumeha - In Madhumeha, the urine is like honey (sweet in taste). Madhumeha is of two kinds. One type of madhumeha is caused by vata increase caused by dhatu ksaya – depletion of tissues. The other type of madhumeha is caused by obstruction of (the channels / passages of) vata by other doshas. (23-24)

आवृतो दोषलिङ्गानि सोऽनिमित्तं प्रदर्शयन् ।
क्षणात् क्षीणः क्षणात् पूर्णो भजते कृच्छ्रसाध्यताम् ॥२५॥
(वा. नि. अ. १०) ।

In case of madhumeha caused by avarana i.e., obstruction of vata by other doshas, the symptoms of doshas which appear are sometimes mild and sometimes severe in nature. Gradually the disease becomes difficult to cure. (25)

Definition of Madhumeha

मधुरं यच्च मेहेषु प्रायो मध्विव मेहति ।
सर्वेऽपि मधुमेहाख्या माधुर्याच्च तनोरतः ॥२६॥
(वा. नि. अ. १०) ।

Any variety of prameha in which the urine is sweet like honey and the whole body also becomes sweet is to be named as Madhumeha. (25-26)

Prameha Pidaka: Diabetic carbuncles

शराविका कच्छपिका जालिनी विनताऽलजी ।
मसूरिका सर्षपिका पुत्रिणी सविदारिका ॥२७॥
विद्रधिश्चेति पिडकाः प्रमेहोपेक्षया दश ।
सन्धिमर्मसु जायन्ते मांसलेषु च धामसु ॥२८॥
(वा. नि. अ. १०) ।

The ten types of carbuncles caused by (related to) prameha are –

1. saravika
2. kacchapika,
3. jalini,
4. vinata
5. alaji,
6. masurika,
7. sarsapika,
8. putrini,
9. vidarika,
10. vidradhika

They appear on joints, vital parts and other fleshy parts of the body. (27-28)

Symptoms of Prameha Pidakas

अन्तोन्नता तु तद्रूपा निम्नमध्या शराविका |
गौरसर्षपसंस्थाना तत्प्रमाणा च सर्षपी ||२९||
सदाहा कूर्मसंस्थाना ज्ञेया कच्छपिका बुधैः |
जालिनी तीव्रदाहा तु मांसजालसमावृता ||३०||
अवगाढरुजाक्लेदा पृष्ठे वाऽप्युदरेऽपि वा |
महती पिडका नीला विनता नाम सा स्मृता ||३१||
महत्यल्पचिता ज्ञेया पिडका चापि पुत्रिणी |
मसूराकृतिसंस्थाना विज्ञेया तु मसूरिका ||३२||
रक्ता सिता स्फोटचिता दारुणा त्वलजी भवेत् |
विदारीकन्दवद्वृत्ता कठिना च विदारिका ||३३||
विद्रधेर्लक्षणैर्युक्ता ज्ञेया विद्रधिका तु सा |३४| (सु. नि. अ. ६) |
ये यन्मयाः स्मृता मेहास्तेषामेतास्तु तन्मयाः ||३४|| (सु. नि. अ. ६) |

Saravika – It resembles a saucer with elevated edges and a depressed centre.
Sarsapika – It is similar to white mustard seeds in colour and size.
Kacchapika – This resembles the shell of a tortoise and is associated with burning sensation.
Jalini – This carbuncle appears like a sieve of muscle fibres and presents with severe burning sensation.
Vinata – It usually appears on the back or abdomen. The carbuncles are hard, blue, blue in colour, big in size and are associated with pain and

exudation.

Putrini – It manifests in the form of a big eruption surrounded by smaller eruptions all around it.

Masurika – It resembles the shape and size of a masura (pea).

Alají – It is surrounded by red or white coloured blisters and is considered to be a dreadful condition.

Vidarika – It is round and hard just like the tuber of Vidari (Pueraria tuberosa).

Vidradhika – This is an eruption (carbuncle) which will present with all the features of an abscess.

These prameha pidakas are also caused by the same doshas which cause the pramehas which are responsible for the manifestation of these pidakas. (The same dosha which causes a particular prameha will also be responsible for the causation of a pidaka resulting from that particular prameha. To put it in simple words, the dosha causing a particular type of prameha and its pidaka is the same.) (29-34)

विना प्रमेहमप्येता जायन्ते दुष्टमेदसः |
तावच्चैता न लक्ष्यन्ते यावद्वास्तुपरिग्रहाः ||३५||
(च. सू. अ. १७) |

The pidakas might also occur without the presence of prameha when the medas i.e. fat / adipose tissue gets severely contaminated (vitiated). (This means that pidakas need not be essentially caused by prameha. Severe vitiation of fat tissue may also cause these pidakas independently). But they cannot be recognized (their specific symptoms will not become evident) until they get localized in specific parts of the body. (35)

गुदे हृदि शिरस्यंस्ये पृष्ठे मर्मसु चोत्थिताः |
सोपद्रवा दुर्बलाग्नेः पिडकाः परिवर्जयेत् ||३६||
(सु. नि. अ. ६) |

The patients who have developed these pidakas in the anal region (rectum), region of the heart, head, shoulders (scapular regions, shoulder blades), back and vital parts of the body, associated with complications and manifesting in those who have poor digestive fire (capacity) are to be refused treatment (because these conditions are incurable). (36)

इति श्रीमाधवकरविरचिते माधवनिदाने प्रमेहप्रमेहपिडकानिदानं समाप्तम् ||३३||

Thus ends the chapter on Prameha Prameha Pidaka Nidanam in Madhava Nidana text written by Acharya Madhavakara.

34

Madhava Nidana Chapter 34 Meda Roga Nidanam

Medo Roga Nidana, Samprapti

अव्यायामदिवास्वप्नश्लेष्मलाहारसेविनः |
मधुरोऽन्नरसः प्रायः स्नेहान्मेदः प्रवर्धयेत् ||१||
मेदसाऽऽवृतमार्गत्वात् पुष्यन्त्यन्ये न धावतः |
मेदस्तु चीयते तस्मादशक्तः सर्वकर्मसु ||२||
क्षुद्रश्वासतृषामोहस्वप्नक्रथनसादनैः |
युक्तः क्षुत्स्वेददुर्गन्धैरल्पप्राणोऽल्पमैथुनः ||३||
मेदस्तु सर्वभूतानामुदरेष्वस्थिषु स्थितम् |
अत एवोदरे वृद्धिः प्रायो मेदस्विनो भवेत् ||४||
मेदसाऽऽवृतमार्गत्वाद्वायुः कोष्ठे विशेषतः |
चरन् सन्धुक्षयत्यग्निमाहारं शोषयत्यपि ||५||
तस्मात् स शीघ्रं जरयत्याहारमभिकाङ्क्षति |
विकारांश्चाप्नुते घोरान् कांश्चित् कालव्यतिक्रमात् ||६||
एतावुपद्रवकरौ विशेषादग्निमारुतौ |
एतौ तु दहतः स्थूलं वनदावो वनं यथा ||७||
मेदस्यतीव संवृद्धे सहसैवानिलादयः |
विकारान् दारुणान् कृत्वा नाशयन्त्याशु जीवितम् ||८||

Important etiological Factors and pathogenesis of Medo Roga -

- Below mentioned are the causative factors of medo roga
- not doing exercises (absence of physical activities, sedentary life)
- excessive sleeping during daytime
- excessive intake of foods which cause aggravation of kapha

Pathogenesis of Medoroga – Due to the above said etiological factors the end product of digestion becomes abnormally sweet and unctuous. This causes an increase of fat. This abnormally increased fat causes obstruction of the nutrient channels of the body. This would supply less or no nutrients to the other tissues of the body. The tissues are not nourished due to the deprivation of nutrition. This further leads to accumulation of only fat tissue in large quantities in the body. This makes the person incapable of doing all activities.

Definition of Atisthula

मेदोमांसातिवृद्धत्वाच्चलस्फिगुदरस्तनः |
अयथोपचयोत्साहो नरोऽतिस्थूल उच्यते ||९|| (च. सू. अ. २१) |

A person is said to be very obese when his buttocks, abdomen and breasts begin to show movement (they sag and are pendulous during activity) due to abnormal increase and accumulation of fat and muscles, and when his muscle mass (body built) and enthusiasm are found to be disproportionate. (9)

इति श्रीमाधवकरविरचिते माधवनिदाने मेदोनिदानं समाप्तम् ||३४||

Thus ends the chapter on Medaroga Nidanam in Madhava Nidana text written by Acharya Madhavakara.

35

Madhava Nidana Chapter 35 Udara Nidanam

Udara Roga Nidana

रोगाः सर्वेऽपि मन्देऽग्नौ सुतरामुदराणि च |
अजीर्णान्मलिनैश्चान्नैर्जायन्ते मलसञ्चयात् ||१||
(वा. नि. अ. १२) |

Etiological Factors for Udara Roga

All diseases in the body, mainly the udara rogas (enlargement of abdomen) are caused by mandāgni (poor digestive fire), indigestion of food, and excessive consumption of dirty or spoiled (contaminated) foods and accumulation of waste products in the body (excreta and other metabolic wastes). (1)

Udara Roga Samprapti

रुद्ध्वा स्वेदाम्बुवाहीनि दोषाः स्रोतांसि सञ्चिताः |
प्राणाग्न्यपानान् सन्दूष्य जनयन्त्युदरं नृणाम् ||२||
(च. चि. अ. १३) |

Pathogenesis of enlargement of abdomen

The doshas undergoing increase and accumulation obstruct the channels of sweat and other body fluids, vitiate prāna, apāna and agni (pitta) and produce Udararoga (enlargement of abdomen). (2)

Udara Samanya Lakshana
आध्मानं गमनेऽशक्तिर्दौर्बल्यं दुर्बलाग्निता |
शोथः सदनमङ्गानां सङ्गो वातपुरीषयोः ||३||
दाहस्तन्द्रा च सर्वेषु जठरेषु भवन्ति हि | (सु. नि. अ. ७) |
General symptoms -

- distension of the abdomen,
- inability to walk,
- weakness,
- weakness of digestive fire (capacity)
- swelling / edema
- looseness / debility in the body parts (extremities)
- obstruction to the movement (expulsion) of flatus and faeces
- burning sensation
- stupor (3-4)

Udara Samkhya
पृथग्दोषैः समस्तैश्च प्लीहबद्धक्षतोदकैः ||४||
सम्भवन्त्युदराण्यष्टौ तेषां लिङ्गं पृथक् शृणु |५|
Types of Udara Roga - Udara is of eight kinds.
one from each doṣha – vataja udara (vatodara), pittaja udara (pittodara) and kaphaja udara (shleshmodara / kaphodara)

1. sannipatodara - one from the combination of all three vitiated doshas
2. pleehodara,
3. baddhodara,
4. kshatodara and
5. udakodara / jalodara

The symptoms of each of these 8 types of udara will be described separately further on. (4)

Vatodara Symptoms
तत्र वातोदरे शोथः पाणिपान्नाभिकुक्षिषु ||५||
कुक्षिपार्श्वोदरकटीपृष्ठरुक् पर्वभेदनम् |

शुष्ककासोऽङ्गमर्दोऽधोगुरुता मलसङ्ग्रहः ||६||
श्यावारुणत्वगादित्वमकस्माद्वृद्धिह्रासवत् |
सतोदभेदमुदरं तनुकृष्णसिराततम् ||७||
आध्मातदृतिवच्छब्दमाहतं प्रकरोति च |
वायुश्चात्र सरुक्शब्दो विचरेत् सर्वतो गतिः ||८||
(वा. नि. अ. १२) |

The symptoms of Vatodara are –

- swelling (oedema) of the hands, feet, umbilicus and lower abdomen;
- pain in the cavity of the abdomen, flanks, abdomen, waist (pelvis), and back and splitting pain in the joints, mainly small joints of the hands and feet (fingers and toes);
- Dry cough, body aches, feeling of heaviness of the lower parts of the body, accumulation of wastes products (excreta) in the body,
- dark brown (bluish) or reddish-brownish (golden yellow) discolouration of skin, etc. (nails, eyes, face, teeth etc),
- sudden increase or decrease of size of the abdomen without any apparent reason,
- pricking, throbbing and other types of pain in the abdomen,
- appearance of thin, black network of veins on the abdomen,
- highly resonant sound elicited on percussion (sound resembling that coming when you tap on a bag / sac filled with air) and the vayu (gases) move all round inside the abdomen (intestines) producing gurgling noises and pain. (5-8)

Pittodara Symptoms

पित्तोदरे ज्वरो मूर्छा दाहस्तृट् कटुकास्यता |
भ्रमोऽतिसारः पीतत्वं त्वगादावुदरं हरित् ||९||
पीतताम्रसिरानद्धं सस्वेदं सोष्म दह्यते |
धूमायते मृदुस्पर्शं क्षिप्रपाकं प्रदूयते ||१०||
(वा. नि. अ. १२) |

Symptoms of Pittodara are –

- fever, loss of consciousness (fainting),
- burning sensation, thirst, manifestation of bitter taste in the mouth,

- giddiness, diarrhoea, yellowish discolouration of skin (nails, eyes, teeth, face) etc.,
- and greenish colour of the abdomen, network of veins of yellow or coppery colour spread out over the abdomen,
- sweating, feeling of excessive heat and burning sensation, sensation of hot smoke or fumes from the surface of the abdomen,
- abdomen is soft to touch and the condition (pittaja udara) undergoes quick suppuration (quickly progresses towards ascites) and there will be severe pain in the abdomen. (9-10)

Kaphodara Symptoms

श्लेष्मोदरेऽङ्गसदनं स्वापश्वयथुगौरवम् |
निद्रोत्क्लेशोऽरुचिः श्वासः कासः शुक्लत्वगादिता ||११||
उदरं स्तिमितं स्निग्धं शुक्लराजीततं महत् |
चिराभिवृद्धं कठिनं शीतस्पर्शं गुरु स्थिरम् ||१२||
(वा. नि. अ. १२)

The symptoms of Kaphodara are -

- debility, loss of activity, oedema and heaviness of the body parts,
- excessive sleep, nausea, loss of taste, dyspnoea (difficulty in breathing),
- cough, whitish discolouration of skin (nails, eyes, teeth, face) etc.
- The abdomen is tense (loss of movements), unctuous, having white striae (covered by long white marks / streak), large in size, increasing slowly, hard, cold to touch, heavy and without movement. (11-12)

Sannipatodara Symptoms

स्त्रियोऽन्नपानं नखलोममूत्रविडार्तवैर्युक्तमसाधुवृत्ताः |
यस्मै प्रयच्छन्त्यरयो गरांश्च दुष्टाम्बुदूषीविषसेवनाद्वा ||१३||
तेनाशु रक्तं कुपिताश्च दोषाः कुर्युः सुघोरं जठरं त्रिलिङ्गम् |
तच्छीतवाते भृशदुर्दिने च विशेषतः कुप्यति दह्यते च ||१४||
स चातुरो मुह्यति हि प्रसक्तं पाण्डुः कृशः शुष्यति तृष्णया च |
दूष्योदरं कीर्तितमेतदेव ...||
(सु. नि. अ. ७) |

Causative factors of Sannipatodara are –

- Ingestion of harmful foods containing (mixed with) nails, body hairs, urine, faeces and menstrual blood etc by women of bad or unappreciable nature (wicked women) or by wicked men or enemies, or
- consumptions of foods mixed with (artificial) poisons served by enemies,
- drinking polluted water
- consumption of slow poisons etc.

Pathogenesis – Due to the consumption of the above said etiological factors, the blood along with the three doshas will get aggravated in quick time and cause tridoshaja udara roga. In this condition the symptoms of all the three doshas will be present together.

Symptoms - This symptom of this condition exacerbates in cold breeze (on days of cold breeze) and overcast conditions (when the sky is enveloped by clouds), and there is severe burning sensation. The person faints frequently, is pale, emaciated, and his mouth gets dried due to severe thirst. This condition is also called as Dusyodara also. (13-14)

Plihodara Symptoms

... प्लीहोदरं कीर्तयतो निबोध ||१५||
विदाह्यभिष्यन्दिरतस्य जन्तोः प्रदुष्टमत्यर्थमसृक् कफश्च |
प्लीहाभिवृद्धिं कुरुतः प्रवृद्धौ प्लीहोत्थमेतज्जठरं वदन्ति ||१६||
तद्वामपार्श्वे परिवृद्धिमेति विशेषतः सीदति चातुरोऽत्र |
मन्दज्वराग्निः कफपित्तलिङ्गैरुपद्रुतः क्षीणबलोऽतिपाण्डुः |

Understand the symptoms of Pleehodara (which has been explained) further -

In persons who indulge in foods which produce burning sensation during digestion and those which block the tissue pores by greasy material, the rakta (blood) and kapha undergo severe aggravation.

They in turn cause enlargement of the spleen and produce plihodara (splenomegaly). In this condition the abdomen is enlarged more towards the left side. The patient is very much debilitated, will have mild fever, poor digestion, symptoms of increased kapha and pitta, loss of strength and severe form of anaemia. (15-16)

Yakrutodaram / Yakruddalyudaram

सव्यान्यपार्श्वे यकृति प्रवृद्धे ज्ञेयं यकृद्दाल्युदरं तदेव ||१७||
(सु. नि. अ. ७) |
If there is such an enlargement on the right side of the abdomen (just like in plihodara) involving the liver, the disease shall be named as Yakrtodara (hepatomegaly). (17)

Dosha symptoms in both Plihodara and Yakrtodara

उदावर्तरुजानाहैर्मोहतृड्दहनज्वरैः |
गौरवारुचिकाठिन्यैर्विद्यात्तत्र मलान् क्रमात् ||१८||
(वा. नि. अ. १२) |
In both these conditions i.e., plihodara and yakrtodara, the dosha involvement should be understood on seeing the associated dosha symptoms –
in association of vata, the symptoms of vata are seen, they are – upward movement of vata, pain in the abdomen and flatulence (distension of abdomen)
in association of pitta, the symptoms of pitta are seen, they are – delusion (loss of consciousness), thirst, burning sensation and fever
in association of kapha, the symptoms of kapha are seen, they are – heaviness in the abdomen, loss of taste in food, and hardness of the abdomen (18)

Baddha Gudodara

यस्यान्त्रमन्नैरुपलेपिभिर्वा बालाश्मभिर्वा पिहितं यथावत् |
सञ्चीयते तस्य मलः सदोषः शनैः शनैः सङ्करवच्च नाड्याम् ||१९||
निरुध्यते तस्य गुदे पुरीषं निरेति कृच्छ्रादपि चाल्पमल्पम् |
हृन्नाभिमध्ये परिवृद्धिमेति तस्योदरं बद्धगुदं वदन्ति ||२०||
(सु. नि. अ. ७) |
Due to the obstruction of the intestines by food materials which are sticky in nature, hairs, stones, etc. the wastes (faeces) along with the three doshas gradually accumulates inside the intestines just like a mixture of dirt (just like the dirt gradually accumulates in a tube or pipe and prevents free flow of water within).
The waste materials thus accumulated in the anus (intestines) get eliminated in small quantities (in the form of small pellets) with great difficulty. In this condition the abdomen is enlarged between the chest and umbilicus. This condition is called Baddha gudodara (intestinal

obstruction). (19-20)

Parisravyudara Symptoms

शल्यं तथाऽन्नोपहितं यदन्त्रं भुक्तं भिनत्त्यागतमन्यथा वा |
तस्मात्स्रुतोऽन्त्रात्सलिलप्रकाशः स्रावः स्रवेद्वै गुदतस्तु भूयः ||२१||
नाभेरधश्चोदरमेति वृद्धिं निस्तुद्यते दाल्यति चातिमात्रम् |
एतत् परिस्राव्युदरं प्रदिष्टं ... |२२| (सु. नि. अ. ७) |

When the foreign bodies (objects) are ingested along with the food or otherwise damages and tears the walls of the intestine or if there is perforation of the wall of the intestine due to any other cause, it will lead to exudation of watery material in large quantities. This watery fluid will accumulate in the abdominal cavity and produce enlargement of the abdomen. Later this fluid will get discharged through the anal route. In this condition the enlargement of the abdomen takes place below the umbilicus. The person will experience pricking or crushing (tearing, bursting) pain in the abdomen. This type of udara is called Parisraaviudara (intestinal perforation and peritonitis). (21-22)

Jalodara symptoms

... दकोदरं कीर्तयतो निबोध ||२२||
यः स्नेहपीतोऽप्यनुवासितो वा वान्तो विरिक्तोऽप्यथवा निरूढः |
पिबेज्जलं शीतलमाशु तस्य स्रोतांसि दूष्यन्ति हि तद्वहानि ||२३||
स्नेहोपलिप्तेष्वथवाऽपि तेषु दकोदरं पूर्ववदभ्युपैति |
स्निग्धं महत्तत्परिवृत्तनाभिसमाततं पूर्णमिवाम्बुना च |
यथा दृतिः क्षुभ्यति कम्पते च शब्दायते चापि दकोदरं तत् ||२४|| (सु. नि. अ. ७) |

Understand the type of udara called as Dakodara now –

When a patient drinks cold water immediately after he has undergone (administered with) therapies like oleation – oral consumption of medicated lipids (oil or ghee) as part of therapy, unctuous (oil or ghee) enema, emesis, purgation or decoction enema, it would cause contamination of the channels of water / fluids. Also when the interior of the water / fluid conveying channels get coated and obstructed by unctuous material (oily material), the fluid gets accumulated in the abdominal cavity as explained in Chidrodara and causes dakodara (ascites).

The abdomen is unctuous (oily appearance) and is greatly enlarged with the umbilicus protruding out. The abdomen trembles (shakes), produces movements and sounds just like a leather bag filled with water. This condition is called Dakodara (enlargement of the abdomen due to the accumulation of the fluid, ascites). (23-24)

Symptoms of incurability of Udara

जन्मनैवोदरं सर्वं प्रायः कृच्छ्रतमं मतम् |
बलिनस्तदजाताम्बु यत्नसाध्यं नवोत्थितम् ||२५||
पक्षाद्बद्धगुदं तूर्ध्वं सर्वं जातोदकं तथा |
प्रायो भवत्यभावाय छिद्रान्त्रं चोदरं नृणाम् ||२६||
(च. चि. अ. १३)० |२७|

Generally, all kinds of udara rogas are difficult to cure right from the time of their onset. This condition can only be cured with great effort in persons who are strong (strong constitution), before the formation of fluid (before fluid accumulates in the abdominal cavity) and when it is of recent onset. Baddha Gudodara will become incurable after the lapse of 15 days (if it cannot be cured within a fortnight it cannot be cured at all). All other types of abdominal enlargements which have progressed to the stage of ascites (accumulation of fluid in the abdominal cavity) are incurable. Parisravi Udara – wherein there is perforation of intestines are going to be fatal and hence incurable. (25-26)

Other symptoms of incurability of udara roga

शूनाक्षं कुटिलोपस्थमुपक्लिन्नतनुत्वचम् |
बलशोणितमांसाग्निपरिक्षीणं च वर्जयेत् ||२७|| (च. चि. अ. १३) |
पार्श्वभङ्गान्नविद्वेषशोथातीसारपीडितम् |
विरिक्तं चाप्युदरिणं पूर्यमाणं विवर्जयेत् ||२८|| (सु. सू. अ. ३३) |

Patients of udara who have developed oedema of the eyes, abnormal curvature of the penis, wet and thin skin, and loss of strength, blood, muscles and digestive capacity are to be refused treatment.

Similarly, when there is compression of the ribs (compression or pain in the flanks), aversion to food, oedema, diarrhoea and fluid accumulating quickly in spite of administering repeated purgation (therapy) are to be rejected. (27-28)

इति श्रीमाधवकरविरचिते माधवनिदाने उदरनिदानं समाप्तम् ||३५||

Thus ends the chapter on Udara Nidanam in Madhava Nidana text written by Acharya Madhavakara.

36

Madhava Nidana Chapter 36Shotha Nidanam

Shotha Samprapti, Bheda

रक्तपित्तकफान् वायुर्दुष्टो दुष्टान् बहिःसिराः ।
नीत्वा रुद्धगतिस्तैर्हि कुर्यात्त्वङ्मांससंश्रयम् ॥१॥
उत्सेधं संहतं शोथं तमाहुर्निचयादतः ।
सर्वं हेतुविशेषैस्तु रूपभेदान्नवात्मकम् ॥२॥
दोषैः पृथग्द्वयैः सर्वैरभिघाताद्विषादपि ।३। (वा. नि. अ. १३) ।

Pathogenesis and types of Shotha

Vaata undergoing increase due to its own etiological factors pushes the vitiated rakta (blood), pitta and kapha into the superficial veins. Therein (inside the veins) the vata gets obstructed by the same blood, pitta and kapha. These three doshas along with the vitiated blood gets accumulated between the skin and muscles and cause swelling. This swelling is called as Shotha.

Types of Shotha – All shothas are of one type seeing that they all present with swelling. But due to different causative factors and symptoms (caused due to different causative factors), shotha is classified into nine types. They are – one each from each dosha (vataja, pittaja and kaphaja), one each from combination of two doshas (vata-pittaja, vata-kaphaja and pitta-kaphaja), one type from the combination of all three doshas (tridoshaja, sannipataja), one from injury (abhighataja) and one from the effect of poisons (vishaja).

(1-2)

Shotha Purvarupa

तत्पूर्वरूपं दवथुः सिरायामोऽङ्गगौरवम् ||३||

(वा. नि. अ. १३) |

Premonitory symptoms of Shotha

Premonitory symptoms of shotha are mild burning sensation of the skin (eyes, nose, etc.), appearance of venous network (engorgement of veins) and feeling of heaviness of the body parts. (3)

Shotha Nidana

शुद्ध्यामयाभुक्तकृशाबलानां क्षाराम्लतीक्ष्णोष्णगुरूपसेवा |
दध्याममृच्छाकविरोधिदुष्टगरोपसृष्टान्ननिषेवणं च ||४||
अर्शांस्यचेष्टा न च देहशुद्धिर्मर्मोपघातो विषमा प्रसूतिः |
मिथ्योपचारः प्रतिकर्मणां च निजस्य हेतुः श्वयथोः प्रदिष्टः ||५|| (च. चि. अ. १२) |

General etiological factors of Shotha

Causes for Nija Shotha (Shotha caused by doshas) –

Excessive administration of foods which are alkaline, sour, strong / deep penetrating, hot (heat producing) or heavy foods (difficult to digest foods), to those who have got emaciated due to (excessive or improper) administration of purificatory therapies (panchakarma therapies like emesis, purgation etc), long standing diseases (fever etc), not eating food / lack of food (starvation) or foods of low quality (and nutrition) and to the weakened persons will cause shotha (by causing aggravation of doshas).

Excessive consumption of curds, uncooked foods, mud, leafy vegetables, mutually incompatible (having opposite qualities and nature) foods, spoilt (contaminated) foods, and gara visha (combination of poisons or foods poisoned by such poisons)

Haemorrhoids

Absence of physical activities

Not administering purificatory measures (panchakarma treatments) in spite of their requirement

Damage to the marmas (vital organs and tissues) by aggravated doshas (disorders of marmas caused by aggravated doshas)

Abnormal delivery in women (miscarriage, abortion)

Improper administration of purificatory therapies (4-5)

Shotha Samanya Lakshana

सगौरवं स्यादनवस्थितत्वं सोत्सेधमूष्माऽथ सिरातनुत्वम् |
सलोमहर्षश्च विवर्णता च सामान्यलिङ्गं श्वयथोः प्रदिष्टम् ||६||

General Symptoms of Shotha

The general symptoms of shotha are - swelling associated with feeling of heaviness, inconsistency i.e., increasing or decreasing frequently, warmth, thinning of the veins, horripilation (hairs standing on ends), and discolouration. (6)

Vataja Shotha

चलस्तनुत्वक् परुषोऽरुणोऽसितः सुषुप्तिहर्षार्तियुतोऽनिमित्ततः |
प्रशाम्यति प्रोन्नमति प्रपीडितो दिवाबली च श्वयथुः समीरणात् ||७|| (च. चि. अ. १२) |

The symptoms of vataja shotha (oedema caused due to increase of vata) are –

the skin over the oedema is movable, thin, rough, golden yellow / brown (reddish brown) or black in colour,
loss of sensation or feeling of pins and needles, horripilations / hyperesthesia,
oedema subsides temporarily without any apparent cause
pits on pressure and when the pressure is released the pit fills up quickly
the swelling increases during daytime (7)

Pittaja Shotha

मृदुः सगन्धोऽसितपीतरागवान् भ्रमज्वरस्वेदतृषामदान्वितः |
य उष्यते स्पष्टरुगक्षिरागकृत् स पित्तशोथो भृशदाहपाकवान् ||८|| (च. चि. अ. १२) |

The symptoms of pittaja shotha (oedema caused due to increase of pitta) are –
the swelling (skin over the swelling) is soft
swelling emits peculiar type of smell
is black, yellow or red in colour
the patient has giddiness, fever, excessive sweating and thirst, intoxication
will have peculiar type of burning sensation in the affected part, clear pain, redness of the eyes
there will be severe burning sensation and quick suppuration of the swelling (8)

Kaphaja Shotha

गुरुः स्थिरः पाण्डुररोचकान्वितः प्रसेकनिद्रावमिवह्निमान्द्यकृत् |
स कृच्छ्रजन्मप्रशमो निपीडितो न चोन्नमेद्रात्रिबली कफात्मकः ||९|| (च. चि. अ. १२) |
The symptoms of Kaphaja shotha (oedema caused due to increase of pitta) are –
the swelling is heavy and immovable (fixed) and pale
the patient has loss of taste, excessive salivation, excessive sleep, poor digestion (weakness of digestive fire or capacity)
the swelling manifests and subsides slowly
the swelling pits on pressure and doesn't fill up quickly after the pressure is released
the swelling is profound (increases) during night time (9)

Dwidoshaja, Tridoshaja Shotha
निदानाकृतिसंसर्गाच्छ्वयथुः स्याद्द्विदोषजः |
सर्वाकृतिः सन्निपाताच्छोथो व्यामिश्रलक्षणः ||१०|| (च. सू. अ. १८) |
Swelling caused by two and three doshas
In dvidosaja shotha there will be presence of combined etiological factors and symptoms of two dosas. On the other hand, in sannipataja shotha the symptoms of all the three doshas are collectively present together. (10)

Abhighataja Shotha
अभिघातेन शस्त्रादिच्छेदभेदक्षतादिभिः |
हिमानिलोदध्यनिलैर्भल्लातकपिकच्छुजैः ||११||
रसैः शूकैश्च संस्पर्शाच्छ्वयथुः स्याद्विसर्पवान् |
भृशोष्मा लोहिताभासः प्रायशः पित्तलक्षणः ||१२||
(वा. नि. अ. १३) |
Assault by weapons causing cutting, breaking or tearing of the parts, assault by snow (frost), breeze, or winds coming from sea (cyclone); contact with fumes or oil of bhallaataka (marking nut) and fine thorns of the pod of kapikacchu (Mucuna pruriens), irritating juices of herbs, etc., bring about an oedema which spreads quickly all around. This condition is associated with severe burning sensation, redness and other symptoms of pitta increase. (11-12)

Vishaja Shotha
विषजः सविषप्राणिपरिसर्पणमूत्रणात् |
दंष्ट्रादन्तनखाघातादविषप्राणिनामपि ||१३||

विण्मूत्रशुक्रोपहतमलवद्वस्त्रसङ्करात् |
विषवृक्षानिलस्पर्शाद्गरयोगावचूर्णनात् ||१४||
मृदुश्चलोऽवलम्बी च शीघ्रो दाहरुजाकरः |१५| (वा. नि. अ. १३) |
Poisonous animals crawling or urinating on the body, stinging, biting with teeth, scratching with nails by non-poisonous animals, contact with faeces, urine, or semen of poisonous animals or coverings / contact with contaminated cloth, contact with poisonous trees, air (gases) and sprinkling or application of artificial poisonous materials also produce oedema. The skin over she swollen part is soft, movable, moves (spreads) quickly in downward direction (to the lower parts of the body) and is associated with burning sensation and pain which manifests quickly. (13-14)

Seat of doshas and shotha
दोषाः श्वयथुमूर्ध्वं हि कुर्वन्त्यामाशयस्थिताः ||१५||
पक्वाशयस्था मध्ये तु वर्चःस्थानगतास्त्वधः |
कृत्स्नदेहमनुप्राप्ताः कुर्युः सर्वसरं तथा ||१६||
(सु. चि. अ. २३) |
Doṣas residing in the stomach produce oedema in the upper part of the body. Doshas residing in the colon (large intestine) produces oedema / swelling in the trunk. The doshas residing in the rectum produce oedema in the lower parts of the body. The doshas which are spread out in the entire body produces swelling / oedema in the entire body (all parts of the body). (15-16)

Symptoms of incurability of Shotha
यो मध्यदेशे श्वयथुः स कष्टः सर्वगश्च यः |
अर्धाङ्गे रिष्टभूतः स्याद्यश्चोर्ध्वं परिसर्पति ||१७||
श्वासः पिपासा छर्दिश्च दौर्बल्यं ज्वर एव च |
यस्य चान्ने रुचिर्नास्ति श्वयथुं तं विवर्जयेत् ||१८|| (सु. चि. अ. २३) |
नवोऽनुपद्रवः शोथः साध्योऽसाध्यः पुरेरितः ||१९|| (वा. नि. अ. १३) |
विवर्जयेत् कुक्ष्युदराश्रितं च तथा गले मर्मणि संश्रितं च |
स्थूलः खरश्चापि भवेद्विवर्ज्यो यश्चापि बालस्थविराबलानाम् ||२०||
Oedema manifesting in the trunk and that which has spread to involve the entire body (all parts of the body) is difficult to cure.
Oedema / swelling occurring in half of the body and also spreads to involve the upper parts of the body are considered to be equal to arista (ominous

signs which indicate that the person is going to die shortly) i.e., it is incurable.

The patients in whom the oedema / swelling is associated with dyspnoea (difficulty in respiration), thirst, vomiting, debility, fever and lack of desire in food should be refused treatment i.e., such a condition of shotha is incurable.

Oedema caused by its own complications which begins in the feet in men should be considered as fatal. Likewise, the swelling which begins in the face and spreads downwards in women should be considered as fatal in women. When the swelling begins in the genitals is considered as fatal in both men and women.

Oedema of recent onset which is not associated with complications is curable and the other type of oedema (explained above) are said to be incurable.

Oedema occurring in the abdominal cavity, abdomen, and neck and located in the vital organs is considered incurable. Similarly, the oedema occurring in children, old aged people and weak (women) people is incurable and hence should not be treated. (17-20)

इति श्रीमाधवकरविरचिते माधवनिदाने शोथनिदानं समाप्तम् ||३६||

Thus ends the chapter on Shotha Nidanam in Madhava Nidana text written by Acharya Madhavakara.

37

Madhava Nidana Chapter 37 Vriddhi Nidanam

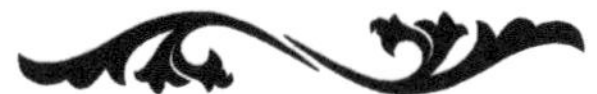

Vriddhi Samprapti, Bheda

क्रुद्धोऽनूर्ध्वगतिर्वायुः शोथशूलकरश्चरन् |
मुष्कौ वङ्क्षणतः प्राप्य फलकोषाभिवाहिनीः ||१||
प्रपीड्य धमनीर्वृद्धिं करोति फलकोषयोः |
दोषास्रमेदोमूत्रान्त्रैः स वृद्धिः सप्तधा गदः ||२||
मूत्रान्त्रजावप्यनिलाद्धेतुभेदस्तु केवलम् |३| (वा. नि. अ. ११) |

Pathogenesis and types of Vriddhi

Pathogenesis - Vaata undergoing increase moves downwards through the groins to the scrotum and causes derangement of the vessels of the scrotum and produces enlargement of the scrotum. This condition is associated with oedema and pain and is called vriddhi.

Types of Vriddhi – Vriddhi is said to be of 7 types – one from each of the three doshas, one from rakta (blood), one from meda (fat), one from mutra (urine) and the seventh one from antra (intestines).

Even the mutraja and antraja are mainly due to vata, though named separately after their causes. (1-2)

Vriddhi Lakshanas

वातपूर्णदृतिस्पर्शो रूक्षो वातादहेतुरुक् ||३||
पक्वोदुम्बरसङ्काशः पित्ताद्दाहोष्मपाकवान्

कफाच्छीतो गुरुः स्निग्धः कण्डूमान् कठिनोऽल्परुक् ||४||
कृष्णस्फोटावृतः पित्तवृद्धिलिङ्गश्च रक्तजः |
कफवन्मेदसा वृद्धिर्मृदुस्तालफलोपमः ||५||
मूत्रधारणशीलस्य मूत्रजः स तु गच्छतः |
अम्भोभिः पूर्णदृतिवत् क्षोभं याति सरुङ्मृदुः ||६||
मूत्रकृच्छ्रमधः स्याच्च चालयन् फलकोषयोः |७| (वा. नि. अ. ११) |

Symptoms of types of Vriddhi

Vataja Vriddhi - In vātaja vriddhi, the scrotum resembles a bag filled with air on touch and is rough. There will be pain without any apparent reason.

Pittaja Vriddhi - In pittaja víddhi, the scrotum resembles a ripe udumbara (wild fig, Ficus glomerata) fruit. The swelling is accompanied with burning sensation, increased heat and tendency to undergo suppuration quickly.

Kaphaja Vriddhi - In kaphaja vriddhi, the scrotum is cold to touch, heavy and unctuous. There is itching, the scrotum is hard on touch and is accompanied with very little pain.

Raktaja Vruddhi – In raktaja vriddhi caused by vitiated blood, the swelling of the scrotum is surrounded by (studded with) black coloured eruptions (blisters). This condition will have all the symptoms of pittaja vriddhi.

Medoja Vriddhi – In Medaja vriddhi caused by vitiated fat, all symptoms of kaphaja vriddhi are seen. The scrotal swelling is soft and resembles (big) a tala fruit (wild palm).

Mutraja Vruddhi – This type of vriddhi occurs in persons who are habituated in suppressing the natural urge of urination. The scrotum is filled with fluid and resembles a water bag filled with fluid and fluctuates while walking. The swelling of the scrotum is soft and is painful. When the scrotum is moved it produces pain similar to that of mutrakrchra (dysuria – difficulty in urination). (3-6)

Antra Vruddhi

वातकोपिभिराहारैः शीततोयावगाहनैः ||७||
धारणेरणभाराध्वविषमाङ्गप्रवर्तनैः |
क्षोभणैः क्षोभितोऽन्यैश्च क्षुद्रान्त्रावयवं यदा ||८||
पवनो विगुणीकृत्य स्वनिवेशादधो नयेत् |
कुर्याद्वङ्क्षणसन्धिस्थो ग्रन्थ्याभं श्वयथुं तदा ||९||
उपेक्ष्यमाणस्य च मुष्कवृद्धिमाध्मानरुक्स्तम्भवतीं स वायुः |
प्रपीडितोऽन्तःस्वनवान् प्रयाति प्रध्मापयन्नेति पुनश्च मुक्तः ||१०||

यस्यान्त्रावयवाश्लेषान्मुष्कयोर्वातसम्भवात् |
अन्त्रवृद्धिरसाध्योऽयं वातवृद्धिसमाकृतिः ||११|| (वा. नि. अ. ११) |
Below mentioned are the etiological factors of antra vriddhi –
Excessive consumption of foods which increase (or tends to increase) vata
Sitting in a tub of cold water regularly and for prolonged periods (tub bath)
Withholding (forcibly controlling) the impending natural body urges or forcibly trying to create the urges which are not present
Carrying heavy loads
Excessive walking for long distances
Abruptly moving the body parts (like doing acrobatics) and such other tiresome activities
Pathogenesis – The vata gets aggravated due to the above said etiological factors. This aggravated vata would constrict a part of the intestine and brings it down into the scrotum causing its enlargement. A swelling resembling a cyst is formed in the groin. When this condition is neglected the vata further gets aggravated and moves the intestine even downwards and causes distension, pain and stiffness in the scrotum. On pressing, the intestine produces sounds and moves back into its position but soon come back into the scrotum once the pressure is released. This condition is called as antraja vriddhi. The symptoms of antra vriddhi are similar to those of vataja vriddhi and this condition is incurable. (7-11)
Thus ends the chapter on Vriddhiroga.

इति श्रीमाधवकरविरचिते माधवनिदाने वृद्धिनिदानं समाप्तम् ||३७||
Thus ends the chapter on Vriddhi Nidanam in Madhava Nidana text written by Acharya Madhavakara.

38

Madhava Nidana Chapter 38 Galaganda, Gandamala, Apachi, Granthi, Arbuda Nidanam

Galaganda Paribhasha

निबद्धः श्वयथुर्यस्य मुष्कवल्लम्बते गले |
महान् वा यदि वा ह्रस्वो गलगण्डं तमादिशेत् ||१||
(सु. नि. अ. ११) |

Word derivation and meaning of the term Galaganda

Galaganda is defined as a swelling (tumour) in the neck, big or small in size, and hanging like the scrotum. (1).

Galaganda Samprapti

वातः कफश्चापि गले प्रदुष्टो मन्ये च संश्रित्य तथैव मेदः |
कुर्वन्ति गण्डं क्रमशः स्वलिङ्गैः समन्वितं तं गलगण्डमाहुः ||२||
(सु. नि. अ. ११) |

Pathogenesis of galaganda

Vaata, kapha and medas (fat) get aggravated in the neck (throat) and reach manya (nape of the neck / side of the neck) and produce ganda i.e., a knot like swelling which grows in size gradually. This condition is called galaganda. In this the symptoms of the involved doshas would manifest (depending on their predominance in the disease). (2)

Vataja Galaganda Symptoms

तोदान्वितः कृष्णसिरावनद्धः श्यावोऽरुणो वा पवनात्मकस्तु |
पारुष्ययुक्तश्चिरवृद्ध्यपाको यदृच्छया पाकमियात्कदाचित् ||३||
वैरस्यमास्यस्य च तस्य जन्तोर्भवेत्तथा तालुगलप्रशोषः |४|
(सु. नि. अ. ११) |

In Vataja Galaganda there will be pricking pain and the swelling will be surrounded by a network of black coloured veins, is blackish brown or golden-brown colour, rough on touch, which grows gradually and doesn't undergo suppuration. By chance if suitable etiological factors are available the swelling may even go suppuration. The patient will also experience bad (opposite) tastes in his mouth and also dryness of the throat and palate. (3)

Kaphaja Galaganda Symptoms

स्थिरः सवर्णो गुरुरुग्रकण्डूः शीतो महांश्चापि कफात्मकस्तु ||४||
चिराभिवृद्धिं भजते चिराद्वा प्रपच्यते मन्दरुजः कदाचित् |
माधुर्यमास्यस्य च तस्य जन्तोर्भवेत्तथा तालुगलप्रलेपः ||५|| (सु. नि. अ. ११) |

In Kaphaja Galaganda, the swelling is immovable, having the same colour as the skin, is heavy, with severe itching, cold to touch, big in size, will grow slowly, will occasionally undergo suppuration slowly, and will be associated with mild pain. The person would experience a sweet taste in the mouth and coating (furring) of the palate and throat. (4-5)

Medoja Galaganda Symptoms

स्निग्धो गुरुः पाण्डुरनिष्टगन्धो मेदोभवः कण्डुयुतोऽल्परुक् च |
प्रलम्बतेऽलाबुवदल्पमूलो देहानुरूपक्षयवृद्धियुक्तः ||६||
स्निग्धास्यता तस्य भवेच्च जन्तोर्गलेऽनुशब्दं कुरुते च नित्यम् |७|
(सु. नि. अ. ११) |

In Medoja Galaganda the swelling will be unctuous, heavy, pale (yellowish white), emit an unpleasant smell, associated with itching and mild pain (one will experience mild pain on scratching). The swelling hangs like an alabu (pitcher gourd) and is attached very loosely. It keeps undergoing increase and decrease (in size) in accordance to the body (health of the body). The inside of the mouth of the patient in this condition will be unctuous (will produce copious salivation) and the patient will make cooing sounds or indistinct sounds from the throat. (6-7)

Symptoms of incurability of Galaganda

कृच्छ्राच्छ्वसन्तं मृदुसर्वगात्रं संवत्सरातीतमरोचकार्तम् ||७||
क्षीणं च वैद्यो गलगण्डयुक्तं भिन्नस्वरं चापि विवर्जयेच्च |८|
(सु. नि. अ. ११) |

The patient of galaganda who has difficulty in breathing, very soft (looseness of) body parts, his swelling persisting for more than one year, is associated with loss of taste, emaciation and broken voice (hoarseness of voice) should be rejected treatment (should not be treated since this condition is incurable). (7-8)

Gandamala

कर्कन्धुकोलामलकप्रमाणैः कक्षांसमन्यागलवङ्क्षणेषु ||८||
मेदःकफाभ्यां चिरमन्दपाकैः स्याद्गण्डमाला बहुभिश्च गण्डैः |९|
(सु. नि. अ. ११) |

More than one ganda (swelling) caused by kapha and medas (fat), appearing in the regions of axilla, shoulders (scapular region), sides of the neck (nape of the neck), front of neck or the groin, varying in size from that of karkandhu and kola (fruit of jujube) to that of amalaka (gooseberry), and undergoing suppuration after long period of time is known as Gandamala (chain of swellings). (8)

Apachi

ते ग्रन्थयः केचिदवाप्तपाकाः स्रवन्ति नश्यन्ति भवन्ति चान्ये ||९||
कालानुबन्धं चिरमादधाति सैवापचीति प्रवदन्ति तज्ज्ञाः |
साध्याः स्मृताः पीनसपार्श्वशूलकासज्वरच्छर्दियुतास्त्ववसाध्याः ||१०||

Some of the swellings undergo suppuration, some more burst open and discharge their contents, some get destroyed or disappear, and some new ones appear. This process continues for a long time. Experts call such conditions as Apaci. This condition is curable. On the other hand, apaci associated with complications like running from the nose, pain in the flanks, cough, fever and vomiting will become incurable. (9-10)

Granthi

वातादयो मांसमसृक् प्रदुष्टाः सन्दूष्य मेदश्च तथा सिराश्च |
वृत्तोन्नतं विग्रथितं च शोथं कुर्वन्त्यतो ग्रन्थिरिति प्रदिष्टः ||११||
(सु. नि. अ. ११) |

Vāta and other two doṣhas (pitta and kapha) undergoing increase, contaminate (bring about abnormalities in the) mamsa (muscles), asrk (blood), meda (fat) and siras (veins) produce round, elevated and cystic swelling. Therefore, these swellings (masses) are called granthi (cyst, tumour). (11)

Vatika Granthi

आयम्यते वृश्च्यति तुद्यते च प्रत्यस्यते मथ्यति भिद्यते च |
कृष्णो मृदुर्बस्तिरिवाततश्च भिन्नः स्रवेच्चानिलजोऽस्रमच्छम् ||१२||
(सु. नि. अ. ११) |

In vataja granthi different kinds of pains are manifested – like pulling / stretching, tearing, throbbing (pricking), pulling, churning, and splitting (cutting) types of pains. The cyst is black in colour, soft, resembles and bulged like a water bag and discharges thin, clear (thin) blood when pricked. (12)

Pittaja Granthi

दन्दह्यते धूप्यति वृश्च्यते च पापच्यते प्रज्वलतीव चापि |
रक्तः सपीतोऽप्यथवाऽपि पित्ताद्भिन्नः स्रवेदुष्णमतीव चास्रम् ||१३||
(सु. नि. अ. ११) |

The symptoms of pittaja granthi include severe burning sensation as if burnt by fire, feeling as if smoke is being eliminated from the swelling / body (raised temperature), pain as if that part of the body is excised, undergoes quick suppuration as if burnt by alkali, and feeling as if the body is burnt into ash. The colour of the cyst is either red or yellow in colour. When the cysts burst open (or pricked), they discharge (exude) large amounts of warm blood. (13)

Kaphaja Granthi

शीतोऽविवर्णोऽल्परुजोऽतिकण्डुः पाषाणवत् संहननोपपन्नः |
चिराभिवृद्धश्च कफप्रकोपाद्भिन्नः स्रवेच्छुक्लघनं च पूयम् ||१४||
(सु. नि. अ. ११) |

In kaphaja granthi, the cyst is cold to touch, will not have any discolouration (or have slight discolouration), will have mild pain and severe itching. The cyst has stone like consistency (hard), grows slowly and when it breaks open it discharges thick and white coloured pus. (14)

Medoja Granthi

शरीरवृद्धिक्षयवृद्धिहानिः स्निग्धो महान् कण्डुयुतोऽरुजश्च |
मेदःकृतो गच्छति चात्र भिन्ने पिण्याकसर्पिःप्रतिमं तु मेदः ||१५||
(सु. नि. अ. ११) |

The cyst of medaja granthi (caused due to vitiated fat) will increase or decrease in size in accordance with that of the body. It is unctuous, big in size, is associated with itching and is painless. When pricked (bursts open), it will discharge thick fatty exudates which resembles the paste of sesame seeds or ghee. (15)

Siraja Granthi

व्यायामजातैरबलस्य तैस्तैराक्षिप्य वायुस्तु सिराप्रतानम् |
सङ्कुच्य सम्पिण्ड्य विशोष्य चापि ग्रन्थिं करोत्युन्नतमाशु वृत्तम् ||१६||
ग्रन्थिः सिराजः स तु कृच्छ्रसाध्यो भवेद्यदि स्यात् सरुजश्चलश्च |
स चारुज श्चाप्यचलो महांश्च मर्मोत्थितश्चापि विवर्जनीयः ||१७||
(सु. नि. अ. ११) |

In persons who are weakened but do excessive indulgence in various kinds of strenuous activities / exercises, vata undergoing increase invades the network of veins, making them constricted, condensed and dried and quickly rolls them into a round big mass. This is known as siraja granthi (cysts or tumours of veins). When there is pain and movement in these granthis it will become difficult to cure. If these cysts are bigger in size and appear on or around the vital organs of the body they are considered as incurable in spite of them being devoid of pain and immobile (fixed). (16-17)

Arbuda

गात्रप्रदेशे क्वचिदेव दोषाः सम्मूर्छिता मांसमसृक् प्रदूष्य |
वृत्तं स्थिरं मन्दरुजं महान्तमनल्पमूलं चिरवृद्ध्यपाकम् ||१८||
कुर्वन्ति मांसोच्छ्रयमत्यगाधं तदर्बुदं शास्त्रविदो वदन्ति |
वातेन पित्तेन कफेन चापि रक्तेन मांसेन च मेदसा वा ||१९||

तज्जायते तस्य च लक्षणानि ग्रन्थेः समानानि तदा भवन्ति |२०|
(सु. नि. अ. ११) |
Pathogenesis of Arbuda - Doshas undergoing increase in any particular part of the body, invade and contaminate the muscle and blood and produce round, immobile, slightly painful, big, deep-seated, slowly increasing tumours which do not suppurate. They appear like balls of muscles (big muscular mass) and are termed by the learned experts as Arbuda (cancer).
Types of Arbuda – Arbuda is of six types. They are – Vataja, Pittaja, Kaphaja, Raktaja, Mamsaja and Medaja. Each of these arbudas will have the symptoms similar to the granthis (granthis formed by the same doshas respectively).
Example – Vataja arbuda will have symptoms similar to vataja granthi, pittaja arbuda will have symptoms similar to pittaja granthi etc. (18-19)

Raktarbuda
दोषः प्रदुष्टो रुधिरं सिराश्च सङ्कुच्य सम्पिण्ड्य ततस्त्वपाकम् ||२०||
सास्रावमुन्नह्यति मांसपिण्डं मांसाङ्कुरैराचितमाशुवृद्धम् |
करोत्यजस्रं रुधिरप्रवृत्तिमसाध्यमेतद्रुधिरात्मकं तु ||२१||
रक्तक्षयोपद्रवपीडितत्वात् पाण्डुर्भवेदर्बुदपीडितस्तु |
(सु. नि. अ. ११) |
The doshas which have undergone increase will contaminate (constrict) and compress the blood and veins. By doing so they would produce a big sized muscular mass (tumour) which does not undergo suppuration (or undergoes less suppuration), is surrounded by (studded all over) many muscular sprouts, grows quickly and has little discharges. Bleeding takes place constantly from such a mass. This is called as raktaja arbuda and it is incurable. Since there is excessive bleeding from the rakta arbuda there would occur severe loss of blood in this condition which would eventually lead to many complications. Due to this the person would quickly become victim of anaemia. (20-21)

Mamsa Arbuda
मुष्टिप्रहारादिभिरर्दितेऽङ्गे मांसं प्रदुष्टं जनयेद्धि शोथम् ||२२||
अवेदनं स्निग्धमनन्यवर्णमपाकमश्मोपममप्रचाल्यम् |
प्रदुष्टमांसस्य नरस्य गाढमेतद्भवेन्मांसपरायणस्य ||२३||
मांसार्बुदं त्वेतदसाध्यमुक्तं... | (सु. नि. अ. ११) |
Assault on the body by the fist, etc.; leads to contamination (derangement)

of the muscles. This leads to causation of a swelling (tumour) which is painless, unctuous, has colour of the skin, does not undergo suppuration, is hard like a stone, and fixed. This condition is called mamsa arbuda. This condition occurs commonly in those who are accustomed and habituated to eating excessive (contaminated) meat (flesh) in their food. This condition should be considered as incurable. (22-23)

Incurability / prognosis of arbuda

...साध्येष्वपीमानि तु वर्जयेच्च |
सम्प्रस्रुतं मर्मणि यच्च जातं स्रोतःसु वा यच्च भवेदचाल्यम् ||२४||
(सु. नि. अ. ११)

|Even among the curable forms of arbuda, the following are to be rejected –
that which has heavy discharges (exudation)
that occurring on or around the vital organs
that occurring on or around the channels including nasal passage etc (and hence imparting pressure on them and obstructing their functioning)
that which is immobile (24)

Adyarbuda / Dwirarbuda

यज्जायतेऽन्यत् खलु पूर्वजाते ज्ञेयं तदद्ध्यर्बुदमर्बुदज्ञैः |
यद्द्वन्द्वजातं युगपत् क्रमाद्वा द्विरर्बुदं तच्च भवेदसाध्यम् ||२५||
(सु. नि. अ. ११) |

यज्जायतेऽन्यत् खलु पूर्वजाते ज्ञेयं तदद्ध्यर्बुदमर्बुदज्ञैः |
यद्द्वन्द्वजातं युगपत् क्रमाद्वा द्विरर्बुदं तच्च भवेदसाध्यम् ||२५||
(सु. नि. अ. ११) |

Adyarbuda - A second arbuda developing over an already existing arbuda (superseding) or after the course of an earlier one (the earlier one being removed) is called Adhyarbuda by the specialists of arbuda.

Dwirarbuda – Arbuda developing alongside yet another arbuda simultaneously or after some time at the same place or at some other place of the body is called as Dvirarbuda.

Both these conditions are incurable. (25)

Why arbudas do not suppurate?

न पाकमायान्ति कफाधिकत्वान्मेदोबहुत्वाच्च विशेषतस्तु |
दोषस्थिरत्वाद्ग्रथनाच्च तेषां सर्वार्बुदान्येव निसर्गतस्तु ||२६||
(सु. नि. अ. ११) |

All arbudas do not suppurate when –
there is predominance of kapha and medas (fat) in them
by the hardness and immobility of doshas
by the very nature of the disease (26)

इति श्रीमाधवकरविरचिते माधवनिदाने गलगण्डगण्डमालापचीग्रन्थ्यर्बुदनिदानं समाप्तम् ||३८||

Thus ends the chapter on Galaganda, Gandamala, Apachi, Granthi, Arbuda Nidanam in Madhava Nidana text written by Acharya Madhavakara.

39

Madhava Nidana Chapter 39 Shlipada Nidanam

Shlipada Samanya Lakshana

यः सज्वरो वङ्क्षणजो भृशार्तिः शोथो नृणां पादगतः क्रमेण |
तच्छ्लीपदं स्यात् करकर्णनेत्रशिश्नौष्ठनासास्वपि केचिदाहुः ||१||

General Symptoms

A swelling starting in the groins and gradually moving towards (involving) the leg, associated with fever and severe pain is known as Shilpada. According to the opinion of others (experts) shlipada may occur even in the hands, ears, eyes, penis, lips and nose. (1)

Symptoms of Doshaja Shlipada

वातजं कृष्णरूक्षं च स्फुटितं तीव्रवेदनम् |
अनिमित्तरुजं तस्य बहुशो ज्वर एव च ||२||
पित्तजं पीतसङ्काशं दाहज्वरयुतं मृदु |
श्लैष्मिकं स्निग्धवर्णं च श्वेतं पाण्डु गुरु स्थिरम् ||३||

Vataja Shlipada - In this condition the swelling is black, dry and has fissures, (cracks). There is severe pain which appears without any apparent reason and is covered with fever.

Pittaja Shlipada – In this condition there is yellowish discolouration. It is associated with burning sensation and fever and the swelling is soft to touch.

Kaphaja Shlipada – Here the swelling is unctuous (oily). It is white or pale in colour, is heavy and fixed (immobile). (2-3)

Asadhya Lakshana

वल्मीकमिव सञ्जातं कण्टकैरुपचीयते |
अब्दात्मकं महत्तच्च वर्जनीयं विशेषतः ||४||

Symptoms of incurability

The swelling of slipada growing upwards like an ant-hill with many small hill-like projections and sprouts (knots), that which exists for more than one year, and that which is very big in size are to be rejected (should not be treated because such shlipada is incurable). (4)

Kapha predominance in all types of Shlipada

त्रीण्यप्येतानि जानीयाच्छ्लीपदानि कफोच्छ्रयात् |
गुरुत्वं च महत्त्वं च यस्मान्नास्ति कफं विना ||५||
(सु. नि. अ. १२) |

In all the three varieties of shlipada, kapha is the predominant doṣha, because heaviness and increase in size cannot be caused without kapha.(5)

Places where Shlipada is prevalent

पुराणोदकभूयिष्ठाः सर्वर्तुषु च शीतलाः |
ये देशास्तेषु जायन्ते श्लीपदानि विशेषतः ||६||
(सु. नि. अ. १२) |

Shlipada is generally prevalent in such places (areas) where there is stagnation of water for a long period of time, in places wherein there is excessive cold in all the seasons of the year. (6)

Other symptoms of incurability of Shlipada

यच्छ्लेष्मलाहारविहारजातं पुंसः प्रकृत्याऽपि कफात्मकस्य |
सास्रावमत्युन्नतसर्वलिङ्गं सकण्डुरं श्लेष्मयुतं विवर्ज्यम् ||७||

Shlipada should be rejected (should not be treated) when it is caused due to excessive indulgence in foods and habits which increase kapha, in those who are of kapha prakriti (whose birth constitution is predominantly kapha) and when the disease presents with exudation, is very big in size, is associated with all the signs and symptoms and has itching. (7)

इति श्रीमाधवकरविरचिते माधवनिदाने श्लीपदनिदानं समाप्तम् ||३९||

`Thus ends the chapter on shlipada Nidanam in Madhava Nidana text written by Acharya Madhavakara.

40

Madhava Nidana Chapter 40 Vidradhi Nidanam

Vidradhi Samprapti, Bheda

त्वग्रक्तमांसमेदांसि सन्दूष्यास्थिसमाश्रिताः |
दोषाः शोथं शनैर्घोरं जनयन्त्युच्छ्रिता भृशम् ||१||
महामूलं रुजावन्तं वृत्तं वाऽप्यथवाऽऽयतम् |
स विद्रधिरिति ख्यातो विज्ञेयः षड्विधश्च सः ||२||
पृथग्दोषैः समस्तैश्च क्षतेनाप्यसृजा तथा |
षण्णामपि हि तेषां तु लक्षणं सम्प्रवक्ष्यते ||३||
(सु. नि. अ. ९) |

Pathogenesis and types of vidradhi

The doshas which have undergone abnormal increase get lodged in the bones and contaminate (bring about abnormal change) skin, blood, muscles and fat gradually (slowly increasing in size) causing localized swelling which is deep seated, painful, round or broad (elongated) in shape. This is known as vidradhi.

This vidradhi is of six types – one from each dosha (vataja, pittaja and kaphaja), one from the combination of all the three doshas (tridoshaja), one from injury (ksataja) and the other one from blood (raktaja). Their features will be described further on. (1-3)

Vataja Vidradhi

कृष्णोऽरुणो वा विषमो भृशमत्यर्थवेदनः |
चित्रोत्थानप्रपाकश्च विद्रधिर्वातसम्भवः ||४||
(सु. नि. अ. ९) |

The vidradhi caused due to increase of vata is black or red (reddish brown) in colour, often increasing or decreasing in size, associated with severe pain, gets manifests and suppurates in many ways (variations are seen in the duration of onset and time of suppuration). (4)

Pittaja Vidradhi

शरावसदृशः पाण्डुः शीतः स्निग्धोऽल्पवेदनः |
चिरोत्थानप्रपाकश्च विद्रधिः कफसम्भवः ||६||
(सु. नि. अ. ९) |

The vidradhi caused due to increase of kapha resembles a big saucer, is pale (yellowish white in colour), cold, unctuous (smooth), associated with mild pain, and is slow in manifesting and suppurating. (6)

Nature of Pus

तनुपीतसिताश्चैषामास्रावाः क्रमशः स्मृताः |७|

Nature of secretions (pus) in the doshaja types of vidradhi -
The pus exuding from the above-mentioned types of doshaja vidradhi will be thin, yellow and white respectively i.e.,
thin in vataja,
yellow in pittaja and
white in kaphaja vidradhi.

Sannipataja Vidradhi

नानावर्णरुजास्रावो घाटालो विषमो महान् ||७||
विषमं पच्यते चापि विद्रधिः सान्निपातिकः |
(सु. नि. अ. ९) |

Sannipaataja vidradhi (due to increase of all the three doshas) will be having different kinds of colours, pain and exudation, with elevated sprout, unsteady in nature, very troublesome and with irregular time of suppuration.(7)

Agantuja Vidradhi

तैस्तैर्भावैरभिहते क्षते वाऽपथ्यकारिणः ||८||

क्षतोष्मा वायुविसृतः सरक्तं पित्तमीरयेत् |
ज्वरस्तृष्णा च दाहश्च जायते तस्य देहिनः ||९||
आगन्तुर्विद्रधिह्येष पित्तविद्रधिलक्षणः |१०|
(सु. नि. अ. ९) |

In persons who are subjected to injury by canes (baton), stones etc. (and other weapons) and also get indulged in unwholesome foods, the heat of the wound being stimulated by vata will also vitiate the blood and pitta. The vidradhi formed as a result of this is called as agantuja vidradhi (abscess caused by external agents / injury). In this condition the person will have fever, thirst and burning sensation. The other symptoms of pittaja vidradhi are also seen in this type of vidradhi. (8-9)

Raktaja Vidradhi

कृष्णस्फोटावृतः श्यावस्तीव्रदाहरुजाकरः ||१०||
पित्तविद्रधिलिङ्गस्तु रक्तविद्रधिरुच्यते |११|
(सु. नि. अ. ९) |

In raktaja vidradhi (abscess caused by aggravated blood) the abscess is enveloped on all sides by black coloured eruptions (boils, blisters), is of blackish blue in colour, causes severe burning sensation and pain and has other symptoms of pittaja vidradhi. (10)

Antarvidradhi (Internal abscess)

पृथक् सम्भूय वा दोषाः कुपिता गुल्मरूपिणम् ||११||
वल्मीकवत् समुन्नद्धमन्तः कुर्वन्ति विद्रधिम् |
गुदे बस्तिमुखे नाभ्यां कुक्षौ वङ्क्षणयोस्तथा ||१२||
वृक्कयोः प्लीह्नि यकृति हृदि वा क्लोम्नि वाऽप्यथ |
तेषामुक्तानि लिङ्गानि बाह्यविद्रधिलक्षणैः ||१३||
अधिष्ठानविशेषेण लिङ्गं शृणु विशेषतः |

The doshas undergoing abnormal increase due to their etiological factors, either individually or in combination, produce vidradhis inside the body, in different organs, resembling a spreading shrub / bush or anthill. Since these abscesses happen inside the body they are called as antarvidradhi.

Places of the body where antarvidradhi develops – The seats of internal abscess include the rectum, opening of urinary bladder, umbilicus, lower part of the abdomen (abdominal cavity), groins, kidneys, spleen, liver, heart, pancreas or any other place in the body i.e., abscesses can occur in these organs or any other organ which has not been mentioned.

General Symptoms – The general symptoms of internal abscesses are similar to the symptoms of external abscesses. Apart from these, the internal abscesses have special symptoms related to the seat in which they get manifested. They will be described here now. (11-14)

Symptoms of Antarvidradi

गुदे वातनिरोधश्च बस्तौ कृच्छ्राल्पमूत्रता ||१४||
नाभ्यां हिक्का तथाऽऽटोपः कुक्षौ मारुतकोपनम् |
कटीपृष्ठग्रहस्तीव्रो वङ्क्षणोत्थे तु विद्रधौ ||१५||
वृक्कयोः पार्श्वसङ्कोचः प्लीहन्युच्छ्वासावरोधनम् |
सर्वाङ्गप्रग्रहस्तीव्रो हृदि कासश्च जायते |
श्वासो यकृति हिक्का च क्लोम्नि पेपीयते पयः ||१६||
(सु. नि. अ. ९) |

Symptoms based on the organs in which they get manifested -

- If the abscess is in the rectum, it causes obstruction to movement of the flatus.
- If the abscess occurs in the urinary bladder, it would cause difficulty in urination and scanty urination.
- The abscess occurring in the umbilicus would cause hiccough and gurgling sounds in the abdomen.
- If the abscess occurs in the abdomen, it would cause the symptoms of vata increase like pain, distension of the abdomen etc.
- If the abscess happens in the groins, it would cause severe stiffness or gripping (catching) pain in the waist or back.
- If the abscess occurs in the kidney, there would be constriction of the flanks.
- If the abscess occurs in the spleen, there will be obstruction or difficulty in breathing.
- If the abscess is found occurring in the heart (region of the heart), there will be catching pain in all the parts of the body and cough.
- If the abscess occurs in the liver it would cause dyspnoea and hiccough.
- If the abscess occurs in the pancreas the person would drink large quantities of water often because in this condition there will be severe thirst. (14-16)

Prognosis of Vidradhi

नाभेरुपरिजाः पक्वा यान्त्यूर्ध्वमितरे त्वधः |१७| (सु. नि. अ. ९) |
अधःस्रुतेषु जीवेत्तु स्रुतेषूर्ध्वं न जीवति ||१७||
हृन्नाभिबस्तिवर्ज्या ये तेषु भिन्नेषु बाह्यतः |
जीवेत् कदाचित् पुरुषो नेतरेषु कदाचन ||१८||
(सु. नि. अ. ९) |

When the vidradhis occurring above the level of umbilicus (organs placed above the level of umbilicus) burst open, they discharge (expel) their contents through an upward route (mouth). On the other hand, when the vidradhis below the level of the umbilicus (organs below the level of umbilicus) burst open, they discharge their content through a downward route (anus or urinary passage – urethra). (The discharges may be in the form of pus or blood).

When the discharges come out in the downward direction the patient will survive. On the other hand, if the discharges occur from the upward routes he will not survive (will die).

The patient in whom the internal abscess, other than those occurring in the region of the heart, umbilicus and urinary bladder burst open towards outside of the body may sometimes survive. (The abscess occurring in the heart, umbilicus and urinary bladder are incurable). Even if the abscess occurring in the region of the heart, umbilicus and urinary bladder open towards outside of the body, the patient would not survive. (17-18)

साध्या विद्रधयः पञ्च विवर्ज्यः सान्निपातिकः |
आमपक्वविदग्धत्वं तेषां शोथवदादिशेत् ||१९||
(वा. नि. अ. ११) |
आध्मातं बद्धनिष्यन्दं छर्दिहिक्कातृषान्वितम् |
रुजाश्वाससमायुक्तं विद्रधिर्नाशयेन्नरम् ||२०||
(सु. सू. अ. ३३) |

Apart from the tridoshaja vidradhi (abscess caused by simultaneous aggravation of all three doshas) the other five kinds of vidradhis are curable. Tridoshaja Vidradhi is incurable. The unripe, ripening and ripened stages of vidradhi are similar to those explained in the context of sotha (inflammatory oedema explained in the next chapter). If the patient of antarvidradhi also has distension of abdomen, obstruction of urination, vomiting, hiccough, thirst, severe pain and difficulty in respiration, the patient will die. (19-20)

इति श्रीमाधवकरविरचिते माधवनिदाने विद्रधिनिदानं समाप्तम् ||४०||

Thus ends the chapter on Vidradhi Nidanam in Madhava Nidana text written by Acharya Madhavakara.

41

Madhava Nidana Chapter 41 Vranashotha Nidanam

एकदेशोत्थितः शोथो व्रणानां पूर्वलक्षणम् |
षड्विधः स्यात् पृथक्सर्वरक्तागन्तुनिमित्तजः ||१||
शोथाः षडेते विज्ञेयाः प्रागुक्तैः शोथलक्षणैः |
विशेषः कथ्यते चैषां पक्वापक्वादिनिश्चये ||२||

A swelling which is localized (and limited to a particular area of the body) becomes the premonitory symptom (stage) of an ulcer and is called as Vrana shopha. In short, Vrana shotha is a localized swelling which occurs prior to the formation of an ulcer. Vrana shopha is of six kinds – one each from each dosha (vataja, pittaja and kaphaja), one caused by combination of all three doshas, one from rakta (blood) and one from external causes (agantu). The symptoms of all these six kinds of vranasotha are similar to those explained in the context of the types of sotha previously.

Now, the special features of unripe and ripened stages of Vrana shopha will be described ahead. (1-2)

Symptoms of Vrana shotha

विषमं पच्यते वातात् पित्तोत्थश्चाचिराच्चिरम् |
कफजः पित्तवच्छोथो रक्तागन्तुसमुद्भवः ||३||

Specific symptoms of the types of Vranashotha

Vātaja type of Vranashotha undergoes ripening inconsistently. Pittaja type of vranashotha will undergo quick suppuration. Kaphaja vranashotha will undergo suppuration very slowly. The raktaja and agantuja vranashothas will have symptoms similar to those of pittaja vranashotha. (3)

Ama (unripe) and Pacyamana (ripening) Vranashotha Symptoms

मन्दोष्मताऽल्पशोथत्वं काठिन्यं त्वक्सवर्णता |
मन्दवेदनता चैतच्छोथानामामलक्षणम् ||४||
दह्यते दहनेनेव क्षारेणेव च पच्यते |
पिपीलिकागणेनेव दश्यते छिद्यते तथा ||५||
भिद्यते चैव शस्त्रेण दण्डेनेव च ताड्यते |
पीड्यते पाणिनेवान्तः सूचीभिरिव तुद्यते ||६||
सोषाचोषो विवर्णः स्यादङ्गुल्येवावघट्यते |
आसने शयने स्थाने शान्तिं वृश्चिकविद्धवत् ||७||
न गच्छेदाततः शोथो भवेदाध्मातबस्तिवत् |
ज्वरस्तृष्णाऽरुचिश्चैव पच्यमानस्य लक्षणम् ||८||

Ama Vranashotha Symptoms – In the unripe stage of Vranashotha the swelling is slightly warm. There is also mild swelling. The swelling is hard, has normal colour of the skin and mild pain.

Pacyamana Vranashotha Symptoms – In the ripening stage of Vranashotha there will be a severe burning sensation as if being burnt by fire or being corroded by strong alkali. The person will feel as if the region of swelling is being bitten by a swarm of ants, being cut or torn by sharp instruments, beaten by a baton, being pressed or squeezed by hands, pricked by (pierced by) needles, is being burnt and as if being burnt in the flanks, discoloration, pain as if being pressed by fingers.

The patient would not find comfort either by sitting, sleeping or standing and will experience continuous pain similar to that of a scorpion sting. The swelling is distended and expanded similar to a urinary bladder filled and distended by urine.

This condition is associated with fever, thirst and loss of taste. (4-8)

Pakva (ripened) Vranashotha Symptoms

वेदनोपशमः शोथोऽलोहितोऽल्पो न चोन्नतः |
प्रादुर्भावो वलीनां च तोदः कण्डूर्मुहुर्मुहुः ||९||
उपद्रवाणां प्रशमो निम्नता स्फुटनं त्वचाम् |
बस्ताविवाम्बुसञ्चारः स्याच्छोथेऽङ्गुलिपीडिते ||१०||

पूयस्य पीडयत्येकमन्तमन्ते च पीडीते |
भक्ताकाङ्क्षा भवेच्चैतच्छोथानां पक्वलक्षणम् ||११||

Pakva Vrana shotha Symptoms - Reduction in the severity of pain, reduction in the size of swelling,

reduction or absence of redness, absence of elevation, appearance of wrinkles on the swelling, repeated episodes of pricking pain and itching, and reduction of complications are seen in the ripened Vrana shopha. The swelling easily pits on pressure with the fingers, cracks appear on the skin, and the movements resembling the movement of water in the bladder or in a water bag are perceived in the swelling when it is pressed with the finger. When the swelling is pressed on one of its edges (side), the pressure of the pus is experienced on the other side of the swelling. The patient would develop a desire for food. (9-11)

Dosha relation during suppuration

नर्तेऽनिलाद्रुङ्न विना च पित्तं पाकः कफं चापि विना न पूयः |
तस्माद्धि सर्वे परिपाककाले पचन्ति शोथांस्त्रय एव दोषाः ||१२||
(सु. सू. अ. १७) |

There is no pain without the involvement of aggravated vata. There will be no suppuration without the involvement of aggravated pitta. There will be no formation of pus without the involvement of aggravated kapha. So, all the three doshas are actively involved during the period of ripening. (12)

Effect of pus which has not been drained

कालान्तरेणाभ्युदितं तु पित्तं कृत्वा वशे वातकफौ प्रसह्य |
पचत्यतः शोणितमेष पाको मतः परेषां विदुषां द्वितीयः ||१३||
कक्षं समासाद्य यथैव वह्निर्वाय्वीरितः सन्दहति प्रसह्य |
तथैव पूयो ह्यविनिःसृतो हि मांसं सिराः स्नायु च खादतीह ||१४||
(सु. सू. अ. १७) |

Just as a small fire hidden inside a haystack (or hearth) activated by the wind burns up the whole mass of hay, the pus too which has not been drained properly would destroy the muscles, veins, tendons etc. (13)

A true physician should know the stages of vranashotha

आमं विदह्यमानं च सम्यक् पक्वं च यो भिषक् |
जानीयात् स भवेद्वैद्यः शेषास्तस्करवृत्तयः ||१५||

Only he who can recognise the unripe, ripening and ripened stages (of the inflammatory swellings) deserves to be called as a physician. All others are only imposters. (14)

यश्छिनत्त्याममज्ञानाद्यो वा पक्वमुपेक्षते |
श्वपचाविव मन्तव्यौ तावनिश्चितकारिणौ ||१६||
(सु. सू. अ. १७) |
He who cuts open the swelling in its unripe stage with ignorance or he who delays its opening though fully ripened-both are to be considered as very mean persons, because they are uncertain in their act.(15)

इति श्रीमाधवकरविरचिते माधवनिदाने व्रणशोथनिदानं समाप्तम् ||४१||
Thus ends the chapter on Vranashota Nidanam in Madhava Nidana text written by Acharya Madhavakara.

42

Madhava Nidana Chapter 42 Shareera Vrana Nidanam

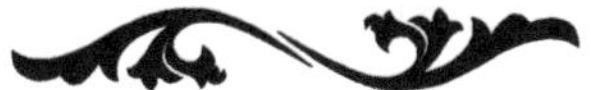

Vrana Bheda

द्विधा व्रणः स विज्ञेयः शारीरागन्तुभेदतः |
दोषैराद्यस्तयोरन्यः शस्त्रादिक्षतसम्भवः ||१||

Types of Vrana

Vraṇas (ulcers) are of two kinds. They are –

1. Sharira Vrana – physical or organic ulcers and
2. Aagantuja Vrana – traumatic ulcers

The first one i.e., sharirika vrana is caused by the doshas. The second type i.e., agantuja vrana is caused by injury caused by weapons, sharp instruments etc. (1)

Lakshanas

स्तब्धः कठिनसंस्पर्शो मन्दस्रावो महारुजः |
तुद्यते स्फुरति श्यावो व्रणो मारुतसम्भवः ||२||
तृष्णामोहज्वरक्लेददाहदुष्ट्यवदारणैः ||
व्रणं पित्तकृतं विद्याद्गन्धैः स्रावैश्च पूतिकैः ||३||
बहुपिच्छो गुरुः स्निग्धः स्तिमितो मन्दवेदनः |

पाण्डुवर्णोऽल्पसङ्क्लेदश्चिरपाकी कफव्रणः ||४|| (च. चि. अ. २५) |
रक्तो रक्तस्रुती रक्ताद्द्विद्वत्रिजः स्यात्तदन्वयैः |५|

Symptoms of types of sarira vranas

Vataja Vrana – The ulcer caused by vitiated vata is immobile (stiff), hard on touch, has less discharges (scanty exudation) and severe pain. The pain is of pricking or pulsating type. The ulcer is of bluish black colour.

Pittaja Vrana – The ulcer caused by vitiated pitta is associated with thirst, delusion (fainting, unconsciousness), fever, wetness (due to secretions), burning sensation, dirty, pain as if being torn (cracking of skin or tendency to burst open quickly), emits bad smell and discharges foul smelling secretions.

Kaphaja Vrana – The ulcer caused by vitiated kapha is excessively sticky, heavy, unctuous (oily), and feels as if covered by wet leather or cloth. The ulcer will be slightly painful, pale (yellowish white) in appearance, less moist, and suppurates slowly.

Raktaja Vrana – The ulcer caused by vitiated blood will be red in colour and will discharge only blood.

Dwija / Dwidoshaja Vraṇa – This is caused by combination of two doshas and will have combined symptoms of those two doshas involved.

Trija / Tridoshaja Vrana – This is caused by a combination of all three vitiated doshas and will have combined symptoms of all three doshas together. (2-4)

Sadhyasadhyata

त्वङ्मांसजः सुखे देशे तरुणस्यानुपद्रवः ||५||
धीमतोऽभिनवः काले सुखे साध्यः सुखं व्रणः |

Prognosis of Sarira Vrana -

Ulcers are curable when they –

- are located in the skin or muscles,
- are located in a convenient place (places of the body other than marmas – vital spots),
- occur in a young person,
- are not associated with complications,
- occur in intelligent persons (those who can discriminate between good and bad)
- are of recent origin,

- occur in appropriate time i.e., favorable season, age etc. (mainly Hemanta and Sisira – late and early winter) (5)

गुणैरन्यतमैर्हीनस्ततः कृच्छ्रो व्रणः स्मृतः ||६||
सर्वैर्विहीनो विज्ञेयस्त्वसाध्यो भूर्युपद्रवः |
(च. चि. अ. २५) |

Those (physical ulcers) which possess a few of the above qualities (few qualities less than those mentioned above – in the curable category) are difficult to cure. On the other hand, those which are devoid of any of the above-mentioned qualities (of curable ulcers) and also associated with many severe complications are incurable. (6)

Dusta Vrana (bad, contaminated ulcer) Symptoms

पूतिः पूयातिदुष्टासृक्स्राव्युत्सङ्गी चिरस्थितिः ||७||
दुष्टो व्रणोऽतिगन्धादिः शुद्धलिङ्गविपर्ययः |८|

Dusta vrana (bad, intractable ulcer) is one which discharges the blood heavily contaminated with foul smelling pus, has sinuses inside it, remains for long periods, has excessive foul smell, discoloration, discharges and pain and possesses opposite qualities of a clean ulcer. (7)

Shuddha Vrana (clean ulcer) Symptoms

जिह्वातलाभोऽतिमृदुः श्लक्ष्णः स्निग्धोऽल्पवेदनः ||८||
सुव्यवस्थो निरास्रावः शुद्धो व्रण इति स्मृतः |९|

A shuddha vraṇa (clean ulcer) is one which is very soft like the upper surface of the tongue, smooth, unctuous (moist), with mild pain, even (without sprouts and sinuses) and without excessive discharges (exudation). (8)

Ruhyamana Vrana (ulcer in the stage of healing) Symptoms

कपोतवर्णप्रतिमा यस्यान्ताः क्लेदवर्जिताः ||९||
स्थिराश्च पिडकावन्तो रोहतीति तमादिशेत् | (सु. सू. अ. २३) |

The edges of a ruhyamana vraṇa (ulcer) i.e., the ulcer in the stage of healing has the colour of a pigeon (slightly blackish white) and is devoid of moistness. The ulcer is fixed and is studded all around by granulations. (9)

Samyak Rudha (ulcer which has healed) Symptoms

रूढवर्त्मानमग्रन्थिमशूनमरुजं व्रणम् ||१०||
त्वक्सवर्णं समतलं सम्यग्रूढं विनिर्दिशेत्| (सु. सू. अ. २३) |
The ulcers in which the edges have closed up (ulcer is filled up with granulation tissue indicating that it is healed), which does not have knots (elevations), which is devoid of swelling or pain, which has attained the normal color of the skin, and that which is levelled is considered to be a samyak rudha vrana i.e., the ulcer which has healed up. (10)

Prognosis of Vranas

कुष्ठिनां विषजुष्टानां शोषिणां मधुमेहिनाम् ||११||
व्रणाः कृच्छ्रेण सिध्यन्ति येषां चापि व्रणे व्रणाः |
वसां मेदोऽथ मज्जानं मस्तुलुङ्गं च यः स्रवेत् ||१२||
आगन्तुजो व्रणः सिद्ध्येन्न सिद्ध्येद्दोषसम्भवः |
(सु. सू. अ. २३) |

Vranas (ulcer) heals with great difficulty in persons who are suffering from leprosy, poisons, tuberculosis and diabetes mellitus. The ulcers in which ulcers develop should also be considered as difficult to cure.

The ulcers which are caused by trauma and discharge muscle fat, fat, bone marrow or brain tissues (brain matter) etc. are curable. On the other hand, if this is caused due to the aggravation of doshas, it is incurable. (11-12)

Arista Lakshanas

मद्यागुर्वाज्यसुमनःपद्मचन्दनचम्पकैः ||१३||
सगन्धा दिव्यगन्धाश्च मुमूर्षूणां व्रणाः स्मृताः |
(सु. सू. अ. २८) |

Signs of ulcer indicating bad prognosis

Vranas (ulcers) which emit a smell similar to alcohol, aguru (Aquilaria agallocha), ghee, flower of jasmine or lotus, sandalwood, campaka flower and such other pleasant / divine smells are going to kill the patient. (13)

Other symptoms of incurability of ulcers

ये च मर्मस्वसम्भूता भवन्त्यत्यर्थवेदनाः ||१४||
दह्यन्ते चान्तरत्यर्थं बहिःशीताश्च ये व्रणाः |
दह्यन्ते बहिरत्यर्थं भवन्त्यन्तश्च शीतलाः ||१५||
प्राणमांसक्षयश्वासकासारोचकपीडिताः |
प्रवृद्धपूयरुधिरा व्रणा येषां च मर्मसु ||१६||

क्रियाभिः सम्यगारब्धा न सिध्यन्ति च ये व्रणाः ।
वर्जयेदपि तान् वैद्यः संरक्षन्नात्मनो यशः ॥१७॥ (सु. सू. अ. २८) ।

Below mentioned are the other symptoms of incurability of ulcers –

- Vranas (ulcers) having severe pain in spite of not manifesting on vital organs,
- Ulcers having severe burning sensation inside and are cold outside
- Ulcers having severe burning sensation outside but are cold inside
- Ulcers manifesting in those having loss of strength, loss of muscles (emaciation), dyspnoea, cough,
- and loss of taste (appetite)
- Ulcers discharging large quantities of pus or blood
- Ulcers occurring on the vital spots of the body
- Ulcers which are not responding to any kind of treatment (ulcers not getting healed in spite of
- administering best of well-planned treatments)
- All these kinds of ulcers shall be rejected (should not be treated) by a physician who does not want his reputation to be damaged. (14-17)

इति श्रीमाधवकरविरचिते माधवनिदाने शारीरव्रणनिदानं समाप्तम् ॥४२॥

Thus ends the chapter on Shareera Vrana Nidanam in Madhava Nidana text written by Acharya Madhavakara.

43

Madhava Nidana Chapter 43 Sadyo Vrana Nidanam

Sadyo Vrana Hetu

नानाधारमुखैः शस्त्रैर्नानास्थाननिपातितैः |
भवन्ति नानाकृतयो व्रणास्तांस्तान्निबोध मे ||१||

Causative factors

Different kinds of ulcers having different shapes, caused by assault with different types of sharp weapons having different kinds of edges, in different places of the body are described further on. (1)

Types of ulcers based on the shapes (appearance)

छिन्नं भिन्नं तथा विद्धं क्षतं पिच्चितमेव च |
घृष्टमाहुस्तथा षष्ठं तेषां वक्ष्यामि लक्षणम् ||२||
(सु. चि. अ. २) |

Below mentioned are the six kinds of ulcers –

1. Chinna - incised wound)
2. Bhinna - puncture wound
3. Viddha – stabbed wound
4. Ḳsata - lacerated wound
5. Piccita - crushed wound and
6. Ghrsta – excoriated

The features of these ulcers shall be henceforth explained. (2)

Chinna Vrana

तिर्यक् छिन्न ऋजुर्वाऽपि यो व्रणस्त्वायतो भवेत् |
गात्रस्य पातनं तद्धि छिन्नमित्यभिधीयते ||३||
(सु. चि. अ. २) |

In Chinnavraṇa the wound is either curved or straight and also wide. The organ or the part of the body which has been mutilated hangs from the wound or even may fall off. (3)

Bhinna Vrana

शक्तिदन्तेषु खड्गाग्रविषाणैराशयो हतः |
यत्किञ्चित् प्रस्रवेत्तद्धि भिन्नलक्षणमुच्यते ||४||
(सु. चि. अ. २) |

Bhinna vraṇa is a puncture wound. It is caused by pointed javelin, teeth / tusk, arrow / spear, the pointed end of the sword or horns of animals. When these enter and damage the interiors of different visceral organs, ulcers (punctured) are formed. This would lead to discharge of various materials depending on the organ which has been punctured. (4)

Definition of Koshta (hollow viscera which would hold many visceral organs) and symptoms of puncture of various visceral organs

स्थानान्यामाग्निपक्वानां मूत्रस्य रुधिरस्य च |
हृदुण्डुकः फुप्फुसश्च कोष्ठ इत्यभिधीयते ||५||
तस्मिन् भिन्ने रक्तपूर्णे ज्वरो दाहश्च जायते |
मूत्रमार्गगुदास्येभ्यो रक्तं घ्राणाच्च गच्छति ||६||
मूर्छा श्वासस्तृषाऽऽध्मानमभक्तच्छन्द एव च |
विण्मूत्रवातसङ्गश्च स्वेदास्रावोऽक्षिरक्तता ||७||
लोहगन्धित्वमास्यस्य गात्रदौर्गन्ध्यमेव च |
हृच्छूलं पार्श्वयोश्चापि विशेषं चात्र मे शृणु ||८||

The organs or seats of ama (undigested food i.e., stomach), agni (digestive juices / enzymes i.e., duodenum, liver, gallbladder and pancreas together), pakva ahara (digested food i.e., intestines / colon), mutra (urine i.e., urinary bladder), and rudhira (blood i.e., liver and spleen), along with hrdaya (heart), unduka (caecum), phuppusa / fupfusa (lungs) are known as kostha (abdominal viscera / visceral space which lodges the mentioned organs). A Puncture wound into the kostha will cause accumulation of blood in the injured organs which leads to manifestation of fever and burning sensation. Bleeding will occur through urethra, anus or nose.

The other general symptoms of puncture to the koshta are fainting (losing consciousness), dyspnoea (increased / difficult respiration), thirst, distension of the abdomen, loss of taste (aversion towards food), obstruction to the movement (expulsion) of urine, faeces and flatus, excessive sweating, redness of the eyes, smell of iron from the mouth, foul smell emitted from the body and pain in the heart and flanks. (5-8)

Symptoms of puncture of specific organs

आमाशयस्थे रुधिरे रुधिरं छर्दयत्यपि |
आध्मानमतिमात्रं च शूलं च भृशदारुणम् ||९||
पक्वाशयगते चापि रुजा गौरवमेव च |
अधःकाये विशेषेण शीतता च भवेदिह ||१०||
(सु. चि. अ. २) |

If amashaya (stomach) is punctured, blood accumulates in the stomach and there will be vomiting of blood, severe distension of abdomen and severe pain in the abdomen.

If pakvaashaya (small and large intestines, mainly colon) is punctured there will be severe pain, heaviness and coldness of the lower extremities. (9-10)

Viddha Vrana

सूक्ष्मास्यशल्याभिहतं यदङ्गं त्वाशयं विना |
उत्तुण्डितं निर्गतं वा तद्विद्धमिति निर्दिशेत् ||११||
(सु. चि. अ. २) |

Viddha vrana (stab / puncture wound) is that caused by a pointed instrument, on other body parts, away from any viscera (viscera not involved). Viddha vrana is of two types – uttundita which presents with swelling around the opening of the wound (due to the instrument lodged inside the wound) or nirgata which presents without swelling, the opening of the wound being depressed (because the instrument causing the wound is not lodged inside the swelling i.e. it has gone out or is extracted). (11)

Ksata Vrana

नातिच्छिन्नं नातिभिन्नमुभयोर्लक्षणान्वितम् |

विषमं व्रणमङ्गे यत्तत् क्षतं त्वभिधीयते ||१२||
(सु. चि. अ. २) |
Kṣata vrana (lacerated wound) is that which is neither deeply incised nor punctured but it does have symptoms of both of them and is irregular in shape. (12)

Picchita Vrana
प्रहारपीडनाभ्यां तु यदङ्गं पृथुतां गतम् |
सास्थि तत् पिच्चितं विद्यान्मज्जरक्तपरिप्लुतम् ||१३||
(सु. चि. अ. २) |
Picchita vrana (crushed wound) is caused by a blow (by a baton, hammer etc) or pressure (by a blunt weapon). Due to this, a part of the body is flattened, the bones also get crushed and blood mixed with bone marrow flows out. (13)

Ghrista Vrana
घर्षणादभिघाताद्वा यदङ्गं विगतत्वचम् |
उषास्रावान्वितं तच्च घृष्टमित्यभिधीयते ||१४||
(सु. चि. अ. २) |
Ghrista vrana (abrasion) is caused by friction with some object or any other kind of trauma / injury. In this condition the skin is peeled off from the body parts. Discharges consistingof hot watery fluids will flow out. (There will be burning sensation and flow of watery fluids). (14)

Ulcers with foreign body
श्यावं सशोथं पिडकाचितं च मुहुर्मुहुः शोणितवाहिनं च |
मृदूद्गतं बुद्बुदतुल्यमांसं व्रणं सशल्यं सरुजं वदन्ति ||१५||
A wound in which the foreign body is hidden inside is bluish black in colour, swollen, studded with eruptions, bleeds frequently, surrounding muscular appearing like soft bubbles (frothy) and is very painful. (15)

Foreign body inside the abdomen
त्वचोऽतीत्य सिरादीनि भित्त्वा वा परिहृत्य वा |
कोष्ठे प्रतिष्ठितं शल्यं कुर्यादुक्तानुपद्रवान् ||१६|| (सु. चि. अ. २) |
तत्रान्तर्लोहितं पाण्डुशीतपादकराननम् |
शीतोच्छ्वासं रक्तनेत्रमानद्धं च विवर्जयेत् ||१७||

A foreign body getting lodged inside the abdomen, after piercing all the layers of the skin and injuring or destroying the veins (blood vessels), muscles, ligaments (and tendons), bones and joints, if not removed at proper time, would cause severe complications like gurgling sounds in the abdomen, flatulence etc explained in pranastashalya vijnaniya chapter. When the blood is filled in the abdomen it would cause pallor and coldness of the feet, hands and face. Such a patient and those having cold breath and redness of the eyes shall be refused treatment. (16-17)

General symptoms of Ksata in muscles, blood vessels (veins), ligaments, bones and joints

भ्रमः प्रलापः पतनं प्रमोहो विचेष्टनं ग्लानिरथोष्णता च |
स्रस्ताङ्गता मूर्छनमूर्ध्ववातस्तीव्रा रुजा वातकृताश्च तास्ताः ||१८||
मांसोदकाभं रुधिरं च गच्छेत् सर्वेन्द्रियार्थोपरमस्तथैव |
दशार्धसङ्ख्येष्वथ विक्षतेषु सामान्यतो मर्मसु लिङ्गमुक्तम् ||१९|| (सु. सू. अ. २५) |

General symptoms of wounds to the five structures (muscles, veins, tendons bony joints and vital organs) are - giddiness, delirium, falling on the ground, unconsciousness (fainting), undesirable movements of the hands and feet, exhaustion, feeling of warmth, laxity or looseness (drooping) of the body parts, perversion of sense organs (abnormal functions), upward movements of vata (inside the abdomen) and severe and many types of pains characteristic of vāta, discharge of blood resembling mutton washed water, and loss of functions of the sense organs. (18-19)

Viddha Lakshanas of Veins etc

सुरेन्द्रगोपप्रतिमं प्रभूतं रक्तं स्रवेत्तत्क्षयजश्च वायुः |
करोति रोगान् विविधान् यथोक्तान् सिरासु विद्धास्वथ वा क्षतासु ||२०||
कौब्ज्यं शरीरावयवावसादः क्रियास्वशक्तिस्तुमुला रुजश्च |
चिराद्व्रणो रोहति यस्य चापि तं स्नायुविद्धं पुरुषं व्यवस्येत् ||२१||

Special symptoms manifesting due to injury of particular structures are as follows -

Sira Viddha Lakshana

If śirās (blood vessels) are injured or punctured, there will be heavy discharge of blood resembling indragopa insects (bright red in colour). The vāta undergoing increase due to the injury (destruction of tissues caused due to injury and subsequent vata increase) would cause a wide array of disorders in later time.

Snayu viddha lakshana

The symptoms of injury / puncture to the tendons (nerves) are - decrease in height (hunchback), looseness or weakness (drooping) of the body parts, loss of functions, very severe pain and wound taking long time to heal.

Sandhi viddha lakshana

शोफाभिवृद्धिस्तुमुला रुजश्च बलक्षयः सर्वत एव शोथः |
क्षतेषु सन्धिष्वचलाचलेषु स्यात् सर्वकर्मोपरमश्च लिङ्गम् ||२२||

Increase of the swelling, severe pain, loss of strength, oedema in other parts of the body and total loss of functions – are the symptoms of injury to mobile or immobile bony joints of the body. (22)

Asthi Viddha Lakshanas

घोरा रुजो यस्य निशादिनेषु सर्वास्ववस्थासु च नैति शान्तिम् |
भिषग्विपश्चिद्विदितार्थसूत्रस्तमस्थिविद्धं पुरुषं व्यवस्येत् ||२३|| (सु. सू. अ. २५) |

The symptoms which would enable an intelligent physician who is well conversant with science (of wounds) to recognize and diagnose that the person is having injury to the bones include very severe pain which is continuously present throughout the day and night (entire day) and not being able to find relief in any posture. (23)

Injury to the Marmas

यथास्वमेतानि विभावयेच्च लिङ्गानि मर्मस्वभिताडितेषु |२४| (सु. सू. अ. २५) |
पाण्डुर्विवर्णः स्पृशितं न वेत्ति यो मांसमर्मण्यभिपीडितः स्यात् ||२४|| (सु. सू. अ. २५) |

Similar symptoms will be found in persons whose vital organs are injured. In case or injury to the vital spots, the same symptoms (mentioned above) should be understood in accordance with the seat of injury (wherein the marma is located).

When the mamsa marmas (vital spots predominantly made up of muscle tissue) are injured, there will be anaemia (pallor) or discoloration. The patient would not appreciate touch sensation (loss of tactile sensation). (24)

Upadrava

विसर्पः पक्षघातश्च सिरास्तम्भोऽपतानकः |
मोहोन्मादव्रणरुजो ज्वरस्तृष्णा हनुग्रहः ||२५||
कासश्छर्दिरतीसारो हिक्का श्वासः सवेपथुः |

षोडशोपद्रवाः प्रोक्ता व्रणानां व्रणचिन्तकैः ||२६|| (च. चि. अ. २५) |

Complications

According to the specialists in the knowledge of wounds the sixteen complications or sequelae of wounds are - erysipelas, hemiplegia, stiffness of the veins, tetanus, delusion, insanity, severe pain in the wound, fever, thirst, lockjaw, cough, vomiting, diarrhoea, hiccough, dyspnoea (difficulty in breathing) and tremors. (25-26)

इति श्रीमाधवकरविरचिते माधवनिदाने सद्योव्रणनिदानं समाप्तम् ||४३||

Thus ends the chapter on Sadhyo Vrana Nidanam in Madhava Nidana text written by Acharya Madhavakara.

44

Madhava Nidana Chapter 44 Bhagna Nidanam

Bhagna Bheda

भग्नं समासाद्द्विविधं हुताश काण्डे च सन्धौ च हि तत्र सन्धौ |
उत्पिष्टविश्लिष्टविवर्तितं च तिर्यग्गतं क्षिप्तमधश्च षट् च ||१||

Types of fractures

Bhagna (fracture) is, in brief, of two kinds;
Kanda Bhagna – that which occurs at the shaft or body of the bones and Sandhi Bhagna – that which occurs at the sandhi – bony joints (meeting place of two bones)
Types of Sandhi Bhagna (fracture at the meeting place of two bones or sutures) – Sandhi Bhagnas are of six types, they are –

1. Utpista
2. Vislista
3. Vivartita
4. Tiryak Ksipta
5. Ksipta and
6. Adhah Ksipta (1)

Sandhi Bhagna Samanya Lakshana

प्रसारणाकुञ्चनवर्तनोग्रा रुक् स्पर्शविद्वेषणमेतदुक्तम् |
सामान्यतः सन्धिगतस्य लिङ्गम्... |२|
General Symptoms of Sandhi Bhagna
The general symptoms of sandhi bhagna are – severe pain during extension, contraction and rotation, and tenderness.

Symptoms of types of Sandhi Bhagna / Sandhi Vislesa
...उत्पिष्टसन्धेः श्वयथुः समन्तात् ||२||
विशेषतो रात्रिभवा रुजा च, विश्लिष्टजे तौ च रुजा च नित्यम् |\
विवर्तिते पार्श्वरुजश्च तीव्रास्तिर्यग्गते तीव्ररुजो भवन्ति ||३||
क्षिप्तेऽतिशूलं विषमत्वमस्थ्नोः क्षिप्ते त्वधो रुग्विघटश्च सन्धेः |
Utpista – In this condition there will be swelling all around the joint and severe pain at nights.
Vislista – This condition will also have the above mentioned two symptoms (swelling around the joint and severe pain at night) but the pain will be constantly present all through the day (day and night), but the swelling will be less
Vivartita – In this type severe pain will be present on both sides of the fracture site (joint)
Tiryak Ksipta – In this type there will be severe pain.
Ksipta – In this type there will be overlapping (overriding) of the bones involved in the fracture leading to curvature of the bones and pain.
Adhah Ksipta – In this type there will be severe pain and abnormal activities (functions) in the joints. According to yet another opinion, the bones at the seat of fracture of joints will slip / slide downwards. (2-3)

Kanda Bhagna
काण्डे त्वतः कर्कटकाश्वकर्णविचूर्णितं पिच्चितमस्थिछल्लिका ||४||
काण्डेषु भग्नं ह्यतिपातितं च मज्जागतं च स्फुटितं च वक्रम् |
छिन्नं द्विधा द्वादशधाऽपि काण्डे स्रस्ताङ्गता शोथरुजातिवृद्धिः ||५||
सम्पीड्यमाने भवतीह शब्दः स्पर्शासहं स्पन्दनतोदशूलाः |
सर्वास्ववस्थासु न शर्मलाभो भग्नस्य काण्डे खलु चिह्नमेतत् ||६||
भग्नं तु काण्डे बहुधा प्रयाति समासतो नामभिरेव तुल्यम् ||७||
Fracture of the bone shaft
Kaanda Bhagna (fracture of shafts or body of bones) is of twelve kinds namely - Karkataka, Ashvakarna, Vichoornita, Piccita, Asthichallikaa, Kaandabhagna, Atipaatita, Majjaagata, Sphutita, Vakra, and two types of

Chinna.

In all these kinds, the general features are – looseness / laxity of the body parts (drooping of the part), swelling and severe pain, crackling sounds at the site of fracture, tenderness, pulsations, pricking pain, pain, and not feeling comfort in any position.

Apart from these twelve types of fractures there might also occur many other types of kanda bhagna i.e., fracture of shafts. They are either included in these types or shall be understood by similarity with its meaning. (4-7)

Symptoms of incurability of Bhagna

अल्पाशिनोऽनात्मवतो जन्तोर्वातात्मकस्य च |
उपद्रवैर्वा जुष्टस्य भग्नं कृच्छ्रेण सिध्यति ||८||
(सु. चि. अ. ३) |

Fractures heal with difficulty in persons who take very little (non-nutritious) quantity of food, in those who do not have self control or those who are habitually indulged in unsuitable foods and activities, in those of vata constitution and in the fractures associated with complications. (8)

Other symptoms of incurability of fractures

भिन्नं कपालं कट्यां तु सन्धिमुक्तं तथा च्युतम् |
जघनं प्रतिपिष्टं च वर्जयेद्धि विचक्षणः ||९||
असंश्लिष्टकपालं च ललाटे चूर्णितं च यत् |
भग्नं स्तनान्तरे पृष्ठे शङ्खे मूर्ध्नि च वर्जयेत् ||१०|| (सु. नि. अ. १५) |

Fracture of the skull / hip bone, fracture of the hip bone, dislocation, Cyuta or Adhahksipta type of fractures, Utpista fracture of hip / pelvic bones (at the sutures of the hip bones), fracture / dislocation of cranial sutures, crushing / cracking of forehead, fracture occurring between the breasts (centre of the chest), fracture of the back, temples and head (skull, vault of the head) are to be rejected considering them as incurable. (9-10)

सम्यक् सन्धितमप्यस्थि दुर्निक्षेपनिबन्धनात् |
सङ्क्षोभाद्वाऽपि यद्गच्छेद्विक्रियां तच्च वर्जयेत् ||११||
(सु. नि. अ. १५) |

Fractures which have once healed but happening again and again due to bad positioning, bandaging or violent activity and creating loss of functions should also be refused treatment since it is incurable. (11)

Fractures presenting in different forms (presentation) in different bones

तरुणास्थीनि नम्यन्ते भिद्यन्ते नलकानि च |

कपालानि विभज्यन्ते स्फुटन्ति रुचकानि च ||१२|| (सु. नि. अ. १५) |

Young bones (cartilages) bend and the long bones break in the middle. Flat bones crack in their body while the teeth (which are also considered as bones in Ayurveda) splinter off. (12)

इति श्रीमाधवकरविरचिते माधवनिदाने भग्ननिदानं समाप्तम् ||४४||

Thus ends the chapter on Bhagna Nidanam in Madhava Nidana text written by Acharya Madhavakara.

45

Madhava Nidana Chapter 45 Nadivrana Nidanam

Nadivrana Nidana, Samprapti

यः शोथमाममतिपक्वमुपेक्षतेऽज्ञो यो वा व्रणं प्रचुरपूयमसाधुवृत्तः |
अभ्यन्तरं प्रविशति प्रविदार्य तस्य स्थानानि पूर्वविहितानि ततः सपूयः ||१||
(सु. नि. अ. १०) |

Etiological Factors and Pathogenesis of Nadivrana

When the ignorant physician who cuts open an unripe swelling or delays draining of a fully ripened swelling (in which the pus has formed completely) or an unscrupulous physician who does not drain out the pus from an ulcer completely, the pus which has been formed makes way into the deeper tissues by making a sinus and piercing into the vrana sthanas (seats of ulcer like skin, muscles etc mentioned by Master Sushruta). (This leads to the formation of nadi vrana) (1).

Nadivrana Nirukti, Bheda

तस्यातिमात्रगमनाद्गतिरिष्यते तु नाडीव यद्वहति तेन मता तु नाडी |२|
(सु. नि. अ. १०) |
दोषैस्त्रिभिर्भवति सा पृथगेकशश्च सम्मूर्छितैरपि च शल्यनिमित्ततोऽन्या ||२|| (सु. नि. अ. १०) |

Definition of the word Nadivrana

Gati – Since there is excessive movement of pus inside the sinus it is called as gati. (gati = movement).

Nadivrana - Since it is in the form of a tube or hollow pipe (because of the formation of hollow passage or sinus) and carries pus in it, this condition is called as nadi vrana.

Types of nadivrana

Nadivrana is of five types, one from each of the three doshas (caused by single dosha predominance – vataja, pittaja and kaphaja), one from the combined vitiation of all the three doshas (tridoshaja, sannipataja) and the other one due to the presence of a foreign body (shalyaja). (2)

1. Vataja Nadivrana
2. Pittaja Nadivrana
3. Kaphaja Nadivrana
4. Sannipataja Nadivrana
5. Shalyaja Nadivrana - caused by foreign bodies such as a sharp instrument

Symptoms of types of nadivrana

Vataja Nadivrana – In this type, the nadi is rough, will have small orifice (opening), is painful, and will have exudation of frothy material especially during cold times and at night.

Pittaja Nadivrana – In this type, the person will have thirst, fever and burning sensation. The sinus will discharge yellowish material (exudates) especially during hot time i.e., daytime (midday).

Kaphaja Nadivrana – In this type, the discharge is copious, excessively thick, white and sticky. The ulcer is hard, has more itching and the pain increases during night time.

Tridoshaja Nadivrana – In this type, there is burning sensation, fever, difficulty in breathing, fainting (loss of consciousness), dryness of the mouth and all symptoms of doshaja nadivranas (vataja, pittaja and kaphaja) explained above mixed together. This condition is said to be fatal and should be considered similar to Kalaratri i.e., sister of God of death in terms of taking away life. (2-5)

तत्रानिलात् परुषसूक्ष्ममुखी सशूला फेनानुविद्धमधिकं स्रवति क्षपासु |३|
(सु. नि. अ. १०) |
पित्तात्तृषाज्वरकरी परिदाहयुक्ता पीतं स्रवत्यधिकमुष्णमहःसु चापि ||३||
(सु. नि. अ. १०) |

ज्ञेया कफाद्बहुघनार्जुनपिच्छिलास्रा स्तब्धा सकण्डुररुजा रजनीप्रवृद्धा |४|
(सु. नि. अ. १०) |
दाहज्वरश्वसनमूर्छनवक्त्रशोषा यस्यां भवन्त्यभिहितानि च लक्षणानि ||४||
तामादिशेत् पवनपित्तकफप्रकोपाद्घोरामसुक्षयकरीमिव कालारात्रिम् |
(सु. नि. अ. १०) |
नष्टं कथञ्चिदनुमार्गमुदीरितेषु स्थानेषु शल्यमचिरेण गतिं करोति ||५||Shalyaja Nadivrana
सा फेनिलं मथितमुष्णमसृग्विमिश्रं स्रावं करोति सहसा सरुजा च नित्यम् |
(सु. नि. अ. १०) |

A foreign body somehow reaching and getting embedded and hidden in the skin, muscle and other seats of vrana (ulcer) will make way into the deeper tissues creating a passage (sinus) and quickly cause nadivrana. From this sinus there is exudation of frothy, as if churned, hot and blood mixed material spontaneously accompanied with pain. This is called as shalyaja nadivrana. (5)

Symptoms of incurability of Nadivrana

नाडी त्रिदोषप्रभवा न सिध्येच्छेषाश्चतस्रः खलु यत्नसाध्याः ||६||
(सु. चि. अ. १७) |

Nadi Vrana (sinus ulcer) of the tridoṣhaja kind does not respond to treatment (it is incurable). The other four types of nadivrana can be treated with difficulty. (6)

इति श्रीमाधवकरविरचिते माधवनिदाने नाडीव्रणनिदानं समाप्तम् ||४५||

Thus ends the chapter on Nadivrana Nidanam in Madhava Nidana text written by Acharya Madhavakara.

46

Madhava Nidana Chapter 46 Bhagandara Nidanam

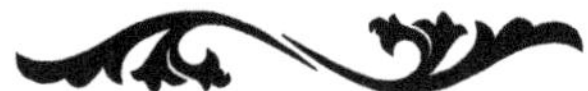

Bhagandara rupa, Sankhya

गुदस्य द्व्यङ्गुले क्षेत्रे पार्श्वतः पिडकाऽऽर्तिकृत् |
भिन्ना भगन्दरो ज्ञेयः स च पञ्चविधो मतः ||१||

Meaning and types of bhagandara

A papule (boil, blister) developing on either side of the anus, within a radius of two angulas accompanied with pain and exudation is known as Bhagandara (fistula-in-ano). It is of five kinds. (1)

Vatika Bhagandara

कषायरूक्षैस्त्वतिकोपितोऽनिलस्त्वपानदेशे पिडकां करोति याम् |
उपेक्षणात्पाकमुपैति दारुणं रुजा च भिन्नाऽरुणफेनवाहिनी ||२||
तत्रागमो मूत्रपुरीषरेतसां व्रणैरनेकैः शतपोनकं वदेत् |३|

Vatika Bhagandara (Shataponaka Bhagandara)

Due to excessive indulgence in foods predominant in astringent taste and dry in nature leads to aggravation of vata.

This aggravated vata causes a papule in the anal region. When it is neglected, it undergoes suppuration and produces severe pain. Many ulcers are formed around the papule. Through these orifices of multiple ulcers, urine, faeces and semen are discharged. Due to multiple ulcers / openings (orifices) vataja bhagandara is also called as sataponaka. (2-3)

Pittaja Bhagandara

प्रकोपणैः पित्तमतिप्रकोपितं करोति रक्तां पिडकां गुदाश्रिताम् ||३||

तदाऽऽशुपाकाऽहिमपूतिवाहिनीं भगन्दरं तूष्ट्रशिरोधरं वदेत् ||४||

Pittaja Bhagandara /Ushtragriva

Pitta undergoing severe increase in a person who has indulged in pitta aggravating etiological factors produces a red coloured pustule in the anal region. This pustule quickly undergoes suppuration. The discharges coming from it are hot and foul smelling. This type of bhagandara is called Ustraśirodhara (ustragrīvā). (4)

Note – Since its shape resembles the neck of the camel, it is called as Ustragriva.

Kaphaja Bagandara

कण्डूयनो घनस्रावी कठिनो मन्दवेदनः |

श्वेतावभासः कफजः परिस्रावी भगन्दरः ||५||

Kaphaja Bhagandara /Parisravi

The bhagandara which is produced by aggravated kapha has itching, thick discharges (exudates), is hard, slightly painful and whitish in colour. This is also called as Parisravi Bhagandara. (5)

Note – Since there are continuous thick discharges taking place from this type of bhagandara it is called parisravi bhagandara.

Sannipataja Bagandara

बहुवर्णरुजास्रावा पिडका गोस्तनोपमा |

शम्बूकावर्तवन्नाडी शम्बूकावर्तको मतः ||६||

Sannipataja Bhagandara / Sambukavarta

These pustules have different kinds of colours and discharges which resemble the teeth of the cow, creating spiral sinuses inside resembling that of seashell or whirls in a river. This is known as Śambūkavārtā (this is produced by increase of all the three doshas together and is associated with many types of pain). (6)

Agantuja Bhagandara

क्षताद्गतिः पायुगता विवर्धते ह्युपेक्षणात् स्युः क्रिमयो विदार्य ते |

प्रकुर्वते मार्गमनेकधा मुखैर्व्रणैस्तदुन्मार्गिभगन्दरं वदेत् ||७||

Agantuja Bhagandara /Unmargini

Injury caused by any foreign object like thorns, etc. at the anus, causes formation of sinus which goes on increasing in size (depth). When this condition is neglected worms (germs) are formed in these sinuses (sinuses get infected with worms / germs). These worms later form many small ulcers with many openings inside the sinuses. This condition is called as unmargi bhagandara. (7)

Symptoms of incurability of Bhagandara

घोराः साधयितुं दुःखाः सर्व एव भगन्दराः |
तेष्वसाध्यस्त्रिदोषोत्थः क्षतजश्च विशेषतः ||८||
(सु. नि. अ. ४) |

All kinds of bhagandara - fistula are dreadful and difficult to cure. Those caused by all the three doshas and injury (by external agents / foreign objects) are mainly incurable. (8)

Other symptoms of incurability of Bhagandara

वातमूत्रपुरीषाणि क्रिमयः शुक्रमेव च |
भगन्दरात् स्रवन्तस्तु नाशयन्ति तमातुरम् ||९|||
(सु. सू. अ. ३३) |

When gas (fart), urine, faeces, worms and semen begin to come out of the fistula, it is going to kill the patient (such fistula is incurable). (9)

इति श्रीमाधवकरविरचिते माधवनिदाने भगन्दरनिदानं समाप्तम् ||४६||

Thus ends the chapter on Bhagandara Nidanam in Madhava Nidana text written by Acharya Madhavakara.

47

Madhava Nidana Chapter 47 Upadamsha Nidanam

Upadamsha Nidana

हस्ताभिघातान्नखदन्तपातादधावनाद्रत्यतिसेवनाद्वा |
योनिप्रदोषाच्च भवन्ति शिश्ने पञ्चोपदंशा विविधापचारैः ||१||

Etiological Factors of Upadamsha

Below mentioned are the etiological factors of upadamsha –
injury to the penis by the hand (masturbation), nails and teeth;
keeping it dirty without washing,
indulging in excessive sexual intercourse,
contact (sexual intercourse) with contaminated or diseased vagina and indulgence in such other bad habits
The above-mentioned etiological factors lead to the causation of the disease upadamsha (venereal disease). Upadamsha is of five types. (1)

Upadamsha Lakshanas

सतोदभेदैः स्फुरणैः सकृष्णैः स्फोटैर्व्यवस्येत् पवनोपदंशम् |
पीतैर्बहुक्लेदयुतैः सदाहैः पित्तेनरक्तात् पिशितावभासैः ||२||
स्फोटैः सकृष्णै रुधिरं स्रवन्तं रक्तात्मकं पित्तसमानलिङ्गम् |
सकण्डुरैः शोथयुतैर्महद्भिः शुक्लैर्घनैः स्रावयुतैः कफेन ||३||
नानाविधस्रावरुजोपपन्नमसाध्यमाहुस्त्रिमलोपदंशम्
विशीर्णमांसं क्रिमिभिः प्रजग्धं मुष्कावशेषं परिवर्जयेच्च ||४||

Symptoms of upadamsha and its types

Vataja Upadamsha – In this type of upadamsha, there will be pricking, cutting and pulsating type of pain. Small papules (eruptions) which are black in colour appear on the penis.

Pittaja Upadamsha – In this type, the papules discharge yellowish fluid, the fluid is large in quantity and the person will also experience a burning sensation.

Raktaja Upadamsha – In this type, the papules resemble muscle, black in colour, bleeds and will have all other symptoms of pittaja upadamsha.

Kaphaja Upadamsha – In this type, the papules are big in size, swollen, have itching and discharges thick white fluid.

Tridoshaja Upadamsha – The upadamsha caused by all the three doshas together will present with different kinds of discharges (exudates) and pains. This condition is incurable.

Symptoms of incurability of Upadamsha

A condition of upadamsha in which the entire fleshy part of the penis has been eroded or eaten away by germs leaving only the scrotum is to be refused treatment (this condition is incurable). (2-4)

Consequence of not treating Upadamsha at right time

सञ्जातमात्रे न करोति मूढः क्रियां नरो यो विषये प्रसक्तः ।
कालेन शोथक्रिमिदाहपाकैर्विशीर्णशिश्नो म्रियते स तेन ॥५॥

Foolish people who are engrossed in excessive sex and do not seek treatment soon after the onset of upadamsha and neglect it, the penis of such a person becomes swollen and gets infected by bacteria. There is also burning sensation, pus formation and destruction (falling off) of penis which eventually leads to the death of the person. (5)

Lingarsha, Lingavarti

अङ्कुरैरिव सङ्घातैरुपर्युपरिसंस्थितैः ।
क्रमेण जायते वर्तिस्ताम्रचूडशिखोपमा ॥६॥
कोषस्याभ्यन्तरे सन्धौ सर्वसन्धिगताऽपि वा ।
(सवेदना पिच्छिला च दुश्चिकित्स्या त्रिदोषजा) ।
लिङ्गवर्तिरभिख्याता लिङ्गार्शं इति चापरे ॥७॥

Sprouts of muscular tissue lying one over the other (superimposed), resembling the crown of a cock, developing inside the prepuce of the penis or at its junction with the penis or nearby, accompanied by pain, discharges which are sticky (sticky exudates) and caused by the combined vitiation of all the tridoshas is called as lingavarti or lingarsha. This condition is difficult to treat. (6-7)

इति श्रीमाधवकरविरचिते माधवनिदाने उपदंशनिदानं समाप्तम् ||४७||

Thus ends the chapter on Upadamsha Nidanam in Madhava Nidana text written by Acharya Madhavakara.

48

Madhava Nidana Chapter 48 Shuka Dosha Nidanam

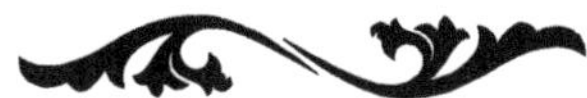

Nidana – Etiological factors

अक्रमाच्छेफसो वृद्धिं योऽभिवाञ्छति मूढधीः ।
व्याधयस्तस्य जायन्ते दश चाष्टौ च शूकजाः ॥१॥

Foolish people who try to increase the size of their penis by unnatural methods (by application of paste of poisonous insects and other materials to the penis) become afflicted with eighteen kinds of diseases (of penis), caused by shukas (poisonous worms and other substances). These diseases are called as suka dosa or suka janya vyadhi. (1)

Sarshapika

गौरसर्षपसंस्थाना शूकदुर्भुग्नहेतुका ।
पिडका श्लेष्मवाताभ्यां ज्ञेया सर्षपिका तु सा ॥२॥
(सु. नि. अ. १४) ।

Sarshapa means mustard. In Sarshapika, vesicles the size of white mustard appear on the penis. This happens due to indiscriminate application of pastes (as mentioned above in the etiological factors). Such pastes cause aggravation of kapha and vata and cause Sarshapika. (2)

Asthilika

कठिना विषमैर्भुग्नैर्वायुनाऽष्ठीलिका भवेत् ।३।

(सु. नि. अ. १४) |

Application of bad and unsuitable suka on the penis indiscriminately leads to abnormal increase of vata. This produces asthilika which is hard and irregular in shape.

Grathita

शूकैर्यत् पूरितं शश्वद्ग्रथितं नाम तत् कफात् ||३||

The eruptions / vesicles which are caused by aggravated vata and appear like nodules (cysts) filled with sukas are called as Gratita Suka Dosha. (3)

Kumbhika

कुम्भिका रक्तपित्तोत्था जाम्बवास्थिनिभाऽशुभा |४|

(सु. नि. अ. १४) |

Kumbhika is produced by abnormally increased rakta (blood) and pitta. It resembles the seeds of jambū fruit (Eugenia jambolina) and is black in colour.

Alaji

तुल्यजां त्वलजीं विद्याद्यथाप्रोक्तां विचक्षणः ||४||

(सु. नि. अ. १४) |

According to Ayurveda experts Alaji Suka Dosa is a condition which resembles a disease of the same name which has been described earlier in the context of prameha pidaka – diabetic carbuncles. (One of the types of prameha pidaka is also named as Alaji. The alaji explained here will have the similar causative factors and symptoms like that of the alaji prameha pidaka). (4)

Mrudita, Sammoodha Pidaka

मृदितं पीडितं यच्च संरब्धं वातकोपतः |५| (सु. नि. अ. १४) |

पाणिभ्यां भृशसम्मूढे सम्मूढपिडका भवेत् ||५|| (सु. नि. अ. १४) |

Mrdita is a swelling of the penis. It is caused by the aggravation of vata caused by rubbing of the penis after application of shuka.

Sammoodha piḍakā is appearance of papules by rubbing the penis briskly after the application of shuka. (This should also be considered as caused by aggravated vata). (5)

Adhimanta

दीर्घा बह्व्यश्च पिडका दीर्यन्ते मध्यतस्तु याः |
सोऽधिमन्थः कफासृग्भ्यां वेदनारोमहर्षकृत् ||६||
(सु. नि. अ. १४) |
In Adhimanta, multiple vesicles which are long are manifested. These vesicles burst open at their center and are accompanied with pain and horripilation. This condition is caused by increased kapha and rakta (blood). (6)

Puskarika
पिडका पिडकाव्याप्ता पित्तशोणितसम्भवा |
पद्मकर्णिकसंस्थाना ज्ञेया पुष्करिका तु सा ||७||
(सु. नि. अ. १४) |
Vesicles caused by increased pitta and rakta, many in number and resembling the sprouts of a lotus flower is known as Pushkarika.(7)

Sparshahani
स्पर्शहानिं तु जनयेच्छोणितं शूकदूषितम् |८|
(सु. नि. अ. १४) |
Sparsahani is a condition caused by rakta infected by suka poison. This infected blood causes loss of (tactile) sensation or sense of touch in the penis.

Uttama
मुद्गमाषोपमा रक्ता रक्तपित्तोद्भवा तु या ||८||
व्याधिरेषोत्तमा नाम शूकाजीर्णनिमित्तजा |
(सु. नि. अ. १४) |
Uttama is the name of the disease in which papules of the size of green gram or black gram appear on the penis. They are red in colour and are caused by vitiated rakta (blood) and pitta. This is caused by repeated application of suka – poisonous paste over the penis. (8)

Shataponaka
छिद्रैरणुमुखैर्लिङ्गं चितं यस्य समन्ततः ||९||
वातशोणितजो व्याधिः स ज्ञेयः शतपोनकः |
(सु. नि. १४) ||११||
The disease in which the penis is studded (enveloped) by many small

openings (holes) all around and is caused by vitiated vata and rakta (blood) is called as Sataponaka. (9)

Tvakpaka

वातपित्तकृतो ज्ञेयस्त्वक्पाको ज्वरदाहकृत् ||१०|| (सु. नि. अ. १४) |

Vata and pitta which are abnormally increased cause ulceration (suppuration) of the skin of the penis, accompanied by fever and burning sensation. This condition is called as Tvakpaka. (10)

Sonitarbuda

कृष्णैः स्फोटैः सरक्ताभिः पिडकाभिर्निपीडितम् |
यस्य वास्तुरुजश्चोग्रा ज्ञेयं तच्छोणितार्बुदम् ||११||
(सु. नि. अ. १४) |

The condition in which black coloured vesicles / blisters or reddish coloured eruptions (papules) appear all over the penis, associated with severe pain is called as Shonitarbuda. (11)

Mamsarbuda, Mamsapaka and Vidradhi

मांसदोषेण जानीयादर्बुदं मांससम्भवम् |१२| (सु. नि. अ. १४) |
शीर्यन्ते यस्य मांसानि यस्य सर्वाश्च वेदनाः ||१२||
विद्यात्तं मांसपाकं तु सर्वदोषकृतं भिषक् | (सु. नि. अ. १४) |
विद्रधिं सन्निपातेन यथोक्तमिति निर्दिशेत् ||१३|| (सु. नि. अ. १४) |

Mamsarbuda should be recognised by involvement of muscle tissue. The muscles are contaminated due to the application of suka poisons leading to the manifestation of this condition.
Mamaspaka is a condition in which the fleshy part of the penis falls off. A wise physician should consider this condition as caused by the vitiation of all the three doshas. As a result, mamsapaka is accompanied by severe kinds of pains caused by all three doshas.
Vidradhi is another condition caused by vitiation of all the three doshas. The signs and symptoms resemble those of sannipataja vidradhi described earlier and presents with different kinds of colours, pains and discharges. (12-13)

Tilakalaka

कृष्णानि चित्राण्यथवा शूकानि सविषाणि वा |
पातितानि पचन्त्याशु मेढ्रं निरवशेषतः ||१४||

कालानि भूत्वा मांसानि शीर्यन्ते यस्य देहिनः |
सन्निपातसमुत्थांस्तु तान् विद्यात्तिलकालकान् ||१५|| (सु. नि. अ. १४) |
When the paste of the highly poisonous insects which are of black colour or of many colours is applied over the penis, it causes quick suppuration of the penis and the entire penis would get detached and fall off without any residue. The muscular part of the penis becomes black in colour and these parts would fall off. This condition is known as Tilakalaka and is caused due to the abnormal increase of all the three doshas together. (It is called as tilakalaka also due to the appearance of warts resembling the black moles of the skin). (14-15)

Asadhyata
तत्र मांसार्बुदं यच्च मांसपाकश्च यः स्मृतः |
विद्रधिश्च न सिद्ध्यन्ति ये च स्युस्तिलकालकाः ||१६|| (सु. नि. अ. १४) |
Symptoms of incurability of suka dosha
Among the above suka dosha diseases, mamsarbuda, mamsapaka, vidradhi and tilákalaka do not respond to treatment i.e. they are incurable. (16)

इति श्रीमाधवकरविरचिते माधवनिदाने शूकदोषनिदानं समाप्तम् ||४८||
Thus ends the chapter on Shuka Dosha Nidanam in Madhava Nidana text written by Acharya Madhavakara.

49

Madhava Nidana Chapter 49 Kushta Nidanam

Nidana, Samprapti

विरोधीन्यन्नपानानि द्रवस्निग्धगुरूणि च |
भजतामागतां छर्दिं वेगांश्चान्यान् प्रतिघ्नताम् ||१||
व्यायाममतिसन्तापमतिभुक्त्वा निषेविणाम् |
घर्मश्रमभयार्तानां द्रुतं शीताम्बुसेविनाम् ||२||
अजीर्णाध्यशिनां चैव पञ्चकर्मापचारिणाम् |
नवान्नदधिमत्स्यातिलवणाम्लनिषेविणाम् ||३||
माषमूलकपिष्टान्नतिलक्षीरगुडाशिनाम् |
व्यवायं चाप्यजीर्णेऽन्ने निद्रां च भजतां दिवा ||४||
विप्रान् गुरून् धर्षयतां पापं कर्म च कुर्वताम् |
वातादयस्त्रयो दुष्टास्त्वग्रक्तं मांसमम्बु च ||५||
दूषयन्ति स कुष्ठानां सप्तको द्रव्यसङ्ग्रहः |
अतः कुष्ठानि जायन्ते सप्त चैकादशैव च ||६||
(च. चि. अ. ७) |

Etiological Factors and Pathogenesis of Kustha

Etiological Factors of Kustha –

- indulgence in incompatible (mutually opposite or antagonistic) foods and drinks,

- excessive intake of foods which are very watery, fatty (unctuous) and heavy (hard to digest),
- suppressing the urges of vomiting and other natural bodily urges,
- doing heavy and excessive physical exercises immediately after taking food and
- too much of exposure to heat (immediately after taking food),
- consuming cold water (immersing in cold water) immediately after exposure to the sunlight (heat of the sun), after doing hard (strenuous) works and after incidents which have caused fear
- use of uncooked foods and over-eating,
- improper methods of administering panchakarma (five purifactory) therapies (emesis, purgation, enema, errhines and bloodletting)
- excessive consumption of fresh grains, curds, fishes, and foods are very salty and sour,
- excessive consumption of black-gram, radish, flours, sesame, milk and jaggery
- indulgence in sexual intercourse while having indigestion
- excessive sleeping during day time (though suffering from indigestion),
- showing disrespect and abusing gods and teachers
- committing many kinds of sinful acts etc.

The above-mentioned etiological factors cause abnormal increase of all the three doshas and derangement (contamination) of skin, blood, muscular tissue and body fluids and produce kustha (leprosy, skin diseases). These seven substances (three doshas and four tissues – skin, blood, muscles and fluid components) together cause seven (major, greater) and eleven (minor, lesser) skin diseases. (1-6)

Seven types of Kustha

कुष्ठानि सप्तधा दोषैः पृथग्द्वन्द्वैः समागतैः |
सर्वेष्वपि त्रिदोषेषु व्यपदेशोऽधिकस्त्वतः ||७||
(वा. नि. अ. १४) |

Kustha (leprosy and other skin disorders) is of seven kinds, one from each dosha, three from the combination of two doshas, and one from the combination of all the three doshas together. Though all the kushtas are tridoshaja (caused due to involvement of all the three doshas), the types of kustha are named as vataja, pittaja etc based on the predominance of any one or two doshas in those types of kustha. (The varieties are named to indicate the predominance of a dosha or doshas in the kustha). (7)

Kustha Purvarupa

अतिश्लक्ष्णखरस्पर्शस्वेदास्वेदविवर्णताः |
दाहः कण्डूस्त्वचि स्वापस्तोदः कोठोन्नतिर्भ्रमः ||८||
व्रणानामधिकं शूलं शीघ्रोत्पत्तिश्चिरस्थितिः |
रूढानामपि रूक्षत्वं निमित्तऽल्पेऽतिकोपनम् ||९||
रोमहर्षोऽसृजः कार्ष्ण्यं कुष्ठलक्षणमग्रजम् |
(वा. नि. अ. १४) |

Premonitory symptoms of Kustha

Below mentioned are the premonitory symptoms of Kustha –

- the skin is either very smooth or rough,
- presence or absence of sweating,
- discolouration,
- burning sensation,
- itching,
- loss of sensation in the skin,
- pricking pain,
- appearance of elevated patches,
- giddiness,
- severe pain in the ulcers,
- ulcers form quickly and remain for long periods (does not heal for long periods of time),
- dryness in those ulcers which have healed,
- severe aggravation (re-appearance) of ulcer with trivial (simplest of or feeble) causes,
- horripilation,
- blackish discolouration of the blood (8-9)

Mahakusta

कृष्णारुणकपालाभं यद्रूक्षं परुषं तनु ||१०||
कापालं तोदबहुलं तत्कुष्ठं विषमं स्मृतम् |
रुग्दाहरागकण्डूभिः परीतं रोमपिञ्जरम् ||११||
उदुम्बरफलाभासं कुष्ठमौदुम्बरं वदेत् |
श्वेतं रक्तं स्थिरं स्त्यानं स्निग्धमुत्सन्नमण्डलम् ||१२||

कृच्छ्रमन्योन्यसंयुक्तं कुष्ठं मण्डलमुच्यते |
कर्कशं रक्तपर्यन्तमन्तःश्यावं सवेदनम् ||१३||
यदृष्यजिह्वसंस्थानमृष्यजिह्वं तदुच्यते |
सश्वेतं रक्तपर्यन्तं पुण्डरीकदलोपमम् ||१४||
सोत्सेधं च सरागं च पुण्डरीकं तदुच्यते |
श्वेतं ताम्रं तनु च यद्रजो घृष्टं विमुञ्चति ||१५||
प्रायश्चोरसि तत् सिध्ममलाबुकुसुमोपमम् |
यत् काकणन्तिकावर्णं सपाकं तीव्रवेदनम् ||१६||
त्रिदोषलिङ्गं तत् कुष्ठं काकणं नैव सिध्यति |
(च. चि. अ. ७) |

Seven types of major skin disorders and their symptoms -

Kapala Kustha – In this condition, the skin resembles a blackish or reddish-brown coloured piece of potsherd (kapala); is dry and rough (coarse) and thin; has severe pricking pain and is intractable.

Udumbara Kustha – This type of kustha resembles the fruit of udumbara (Ficus infectoria) and hence the name. It presents with pain, burning sensation, redness, itching and hairs turned to pink colour.

Mandala Kustha – In this condition, the skin is white or red in colour, tight (hard), moist (wet) and unctuous (oily). It has round and elevated patches which are joined to one another and is difficult to treat.

Rishyajihva Kustha – In this type of Mahakustha, the skin is very rough, is red in colour outside and black inside, and is associated with pain. It resembles the tongue of a black deer (Rishya) and hence the name.

Pundarika Kustha – In this, the skin is white at the centre and red at the edges resembling the petals of the lotus flower, with elevated patches which are red in colour.

Sidhma Kustha – The skin in this condition is white or coppery red in colour. It has thin scales which come off on scratching and are found mainly on the chest. They resemble the flowers of pitcher gourd.

Kakana Kustha – This type of mahakustha has the colour of gunja (Abrus precatorius), undergoing suppuration (pus formation), very painful and caused by all the three doshas and which does not respond to any kind of treatment (incurable). (10-16)

Kshudra kushta

अस्वेदनं महावास्तु यन्मत्स्यशकलोपमम् ||१७||
तदेककुष्ठं, चर्माख्यं बहलं हस्तिचर्मवत् |

श्यावं किणखरस्पर्शं परुषं किटिभं स्मृतम् ||१८||
वैपादिकं पाणिपादस्फुटनं तीव्रवेदनम् |
कण्डूमद्भिः सरागैश्चः गण्डैरलसकं चितम् ||१९||
सकण्डूरागपिडकं दद्रुमण्डलमुद्गतम् |
रक्तं सशूलं कण्डूमत् सस्फोटं यद्गलत्यपि |
तच्चर्मदलमाख्यातं संस्पर्शासहमुच्यते ||२०|| (च. चि. अ. ७) |
सूक्ष्मा बह्व्यः पिडकाः स्राववत्यः पामेत्युक्ताः कण्डुमत्यः सदाहाः |
सैव स्फोटैस्तीव्रदाहैरुपेता ज्ञेया पाण्योः कच्छुरुग्रा स्फिचोश्च ||२१||
स्फोटाः श्यावारुणाभासा विस्फोटाः स्युस्तनुत्वचः |
रक्तं श्यावं सदाहार्ति शतारुः स्याद्बहुव्रणम् ||२२||
सकण्डूः पिडका श्यावा बहुस्रावा विचर्चिका |
(च. चि. अ. ७) |

Seven types of minor skin disorders and their symptoms

Ekakustha – In this, there is no sweating, the area of skin involved is large, and the skin resembles the scales of a fish.

Carmakhya Kustha – In this condition, the skin becomes thick like that of an elephant skin.

Kitibha Kustha – The skin in this condition is blackish, rough and coarse just like the scar of a wound (granulation).

Vaipadika Kustha – This type of kshudra kustha presents with cracks and fissures formed on the hands and feet associated with severe pain.

Alasaka Kustha – This presents with nodules which are red in colour and associated with itching.

Dadru Mandala Kustha – In this condition there are raised patches studded with small, itching, reddish papules

Carmadala Kustha – It is a condition in which the skin is studded with red coloured nodules in which there is pain and itching. They burst open and fall off and are sensitive to touch (do not tolerate when touched).

Pama – It presents in the form of small and plentiful pustules from which discharges (exudates) take place. Itching and burning sensation are also present.

Kacchu – This is a condition in which the same pustules (as explained in pama) appear on the hands and on the buttocks associated with burning sensation.

Visphota – This condition presents with boils on the skin which are bluish black or brownish red in colour. It is called Visphota in which the skin becomes thin.

Shataru – This type of kshudra kustha presents with innumerable small ulcers which are red or blackish blue in colour and are associated with severe burning sensation and pain.
Vicharchika – In this condition, black coloured nodules are found from which plenty of copious exudates are discharged. This condition is also associated with itching. (17-22)
(The above eleven kinds are known as Kshudra kusthas i.e. minor leprosies / skin diseases).

Symptoms of Kushta based on the predominance of dosha

खरं श्यावारुणं रूक्षं वातात् कुष्ठं सवेदनम् ||२३||
पित्तात् प्रक्वथितं दाहरागस्रावान्वितं मतम् |
कफात् क्लेदि घनं स्निग्धं सकण्डूशैत्यगौरवम् ||२४||
द्विलिङ्गं द्वन्द्वजं कुष्ठं, त्रिलिङ्गं सान्निपातिकम् |२५|

Symptoms of vata predominance in all kinds of Kustha include – manifestation of roughness, bluish black or brownish red colour, dryness and pain.
Symptoms of pitta predominance in all kinds of Kustha include – manifestation of putrefaction, burning sensathion, redness and exudation (discharges).
Symptoms of kapha predominance in all kinds of Kustha include – manifestation of moistness (wetness), thickness, unctuousness (greasiness), itching, coldness and heaviness.
In dwandwaja Kustha – symptoms of two doshas are manifested together.
In sannipataja Kustha – symptoms of all three doshas are present together. (23-24)

Dhatugata Kustha Symptoms

त्वक्स्थे वैवर्ण्यमङ्गेषु कुष्ठे रौक्ष्यं च जायते ||२५||
त्वक्स्वापो रोमहर्षश्च स्वेदस्यातिप्रवर्तनम् |
कण्डूर्विपूयकश्चैव कुष्ठे शोणितसंश्रिते ||२६||
बाहुल्यं वक्त्रशोषश्च कार्कश्यं पिडकोद्गमः |
तोदः स्फोटः स्थिरत्वं च कुष्ठे मांससमाश्रिते ||२७||
कौण्यं गतिक्षयोऽङ्गानां सम्भेदः क्षतसर्पणम् |
मेदःस्थानगते लिङ्गं प्रागुक्तानि तथैव च ||२८||
नासाभङ्गोऽक्षिरागश्च क्षतेषु क्रिमिसम्भवः |

स्वरोपघातश्च भवेदस्थिमज्जसमाश्रिते ||२९||
दम्पत्योः कुष्ठबाहुल्याद्दुष्टशोणितशुक्रयोः |
यदपत्यं तयोर्जातं ज्ञेयं तदपि कुष्ठितम् ||३०||
(सु. नि. अ. ५) |

Twakgata Kustha – When kustha is located in the skin (rasa tissue) there will be discolouration of the skin, roughness, loss of sensation, horripilation and profuse sweating.

Raktagata Kustha – When kustha is located in the blood, there will be itching and the appearance of pustules in large numbers / foul smelling pus formation.

Mamsagata Kustha – When kustha is located in the muscle tissue, there will be the appearance of thick elevated patches, dryness of the mouth, roughness, appearance of nodules, pricking pain, boils / blisters and tightness of the skin.

Medogata Kustha – When kustha is located in the fat tissue, the fingers will fall off, and there will be loss of movements in the body parts (inability to walk), splitting pain and spreading of ulcer.

Asthi-Majjagata Kustha – When kustha is located in the bones and bone marrow, there is loss of / falling of nose, redness of the eyes, appearance of worms in the ulcers and loss of voice.

Shukragata Kustha – When the couple suffer from kustha, the child produced by them will also be born with kustha since both sperm (of the man) and ovum (of the woman) are both affected by kustha. (25-30)

Prognosis of Kushta

साध्यं त्वग्रक्तमांसस्थं वातश्लेष्माधिकं च यत् |
मेदसि द्वन्द्वजं याप्यं वर्ज्यं मज्जास्थिसंश्रितम् ||३१||

Kustha is located (invading) in skin, blood and muscle tissues and those varieties which are caused by the predominance of vata and kapha are easy to cure.

Kushta located (invading) the fat tissue and those caused by combination of two doshas together become manageable (chronic – curable but needs treatment throughout the life).

Kustha is located (invading) in the bone marrow and bones should not be treated (because they are incurable). (31)

Symptoms which are fatal in Kusta

क्रिमितृड्दाहमन्दाग्निसंयुक्तं यत्त्रिदोषजम् |
प्रभिन्नं प्रस्रुताङ्गं च रक्तनेत्रं हतस्वरम् ||३२||
पञ्चकर्मगुणातीतं कुष्ठं हन्तीह मानवम् |
(सु. सू. अ. ३३) |

Kustha is going to kill the patient in the presence of the below mentioned symptoms / conditions –

- presence of worms in the ulcers,
- thirst,
- burning sensation,
- poor digestive capacity
- involvement of all the three doshas together (in the causation of kustha – tridoshaja kustha)
- mutilation, loss of and decaying of body parts
- redness of the eyes
- loss of voice

If the cure is beyond the capacity of panchakarma (cannot be cured in spite of administering the five purifactory therapies or the patients not suitable to undergo these therapies which are otherwise highly beneficial) (32)

Dosha relation in each kustha

वातेन कुष्ठं कापालं पितेनौदुम्बरं कफात् ||३३||
मण्डलाख्यं विचर्ची च ऋष्याख्यं वातपित्तजम् |
चर्मैककुष्ठं किटिभं सिध्मालसविपादिकाः ||३४||
वातश्लेष्मोद्भवाः श्लेष्मपित्ताद्दद्रुशतारुषी |
पुण्डरीकं सविस्फोटं पामा चर्मदलं तथा ||३५||
सर्वैः स्यात् काकणं पूर्वत्रिकं दद्रु सकाकणम् |
पुण्डरीकर्ष्यजिह्वे च महाकुष्ठानि सप्त तु ||३६|| (वा. नि. अ. १४) |

Kapala kustha is produced by **vata** predominance.
Udumbara Kustha is caused by pitta predominance.
Mandala Kustha and Vicarcika Kustha are caused by kapha predominance.
Rsyajihva Kustha is caused by predominance of vata and pitta together.
Carmakhya Kustha, Eka Kustha, Kitibha Kustha, Sidhma Kustha, Alasa Kustha, Vipadika Kustha – all these are caused by predominant vitiation of both vata and kapha together.

Dadru Kustha, Sataru Kustha, Pundarika Kustha, Visphota Kustha, Pama Kustha and Carmadala Kustha – all these are caused by predominance of both kapha and pitta together.

Kakana Kustha is caused by vitiation of all the three doshas together.

The first three types of Kustha i.e. Kapala, Udumbara and Mandala and Dadru, Kakana, Pundarika and Rsyajihva – these seven types are called as Mahakusthas. (33-36)

Kilasa Kustha

कुष्ठैकसम्भवं श्वित्रं किलासं वारुणं भवेत् |
निर्दिष्टमपरिस्रावि त्रिधातूद्भवसंश्रयम् ||३७||
वाताद्रूक्षारुणं, पित्तात्ताम्रं कमलपत्रवत् |
सदाहं रोमविध्वंसि कफाच्छ्वेतं घनं गुरु ||३८||
सकण्डूरं क्रमाद्रक्तमांसमेदःसु चादिशेत् |
वर्णैनैवेद्दगुभयं कृच्छ्रं तच्चोत्तरोत्तरम् ||३९|| (वा. नि. अ. १४) |

Svitra, Kiläsa and Aruna are the variants of Kustha. They are produced by the same causative factors which cause kustha (leprosy).

There is no production of exudates in this condition (no discharges) and are caused by vitiation of all the three doshas together.

Vata predominance in these conditions causes roughness and pinkish discolouration.

Pitta predominance would present with lesions which are red like the petals of a lotus, associated with burning sensation and destruction (loss) of body hairs.

Kapha predominance in these conditions causes whitish discolouration, thickness, feeling of heaviness and itching.

Kilasa is of three types – Aruna, Tamra and Sveta. They are manifested in the blood, muscles and fat tissues respectively. (Involvement of blood causes aruna with pinkish or brownish red or golden yellow discolouration, Involvement of muscles causes tamra i.e., coppery discoloration and involvement of fat tissue will cause sveta i.e., whitish discoloration). The successive kinds are more dreadful than their preceding ones. Kilasa caused by ulcers and doshas will become incurable in successive (deeper) tissues. (37-39)

Prognosis of Svitra / Kilasa

अशुक्लरोमाऽबहुलमसंश्लिष्टमथो नवम् |

अनग्निदग्धजं साध्यं श्वित्रं वर्ज्यमतोऽन्यथा ||४०||
गुह्यपाणितलौष्ठेषु जातमप्यचिरन्तनम् |
वर्जनीयं विशेषेण किलासं सिद्धिमिच्छता ||४१||
(अ. सं. नि. अ. १४) |

Svitra (leucoderma) in which the hairs are not white; the skin is not thick, the patches are not joined together, which is of recent origin and that which has not been caused by burns are curable. Those having symptoms opposite to these are said to be incurable.

The physician desirous of success should refuse treating kilasa which has been manifested over the genitals, palms of the hands, soles of the food and lips and those which have persisted for a long time (chronic cases). (40-41)

Aupasargika Roga

प्रसङ्गाद्गात्रसंस्पर्शान्निःश्वासात् सहभोजनत् |
एकशय्यासनाच्चैव वस्त्रमाल्यानुपलेनात् ||४२||
कुष्ठं ज्वरश्च शोषश्च नेत्राभिष्यन्द एव च |
औपसर्गिकरोगाश्च सङ्क्रामन्ति नरान्नरम् ||४३||
(सु. नि. अ. ५) |

Sexual intercourse, physical contact, contact with expired air, dining together, sleeping together, and sharing the dress and garlands / ornaments, diseases like leprosy (skin diseases), fever, tuberculosis and conjunctivitis and many other diseases are transmitted from one person to the other. These diseases are called Aupasargika Rogas (infectious / contagious diseases). (42-44)

इति श्रीमाधवकरविरचिते माधवनिदाने कुष्ठनिदानं समाप्तम् ||४९||

Thus ends the chapter on Kustha Nidanam in Madhava Nidana text written by Acharya Madhavakara.

50

Madhava Nidana Chapter 50 Sheetapitta, Udarda, Kotha Nidanam

Samanya Nidana

शीतमारुतसंस्पर्शात् प्रदुष्टौ कफमारुतौ |
पित्तेन सह सम्भूय बहिरन्तर्विसर्पतः ||१||

General causes for Sitapitta, Udarda, Kotha

By contact with a very cold breeze, kapha and vata get increase. These doshas get associated with pitta (increased by its etiological factors) spreads out externally (towards the skin) and internally (into blood and other tissues) and produces sitapitta, udarda and kotha. (1)

Purvarupa

पिपासारुचिहृल्लासदेहसादाङ्गगौरवम् |
रक्तलोचनता तेषां पूर्वरूपस्य लक्षणम् ||२||

Premonitory symptoms

The premonitory symptoms of the above-mentioned conditions are – thirst, loss of taste, nausea, debility in the body parts, and feeling of heaviness in the body and redness of the eyes. (2)

Udarda Lakshana

वरटीदष्टसंस्थानः शोथः सञ्जायते बहिः |
सकण्डूस्तोदबहुलश्छर्दिज्वरविदाहवान् ||३||
उदर्दमिति तं विद्याच्छीतपित्तमथापरे |
वाताधिकं शीतपित्तमुदर्दस्तु कफाधिकः ||४||

Symptoms of Udarda

Swelling / elevated patches (rashes) resembling the rashes produced by the sting of the wasp produced on the skin, associated with itching and severe pricking pain, vomiting, fever and feeling of burning sensation are the characteristic features of Udarda. This condition is called Sitapitta by other experts. The difference in these two conditions is that in Sitapitta, vata is predominant and in udarda, kapha is predominant. (3-4)

Other form and presentation of Udarda

सोत्सङ्गैश्च सरागैश्च कण्डूमद्भिश्च मण्डलैः |
शैशिरः कफजो व्याधिरुदर्द इति कीर्तितः ||५||

A condition manifesting with elevated patches which are reddish, have severe itching, caused by vitiated kapha during sisira rtu (late winter) is also known as udarda. (5)

Kotha

असम्यग्वमनोदीर्णपित्तश्लेष्मान्ननिग्रहैः |
मण्डलानि सकण्डूनि रागवन्ति बहूनि च |
उत्कोठः सानुबन्धश्च कोठ इत्यभिधीयते ||६||

Incomplete / inadequate or erroneous administration of emesis therapy (improper administration of emetics and other treatments), and suppression (obstruction) of the movement of pitta, kapha and anna (food) leads to the appearance of innumerable rashes, red in colour and highly itching is called as Kotha. If the same condition repeats (relapses) again and again, many times, it is called as Utkotha. (6)

इति श्रीमाधवकरविरचिते माधवनिदाने शीतपित्तोदर्दकोठानिदानं समाप्तम् ||५०||

Thus ends the chapter on Sheetapitta Udarda Kotha Nidanam in Madhava Nidana text written by Acharya Madhavakara.

51

Madhava Nidana Chapter 51 Amlapitta Nidanam

Nidana, Samprapti

विरुद्धदुष्टाम्लविदाहिपित्तप्रकोपिपानान्नभुजो विदग्धम् |
पित्तं स्वहेतूपचितं पुरा यत्तदम्लपित्तं प्रवदन्ति सन्तः ||१||

Etiological Factors and Pathogenesis of Amlapitta

In persons in whom pitta has already undergone increase and excessive sourness; excessive indulgence in foods which are of incompatible combinations, spoiled, very sour, those causing burning sensation inside and such other foods and drinks which cause increase of pitta, produce Amlapitta, so say the wise. (1)

Amlapitta Lakshana

अविपाकक्लमोत्क्लेशतिक्ताम्लोद्गारगौरवैः |
हृत्कण्ठदाहारुचिभिश्चाम्लपित्तं वदेद्भिषक् ||२||

Symptoms of amlapitta

The disease in which the patient has indigestion, exhaustion without any exertion, nausea, eructation (belching) with bitter or sour taste, feeling of heaviness of the body, burning sensation in the chest and throat and loss of taste - is to be called as Amlapitta. (2)

Adhoga Amlapitta Symptoms

तृड्दाहमूर्छाभ्रममोहकारि प्रयात्यधो वा विविधप्रकारम् |
हृल्लासकोठानलसादहर्षस्वेदाङ्गपीतत्वकरं कदाचित् ||३||

The symptoms of adhoga (downward) amlapitta are - thirst, burning sensation, fainting, giddiness, delusion, movement downwards of different kinds (of diarrhoea), nausea (occasional oppression in the chest), rashes on the skin, poor digestion, horripilation, excessive perspiration and yellowish skin (of parts of the body). (3)

Urdhwaga Amlapitta Symptoms

वान्तं हरित्पीतकनीलकृष्णमारक्तरक्ताभमतीव चाम्लम् |
मांसोदकाभं त्वतिपिच्छिलाच्छं श्लेष्मानुजातं विविधं रसेन ||४||
भुक्ते विदग्धे त्वथवाऽप्यभुक्ते करोति तिक्ताम्लवमिं कदाचित् |
उद्गारमेवंविधमेव कण्ठहृत्कुक्षिदाहं शिरसो रुजं च ||५||
करचरणदाहमौष्ण्यं महतीमरुचिं ज्वरं च कफपित्तम् |
जनयति कण्डूमण्डलपिडकाशतनिचितगात्ररोगचयम् ||६||

Symptoms of ūrdhvaga (upward) amlapitta - vomiting of green, yellow, blue, black, slightly red or bright red coloured very sour materials, resembling mutton wash, very sticky, thin, followed by kapha (expulsion of kapha) and of different tastes (salty, pungent, bitter etc). Vomiting having a bitter or sour taste occurs during digestion of food or even on an empty stomach, occasionally.

Belching is also of similar nature (as that of vomiting). Burning sensation in the throat, chest and upper abdomen and headache are also present. Apart from this there is burning sensation in the palms and soles, feeling of great heat, severe loss of taste, fever of kapha-pitta type, itching, appearance of circular rashes, studded with numerous small vesicles on the skin, indigestion, watery secretions in the mouth and other troubles of the body. (4-6)

Prognosis of Amlapitta

रोगोऽयमम्लपित्ताख्यो यत्नात् संसाध्यते नवः |
चिरोत्थितो भवेद्याप्यः, कृच्छ्रसाध्यः स कस्यचित् ||७||

This disease amlapitta - which is of recent onset, responds to treatment with difficulty. The amlapitta which is of long duration will be chronic or curable with difficulty in a few people. (7)

Amlapitta Samsarga

सानिलं सानिलकफं सकफं तच्च लक्षयेत् |
दोषलिङ्गेन मतिमान् भिषङ्मोहकरं हि तत् ||८||
कम्पप्रलापमूर्छाचिमिचिमिगात्रावसादशूलानि |
तमसो दर्शनविभ्रमविमोहहर्षाण्यनिलकोपात् ||९||
कफनिष्ठीवनगौरवजडतारुचिशीतसादवमिलेपाः |
दहनबलसादकण्डूनिद्राश्चिह्नं कफानुगते ||१०||
उभयमिदमेव चिह्नं मारुतकफसम्भवे भवत्यम्ले |
तिक्ताम्लकटुकोद्गारहृत्कुक्षिकण्ठदाहकृत् ||११||
भ्रमो मूर्छारुचिश्छर्दिरालस्यं च शिरोरुजा |
प्रसेको मुखमाधुर्यं श्लेष्मपित्तस्य लक्षणम् ||१२||

The physician should clearly recognise the symptoms of amlapitta caused by vata, vata kapha and kapha as they are likely to create confusion to him (and hence the mastery in understanding these conditions is a must).

Vata symptoms – Symptoms caused by vata are - tremors, delirium, fainting, feeling of pins and needles, weakness of the body parts, pain, appearance of darkness before the eyes, giddiness, delusion, horripilation.

Kapha symptoms – Symptoms of kapha are - expectoration of thick phlegm, feeling of heaviness, lassitude, loss of taste, coldness, weakness, vomiting, and coating on the tongue, decrease of digestive strength, itching and excessive sleep.

Appearance of both the above symptoms together is seen in amlapitta in which both vata and kapha are associated.

(Eructation / belching having bitter, sour and pungent tastes, burning sensation in the chest, upper abdomen and throat, giddiness, fainting, loss of taste, vomiting, lassitude, headache, excessive salivation, sweet taste in the mouth are the symptoms of amla-pitta caused by kapha and pitta together.(8-12)

इति श्रीमाधवकरविरचिते माधवनिदानेऽम्लपित्तनिदानं समाप्तम् ||५१||

Thus ends the chapter on Amlapitta Nidanam in Madhava Nidana text written by Acharya Madhavakara.

52

Madhava Nidana Chapter 52 Visarpa Nidanam

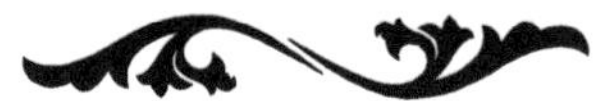

Visarpa Nidana

लवणाम्लकटूष्णादिसंसेवादोषकोपतः |
विसर्पः सप्तधा ज्ञेयः सर्वतः परिसर्पणात् ||१||

Etiological factors of Visarpa

Ingestion of too much of salty, sour, pungent and hot foods and such other factors would lead to abnormal increase of all the three doshas. These vitiated doshas produce seven types of visarpa. Visarpa is called so because of its nature of spreading all over the body. (1)

Types of Visarpa

पृथक् त्रयस्त्रिभिश्चैको विसर्पा द्वन्द्वजास्त्रयः |
वातिकः पैत्तिकश्चैव कफजः सान्निपातिकः ||२||
चत्वार एते वीसर्पा वक्ष्यन्ते द्वन्द्वजास्त्रयः |
आग्नेयो वातपित्ताभ्यां ग्रन्थ्याख्यः कफवातजः ||३||
यस्तु कर्दमको घोरः स पित्तकफसम्भवः |४|
(च. चि. अ. २१) |

There are seven kinds of visarpa – one from each dosha, one from all three doshas mixed together and three from combination of two doshas. They are –

- Vataja Visarpa
- Pittaja Visarpa
- Kaphaja Visarpa
- Sannipataja Visarpa
- Agneya Visarpa – from the combination of vata and pitta
- Granthi Visarpa – from the combination of kapha and vata
- Kardama Visarpa – from the combination of pitta and kapha, which is considered dreadful (2-3)

Hetu – Sapta Dhatu
रक्तं लसीका त्वङ्मांसं दूष्यं दोषास्त्रयो मलाः ||४||
विसर्पाणां समुत्पत्तौ विज्ञेयाः सप्त धातवः |
(च. चि. अ. २१)
7 body components involved in the causation of visarp
The seven factors involved in the causation of visarpa are –
Dushyas / tissues (4 in number) - Rakta (blood), Lasīkā (lymph), Tvak (skin) and Mamsa (muscles) are the düsyas (tissues involved) and
Doshas (3 in number) – all the three doshas are involved in the causation of visarpa
The 4 tissues and 3 doshas put together form the seven important (and mandatory) factors responsible for causation of visarpa. (4)

Symptoms of Doshaja Visarpa
तत्र वातात् स वीसर्पो वातज्वरसमव्यथः ||५||
शोथस्फुरणनिस्तोदभेदायासार्तिहर्षवान् |
पित्ताद्द्रुतगतिः पित्तज्वरलिङ्गोऽतिलोहितः ||६||
कफात् कण्डूयुतः स्निग्धः कफज्वरसमानरुक् | (वा. नि. अ. १३) |
सन्निपातसमुत्थश्च सर्वलिङ्गसमन्वितः ||७||
Vataja visarpa – This type of visarpa has identical symptoms as found in vāta jwara (fever). Along with these there will also be the presence of swelling, pulsations, pricking or splitting (cutting) types of pain, tiredness, body aches and horripilation.
Pittaja visarpa – This type of visarpa would progress quickly and has similar symptoms to those of pittaja jwara and the lesions are dark red in colour.
Kaphaja visarpa – This type of visarpa would have itching and

unctuousness of the lesions and its symptoms will be similar to those of kaphaja jwara.

Sannipataja Visarpa – In this type of visarpa caused by aggravation of all the three doshas, all the symptoms of individual doshaja visarpa will be seen together. (5-7)

Agneya Visarpa:Vata Pittaja Visarpa

वातपित्ताज्ज्वरच्छर्दिमूर्छातीसारतृड्भ्रमैः |
ग्रन्थिभेदाग्निसदनतमकारोचकैर्युतः ||८||
करोति सर्वमङ्गं च दीप्ताङ्गारावकीर्णवत् |
यं यं देशं विसर्पश्च विसर्पति भवेत् स सः ||९||
शान्ताङ्गारासितो नीलो रक्तो वाऽऽशु च चीयते |
अग्निदग्ध इव स्फोटैः शीघ्रगत्वाद्द्रुतं स च ||१०||
मर्मानुसारी वीसर्पः स्याद्वातोऽतिबलस्ततः |
व्यथतेऽङ्गं हरेत् सञ्ज्ञां निद्रां च श्वासमीरयेत् ||११||
हिक्कां च स गतोऽवस्थामीदृशीं लभते न ना |
क्वचिच्छर्मारतिग्रस्तो भूमिशय्यासनादिषु ||१२||
चेष्टमानस्ततः क्लिष्टो मनोदेहप्रमोहवान् |
दुष्प्रबोधोऽश्नुते निद्रां सोऽग्निवीसर्प उच्यते ||१३||
(वा. नि. अ. १३) |

Visarpa caused by combination of increased väta and pitta will have the following symptoms –
fever, vomiting, fainting, diarrhea, thirst, giddiness,
bursting pain in the glands or joints
poor digestion capacity
experiencing darkness before the eyes
loss of taste
feeling as if the whole body, mainly the affected part of the body has been covered by and is in contact with burning charcoal,
the skin of the part or parts of the body to which visarpa spreads becomes black or blue just like burning coal which has calmed down and that area quickly gets covered by blebs resembling fire burns, the lesions quickly spread out to other places,
visarpa gets located in the vital spots or organs (marma) quickly due to the quick spreading nature of the disease,
(due to this) the vata gets aggravated and produces pain and trouble in the

affected parts, and causes loss of consciousness and sleep, hiccough and dyspnoea (difficulty in breathing)
the patient having reached this condition does not find even slightest of relief with anything and anywhere, he becomes restless sleeps (lays) or sits on the ground repeatedly, while doing so he would faint becoming severely distressed and would enter into a deep sleep (which is equivalent to death) from which he cannot wake up again (dies). This type of visarpa is known as Agni Visarpa. (8-13)

Granthi Visarpa: Vata Kaphaja Visarpa

कफेन रुद्धः पवनो भित्त्वा तं बहुधा कफम् |
रक्तं वा वृद्धरक्तस्य त्वक्सिरास्नायुमांसगम् ||१४||
दूषयित्वा तु दीर्घाणुवृत्तस्थूलखरात्मनाम् |
ग्रन्थीनां कुरुते मालां सरक्तां तीव्ररुग्ज्वराम् ||१५||
श्वासकासातिसारास्यशोषहिक्कावमिभ्रमैः |
मोहवैवर्ण्यमूर्छाङ्गभङ्गाग्निसदनैर्युताम् ||१६||
इत्ययं ग्रन्थिवीसर्पः कफमारुतकोपजः |१७|
(वा. नि. अ. १३) |

Visarpa caused by combination of increased vata and kapha will have the following symptoms –
Vata getting obstructed by kapha in turn spreads the kapha immensely in the body. Or in a person in whom the blood has already undergone abnormal increase, vata would vitiate the blood located in the skin, veins, ligaments (and tendons) and muscles. Following these events vata would produce chains of tumours (cystic swellings) which are elongated, small, round, hard or rough. These cysts are red in colour, painful and associated with fever. Other symptoms include dyspnoea (difficulty in breathing), cough, diarrhoea, dryness of the mouth, hiccough, vomiting, giddiness, delusion, discolouration, fainting, pain all over the body and poor digestion. This disease caused by vitiated vata and kapha together is called as Granthi Visarpa. (14-16)

Kardama Visarpa:Kapha Pittaja Visarpa

कफपित्ताज्ज्वरः स्तम्भो निद्रा तन्द्रा शिरोरुजा ||१७||
अङ्गावसादविक्षेपौ प्रलेपारोचकभ्रमाः |
मूर्छाग्निहानिर्भेदोऽस्थ्नां पिपासेन्द्रियगौरवम् ||१८||
आमोपवेशनं लेपः स्रोतसां स च सर्पति |

प्रायेणामाशयं गृह्णन्नेकदेशं न चातिरुक् ||१९||
पिडकैरवकीर्णोऽतिपीतलोहितपाण्डुरैः |
स्निग्धोऽसितो मेचकाभो मलिनः शोथवान् गुरुः ||२०||
गम्भीरपाकः प्राज्योष्मा स्पृष्टः क्लिन्नोऽवदीर्यते |
पङ्कवच्छीर्णमांसश्च स्पष्टस्नायुसिरागणः ||२१||
शवगन्धी च वीसर्पः कर्दमाख्यमुशन्ति तम् |२२| (वा. नि. अ. १३) ||

Visarpa caused by combination of increased kapha and pitta will have the following symptoms –

fever, stiffness of the body parts, stupor, sleep, headache,

weakness of the body parts, involuntary movements of the body parts, coating of the tongue, loss of taste, giddiness,

fainting, destruction of digestive fire (loss of digestive functions), splitting pain in the bones, thirst, dullness (heaviness) of the sense organs,

excretion of faeces mixed with ama (inadequately formed faeces or faeces mixed with undigested portions of foods)

coating of thick material which leads to obstruction in the channels of the body (orifices, cell pores, tissue spaces, passages of transportation etc)

this type of visarpa probably invades the stomach or one side of the body and presents with mild pain,

it is surrounded by small tumours which are of deep yellow, red, pale, unctuous, black, dark black like collyrium and dirty

they are swollen, heavy, undergoes suppuration deep within (pus is formed inside) and excessively hot,

since the lesions are filled with fluids, they mostly burst out discharging the pus on touching them

the muscles become loose, semi-liquid like silt and fall off exposing the network of tendons and veins and emits smell resembling that of a dead body

This type of visarpa is called as Kardama Visarpa. (17-21)

Kshata Visarpa

बाह्यहेतोः क्षतात् क्रुद्धः सरक्तं पित्तमीरयन् ||२२||
वीसर्पं मारुतः कुर्यात् कुलत्थसदृशैश्चितम् |
स्फोटैः शोथज्वररुजादाहाढ्यं श्यावशोणितम् ||२३|| (वा. नि. अ. १३) |

Another variety of visarpa is caused by ksata (external injury). Vata aggravated due to external injury would provoke blood along with pitta and cause visarpa. In this, vesicles of the size of horse gram appear all over the body and are associated with swelling, fever, pain and burning sensation. The lesions have blackish blue or blood colour. (22-23)

Complications of Visarpam

ज्वरातिसारौ वमथुस्त्वङ्मांसदरणं क्लमः |
अरोचकाविपाकौ च विसर्पाणामुपद्रवाः ||२४||

The complications of visarpa are fever, diarrhea, vomiting, cracking / fissuring of skin and muscles, exhaustion, loss of taste and indigestion are the complications of visarpa. (24)

Prognosis of Visarp

सिध्यन्ति वातकफपित्तकृता विसर्पाः सर्वात्मकः क्षतकृतश्च न सिद्धिमेति |
पित्तात्मकोऽञ्जनवपुश्च भवेदसाध्यः कृच्छ्राश्च मर्मसु भवन्ति हि सर्व एव ||२५||
(सु. नि. अ. १०) |

Visarpas produced by anyone dosha – i.e., vata, kapha and pitta are curable.
The tridoshaja and ksataja visarpas do not respond to the treatment.
Visarpa produced by pitta and that in which the body becomes black like anjana (eye salve, collyrium) are incurable.
Visarpa which occurs on the vital spots / organs are difficult to cure. (25)

इति श्रीमाधवकरविरचिते माधवनिदाने विसर्पनिदानं समाप्तम् ||५२||

Thus ends the chapter on Visarpa Nidanam in Madhava Nidana text written by Acharya Madhavakara.

53

Madhava Nidana Chapter 53 Visphota Nidanam

Nidana, Samprapti

कट्वम्लतीक्ष्णोष्णविदाहिरूक्षक्षारैरजीर्णाध्यशनातपैश्च |
तथर्तुदोषेण विपर्ययेण कुप्यन्ति दोषाः पवनादयस्तु ||१||
त्वचमाश्रित्य ते रक्तमांसास्थीनि प्रदूष्य च |
घोरान् कुर्वन्ति विस्फोटान् सर्वान् ज्वरपुरःसरान् ||२||
कट्वम्लतीक्ष्णोष्णविदाहिरूक्षक्षारैरजीर्णाध्यशनातपैश्च |
तथर्तुदोषेण विपर्ययेण कुप्यन्ति दोषाः पवनादयस्तु ||१||
त्वचमाश्रित्य ते रक्तमांसास्थीनि प्रदूष्य च |
घोरान् कुर्वन्ति विस्फोटान् सर्वान् ज्वरपुरःसरान् ||२||

Etiological factors and pathogenesis of Visphota

Etiological Factors – excessive indulgence in foods which are pungent and sour in taste, penetrating, hot, those producing burning sensation (corrosive), dry, alkaline, uncooked and in excessive quantity, exposure to sun-light, bad effects of seasons (due to exposure to excessive heat, wind, cold etc.) and abnormal seasons (excessive cold in summer, excessive cold in summer etc.) are the etiological factors of visphota.

Pathogenesis – The above said etiological factors cause aggravation of vata and other doshas (pitta, kapha). These doshas in turn get lodged in the skin and contaminate blood, muscles and bones and produce many dreadful vesicles on the skin preceded by fever. (This condition is called visphota).

(1-2)

Nature of Visphot

अग्निदग्धनिभाः स्फोटाः सज्वरा रक्तपित्तजाः |
क्वचित् सर्वत्र वा देहे विस्फोटा इति ते स्मृताः ||३|| (सु. नि. अ. १३) |

Vesicles resembling boils formed by the touch of fire (boils which occur due to fire burns), caused by aggravation of blood and pitta, associated with fever, occurring in some or all the parts of the body is known as Visphota. (3)

Symptoms of doshaja visphota

शिरोरुक् शूलभूयिष्ठं ज्वरस्तृट् पर्वभेदनम् |
सकृष्णवर्णता चेति वातविस्फोटलक्षणम् ||४||
ज्वरदाहरुजास्रावपाकतृष्णाभिरन्वितम् |
पीतलोहितवर्णं च पित्तविस्फोटलक्षणम् ||५||
छर्द्यरोचकजाड्यानि कण्डूकाठिन्यपाण्डुताः |
अवेदनश्चिरात्पाकी स विस्फोटः कफात्मकः ||६||
वातपित्तकृतो यस्तु कुरुते तीव्रवेदनाम् |
कण्डूस्तैमित्यगुरुभिर्जानीयात् कफवातिकम् ||७||
कण्डूर्दाहो ज्वरश्छर्दिरेतैस्तु कफपैत्तिकः |८|

Vataja Visphota – The symptoms of visphota caused by predominance of vata are headache, severe pain, fever, thirst, splitting pain in the small joints of the hands and feet and the manifestation of vesicles which are black in colour.

Pittaja Visphota – The symptoms of visphota caused by predominance of pitta are – fever, burning sensation, pain, discharges (exudates), suppuration (formation of pus), thirst and formation of vesicles which are yellow or red in colour.

Kaphaja Visphota – The symptoms of visphota caused by predominance of kapha are – vomiting, loss of taste, lassitude, itching, hardness, pallor, lack of pain and formation of vesicles which undergo slow suppuration.

Vata-pittaja Visphota – presents with severe pain.

Vata-kaphaja Visphota – presents with itching, feeling of being covered with wet leather or cloth and heaviness.

Kapha-pittaja Visphota – presents with itching, burning sensation, fever and vomiting. (4-7)

Sannipataja Visphota

मध्ये निम्नोन्नतोऽन्ते च कठिनोऽल्पप्रपाकवान् ||८||
दाहरागतृषामोहच्छर्दिमूर्छारुजाज्वराः |
प्रलापो वेपथुस्तन्द्रा सोऽसाध्यः स्यात्त्रिदोषजः ||९||

The visphota (vesicles) caused by simultaneous aggravation of all the three doshas will have depression in the centre and are elevated at the edges, are hard and undergo less suppuration (with little quantity of pus in them). This condition is associated with burning sensation, redness, thirst, delusion, vomiting, fainting, pain, fever, delirium, tremors, and stupor. This condition is incurable. (8-9)

Raktaja Visphota

रक्ता रक्तसमुत्थाना गुञ्जाविद्रुमसन्निभाः |
वेदितव्यास्तु रक्तेन पैत्तिकेन च हेतुना ||१०||
न ते सिद्धिं समायान्ति सिद्धैर्योगशतैरपि |

Visphota caused by rakta (vitiated blood) will have vesicles which are red in colour resembling guñjā seed (Abrus precatorius) or coral bead. They are caused by blood vitiated by pitta aggravating etiological factors. They do not respond to any kinds of treatments even by administering hundreds of efficient recipes. (10)

Prognosis of Visphot

एकदोषोत्थितः साध्यः कृच्छ्रसाध्यो द्विदोषजः |
सर्वदोषोत्थितो घोरस्त्वसाध्यो भूर्युपद्रवः ||११||

Visphota caused by single dosha is curable.

Visphota caused by simultaneous aggravation of two doshas is curable with difficulty.

Visphota caused by simultaneous aggravation of all the three doshas and that which is associated with complications is incurable. (11)

इति श्रीमाधवकरविरचिते माधवनिदाने विस्फोटनिदानं समाप्तम् ||५३||

Thus ends the chapter on Visphota Nidanam in Madhava Nidana text written by Acharya Madhavakara.

54

Madhava Nidana Chapter 54 Masurika Nidanam

Masoorika Nidana

कट्वम्ललवणक्षारविरुद्धाध्यशनाशनैः ।
दुष्टनिष्पावशाकाद्यैः प्रदुष्टपवनोदकैः ॥१॥
क्रूरग्रहेक्षणाच्चापि देशे दोषाः समुद्धताः ।
जनयन्ति शरीरेऽस्मिन् दुष्टरक्तेन सङ्गताः ॥२॥
मसूराकृतिसंस्थानाः पिडकाः स्युर्मसूरिकाः ।

Etiological factors of Masurika

Below mentioned are the causative factors of masurika –

excessive indulgence in foods which are pungent, sour, salty, alkaline and of incompatible nature (mutually opposite / antagonist foods)

intake of foods in large quantities too frequently

excessive consumption of contaminated foods, beans, and leafy vegetables

excessive and repeated exposure to contaminated air and water

influence of bad planetary positions (seeing bad planets which influences on certain areas of the country (in community of people)

Pathogenesis – Due to the above said etiological factors the doshas get aggravated in the entire body. These doshas get associated with the contaminated blood and produce eruptions on the body which resemble masura – lentils in shape and size and hence the name masurika. (1-2)

Masurika Purvarupa

तासां पूर्वं ज्वरः कण्डूर्गात्रभङ्गोऽरतिर्भ्रमः ||३||
त्वचि शोथः सवैवर्ण्यो नेत्ररागश्च जायते |४|

Premonitory symptoms of Masurika

The premonitory symptoms of masurika include fever, itching, breaking pain all over the body, restlessness, giddiness, swelling in the skin, discolouration of skin and redness of the eyes. (3)

Vataja Masoorika

स्फोटाः श्यावारुणा रूक्षास्तीव्रवेदनयाऽन्विताः ||४||
कठिनाश्चिरपाकाश्च भवन्त्यनिलसम्भवाः |
सन्ध्यस्थिपर्वणां भेदः कासः कम्पोऽरतिः क्लमः ||५||
शोषस्ताल्वोष्ठजिह्वानां तृष्णा चारुचिसंयुता |६|

The symptoms of masurika caused by predominant vitiation of vata are – manifestation of eruptions which are black or crimson in color, dry, severely painful, hard and undergo slow suppuration. This condition is also associated with splitting pain in the joints, bones and small joints of the hands and feet, cough, tremors, restlessness, exhaustion, dryness of the palate, lips and tongue, thirst and loss of taste. (4-5)

Pittaja Masurika

रक्ताः पीतासिताः स्फोटाः सदाहास्तीव्रवेदनाः ||६||
भवन्त्यचिरपाकाश्च पित्तकोपसमुद्भवाः |
विड्भेदश्चाङ्गमर्दश्च दाहस्तृष्णाऽरुचिस्तथा ||७||
मुखपाकोऽक्षिरागश्च ज्वरस्तीव्रः सुदारुणः |८|

The symptoms of masurika caused by predominant vitiation of pitta are – manifestation of eruptions which are red or yellowish white in colour associated with severe burning sensation and pain. These eruptions will undergo suppuration quickly. The patient would also have diarrhoea, pain as if someone has beaten all over the body, burning sensation, thirst, loss of taste, stomatitis (ulcerations in the mouth), redness of the eyes, very high fever and great distress. (6-7)

Raktaja Masurika

रक्तजायां भवन्त्येते विकाराः पित्तलक्षणाः ||८||

The symptoms of masurika caused by predominant vitiation of rakta (blood) are similar to those of pittaja masurika. (8)

Kaphaja Masurika
कफप्रसेकः स्तैमित्यं शिरोरुग् गात्रगौरवम् |
हृल्लासः सारुचिर्निद्रा तन्द्रालस्यसमन्विताः ||९||
श्वेताः स्निग्धा भृशं स्थूलाः कण्डूरा मन्दवेदनाः |
मसूरिकाः कफोत्थाश्च चिरपाकाः प्रकीर्तिताः ||१०||
The symptoms of masurika caused by predominant vitiation of kapha are – excessive salivation (watery discharges from the mouth), feeling as though the body has been covered by wet leather or cloth, headache, heaviness of the body, nausea, loss of taste, excessive sleep, stupor and lassitude. The eruptions are white in colour, are unctuous, big in size, and are associated with itching and mild pain. In these eruptions the suppuration is slow. (9-10)

Sannipataja Masoorika
नीलाश्चिपिटविस्तीर्णा मध्ये निम्ना महारुजाः |
चिरपाकाः पूतिस्रावाः प्रभूताः सर्वदोषजाः ||११||
कण्ठरोधारुचिस्तम्भप्रलापारतिसंयुताः |
दुश्चिकित्स्याः समुद्दिष्टाः पिडकाश्चर्मसञ्ज्ञिताः ||१२||
The symptoms of masurika caused by predominant vitiation of all three doshas together are – manifestation of eruptions which are blue in colour, flat, broad, depressed in the centre (and elevated at its edges) and severely painful. There is slow suppuration in these eruptions. Large quantities of foul smelling discharges come out of the eruptions (pus with offensive smell). There is also obstruction in the throat, loss of taste, stiffness of the body, delirium and restlessness. This condition is also called Carmapidaka. This condition caused by aggravation of all the three doshas together is difficult to treat. (11-12)

Romantika
रोमकूपोन्नतिसमा रागिण्यः कफपित्तजाः |
कासारोचकसंयुक्ता रोमान्त्यो ज्वरपूर्विकाः ||१३||
Small, red eruptions occurring at the roots of the hairs making slight elevations which appear like raised sweat glands / pores, caused by abnormal increase of kapha and pitta are called Romantika (measles). This condition is associated with cough, loss of taste and preceded by fever. (13)

Dhatugata Masoorika

तोयबुद्बुदसङ्काशास्त्वग्गतास्तु मसूरिकाः |
स्वल्पदोषाः प्रजायन्ते भिन्नास्तोयं स्रवन्ति च ||१४||
रक्तस्था लोहिताकाराः शीघ्रपाकास्तनुत्वचः |
साध्या नात्यर्थदुष्टाश्च भिन्ना रक्तं स्रवन्ति च ||१५||
मांसस्थाः कठिनाः स्निग्धाश्चिरपाका घनत्वचः |
गात्रशूलतृषाकण्डूज्वरारतिसमन्विताः ||१६||
मेदोजा मण्डलाकारा मृदवः किञ्चिदुन्नताः |
घोरज्वरपरीताश्च स्थूलाः स्निग्धाः सवेदनाः ||१७||
सम्मोहारतिसन्तापाः कश्चिदाभ्यो विनिस्तरेत् |
क्षुद्रा गात्रसमा रूक्षाश्चिपिटाः किञ्चिदुन्नताः ||१८||
मज्जोत्था भृशसम्मोहवेदनारतिसंयुताः |
छिन्दन्ति मर्मधामानि प्राणानाशु हरन्ति हि ||१९||
भ्रमरेणेव विद्धानि कुर्वन्त्यस्थीनि सर्वतः |
पक्वाभाः पिडकाः स्निग्धाः सूक्ष्माश्चात्यर्थवेदनाः ||२०||
स्तैमित्यारतिसम्मोहदाहोन्मादसमन्विताः |
शुक्रजायां मसूर्यां तु लक्षणानि भवन्ति हि ||२१||
निर्दिष्टं केवलं चिह्नं दृश्यते न तु जीवितम् |
दोषमिश्रास्तु सप्तैता द्रष्टव्या दोषलक्षणैः ||२२||
त्वग्गता रक्तजाश्चैव पित्तजाः श्लेष्मजास्तथा |
श्लेष्मपित्तकृताश्चैव सुखसाध्या मसूरिकाः ||२३||

Twak-gata Masurika – When masurika is localised in the skin (affecting the rasa tissue), the eruptions would appear like water bubbles, discharge thin watery fluid on pricking and will have mild aggravation of doshas.

Raktagata Masurika - If Masurika is localized in the blood tissue, the eruptions would be red in colour, suppurates quickly, with thin skin. These are curable when they do not have severe vitiation of doshas. When these eruptions are pricked, they discharge blood.

Mamsagata Masurika – When the disease is localized in the muscle tissue, the eruptions are hard, unctuous, undergo suppuration slowly, and are covered with a thick layer of skin. This condition is associated with pain all over the body, thirst, itching, fever and restlessness.

Medogata Masurika – If the disease masurika invades and gets localized in the fat tissue there is manifestation of eruptions which are in the form of round patches, soft and slightly elevated, large, unctuous (greasy), painful and accompanied with very high fever, delusion, restlessness and distress (raised heat in the body and mind). Few people would get over these conditions.

Majjagata Masurika – If masurika is localized in the bone marrow there is manifestation of eruptions which are small in size, have the same colour as that of the skin, dry, flat or slightly elevated. It is associated with severe delusion, pain, and restlessness.

Asthigata Masurika - If masurika is localized in the bones, there will be cutting pain in the marmas i.e., vital organs which would pose threat to life. The bones would appear as though many bees have made many holes (perforations) in the bones (pain in the bones as though stung by bees).

Shukragata Masurika – When masurika gets lodged in the semen, there is a manifestation of eruptions which are ripened, unctuous (greasy, waxy), small in size, severely painful. The person would feel as if covered by wet leather or cloth and will also experience restlessness, delusion, burning sensation and insanity (intoxication). The symptoms of this condition are formally explained. In any case, the patient would lose his life quickly.

These (above said) seven types of masurika located in the tissues are always associated with vata and other (pitta, kapha) doshas. Therefore, they might have symptoms of one or more of the increased doshas. They should be understood on the basis of the symptoms of increased doshas associated with masurika located in the tissues.

Masurika resides in the skin and blood, and those caused by vitiated pitta, kapha and kapha-pitta are easy to cure. (14-23)

Prognosis of Masurika

वातजा वातपित्तोत्थाः श्लेष्मवातकृताश्च याः |
कृच्छ्रसाध्यतमास्तस्माद्यत्नादेता उपाचरेत् ||२४||
असाध्याः सन्निपातोत्थास्तासां वक्ष्यामि लक्षणम् |
प्रवालसदृशाः काश्चित् काश्चिज्जम्बूफलोपमाः ||२५||
लोहजालसमाः काश्चिदतसीफलसन्निभाः |
आसां बहुविधा वर्णा जायन्ते दोषभेदतः ||२६||

Masurika caused by vata, vāta-pitta, kapha-vata are very difficult to cure. Therefore, they shall be treated with great care and effort.

Masurika caused by sannipata i.e., all the vitiated doshas combined together is incurable. Their symptoms are hereby explained. The eruptions resemble coral beads in colour, and some resemble fruits of jambu (Eugenia jambolana) and some others appear like an iron sieve. Some others

resemble fruits of atasi (linseed).
The eruptions of masurika will also have many other colours depending on the type of dosha or doshas involved therein. (24-26)

Other symptoms of incurability of masurika

कासो हिक्का प्रमेहश्च ज्वरस्तीव्रः सुदारुणः |
प्रलापश्चारतिर्मूर्छा तृष्णा दाहोऽतिघूर्णता ||२७||
मुखेन प्रस्रवेद्रक्तं तथा घ्राणेन चक्षुषा |
कण्ठे घुर्घुरकं कृत्वा श्वसित्यत्यर्थवेदनम् ||२८||
मसूरिकाभिभूतस्य यस्यैतानि भिषग्वरैः |
लक्षणानि च दृश्यन्ते न दद्यादत्र भेषजम् ||२९||

When the below mentioned symptoms are found in a patient suffering from masurika he should not be administered with medicines and should be refused treatment (since it indicates that masurika associated with these symptoms is incurable) –
cough,
hiccough,
diabetes,
high fever,
severe delirium,
restlessness,
fainting,
thirst,
burning sensation,
excessive curvature of the body (cramps, excessive yawning)
bleeding from the mouth, nose and eyes
patient breathes with severe pain and difficulty while making cooing sounds in the throat (27-29)

Other symptoms of incurability

मसूरिकाभिभूतो यो भृशं घ्राणेन निःश्वसेत् |
स भृशं त्यजति प्राणांस्तृषार्तो वायुदूषितः ||३०||

The patient of masurika who is breathing only through his nose (very shallow breathing), has severe thirst and whose vata is severely aggravated, is definitely going to die soon. (30)

Upadrava

मसूरिकान्ते शोथः स्यात् कूर्परे मणिबन्धके |
तथांऽसफलके चापि दुश्चिकित्स्यः सुदारुणः ||३१||

Complications of masurika

When at the end of masurika (last stages of masurika), if the patient develops profound swelling in the elbow, wrist and shoulder joints (shoulder blades, scapulae), the disease should be considered as incurable. (31)

इति श्रीमाधवकरविरचिते माधवनिदाने मसूरिकानिदानं समाप्तम् ||५४||

Thus ends the chapter on Masurika Nidanam in Madhava Nidana text written by Acharya Madhavakara.

55

Madhava Nidana Chapter 55 Kshudra Roga Nidanam

Ajagallika

स्निग्धाः सवर्णा ग्रन्थिता नीरुजो मुद्‌गसन्निभाः |
कफवातोत्थिता ज्ञेया बालानामजगल्लिकाः ||१||
(सु. नि. अ. १३) ||

A disease characterised by appearance of papules which are unctuous (waxy, oily), having the same colour of the skin (not discoloured), having cystic appearance (nodular), devoid of pain and resemble green gram (in size and appearance), caused by abnormal increase of kapha and vata together, especially occurring in children, is called by the name ajagallika. (1)

Yavaprakhya

यवाकारा सुकठिना ग्रथिता मांससंश्रिता |
पिडका कफवाताभ्यां यवप्रख्येति सोच्यते ||२||
(सु. नि. अ. १३) |

Papules of the size of barley, hard, nodular, localized in the muscles and caused by combined vitiation of kapha and vata is known as Yavaprakhya. (2)

Antralaji

घनामवक्त्रां पिडकामुन्नतां परिमण्डलाम् |
अन्त्रालजीमल्पपूयां तां विद्यात् कफवातजाम् ||३||
(सु. नि. अ. १३) |
A big (stout) papule without an opening, raised, round in shape, having less quantity of pus in it and caused by simultaneous aggravation of kapha and vata is known as Antralaji (or Andhalaji). (3)

Vivruta
विवृतास्यां महादाहां पक्वोदुम्बरसन्निभाम् |
विवृतामिति तां विद्यात् पित्तोत्थां परिमण्डलाम् ||४||
(सु. नि. अ. १३) |
That which has a wide opening, is associated with severe burning sensation, is of the colour (size) of a ripened udumbara fruit (Ficus glomerata), round in shape, and produced by increased pitta is known as Vivrta. (4)

Kacchapika
ग्रथिताः पञ्च वा षड्वा दारुणाः कच्छपोपमाः |
कफानिलाभ्यां पिडका ज्ञेयाः कच्छपिका बुधैः ||५||
(सु. नि. अ. १३) |
Five or six piḍakaas (papules), nodular (hard), resembling the shell of a tortoise caused by increased kapha and vaata together is named as Kacchapika by the wise. (5)

Valmika
ग्रीवांसकक्षाकरपाददेशे सन्धौ गले वा त्रिभिरेव दोषैः |
ग्रन्थिः स वल्मीकवदक्रियाणां जातः क्रमेणैव गतः प्रवृद्धिम् ||६||
मुखैरनेकैः स्रुतितोदवद्भिर्विसर्पवत् सर्पति चोन्नताग्रैः |
वल्मीकमाहुर्भिषजो विकारं निष्प्रत्यनीकं चिरजं विशेषात् ||७||
A granthi (tumour / cystic swelling) caused by increase of all the three doshas together, resembling an ants' hill, appear in the neck, shoulder (shoulder blade, scapular region), axilla (arm pits), hands, feet, bony joints or throat regions. If this is not treated properly on time, it gradually increases in size. It will have many mouths (openings) discharging fluids, with pricking pain, spreading to other parts of the body like visarpa (erysipelas), with pointed sprouts. Such a chronic disease (which has not been treated for a long time) is incurable and has been named as Valmika by

the wise physicians. (6-7)

Indraviddha

पद्मकर्णिकवन्मध्ये पिडकाभिः समाचिताम् |
इन्द्रविद्धां तु तां विद्याद्वातपित्तोत्थितां भिषक् ||८||
(सु. नि. अ. १३) |

Small pidakaas (papules) spread out in the centre, resembling the central part of a lotus flower – which consists of seeds of lotus centered in a capsule, caused by increased vata and pitta together is known to physicians as Indraviddha. (8)

Gardhabhika

मण्डलं वृत्तमुत्सन्नं सरक्तं पिडकाचितम् |
रुजाकरीं गर्दभिकां तां विद्याद्वातपित्तजाम् ||९||

Round, elevated, red mandalas (patches), studded with small pidakas (papules) causing pain is known as Gardhabhika. This condition is caused by vatapitta – vata and pitta increased together. (9)

Pasanagardabha

वातश्लेष्मसमुद्भूतः श्वयथुर्हनुसन्धिजः |
स्थिरो मन्दरुजः स्निग्धो ज्ञेयः पाषाणगर्दभः ||१०||

A sotha (swelling) which is caused due to simultaneous vitiation of vata and kapha, manifesting in the joint of the lower jaw, which is fixed (hard), has mild pain and is unctuous (greasy, oily appearance) is known as Paasanagardabha (10).

Panasika

कर्णस्याभ्यन्तरे जातां पिडकामुग्रवेदनाम् |
स्थिरां पनसिकां तां तु विद्याद्वातकफोत्थिताम् ||११||

A pidaka (papule) occurring inside the ear, associated with severe pain, is fixed (hard) and caused by increased vata and kapha together is known as Panasika. (11)

Jalagardabha

विसर्पवत् सर्पति यः शोथस्तनुरपाकवान् |
दाहज्वरकरः पित्तात् स ज्ञेयो जालगर्दभः ||१२||
(सु. नि. अ. १३) |

A thin swelling which spreads quickly like visarpa (herpes, erysipelas), without undergoing suppuration (without pus being formed) and associated with burning sensation and fever, caused by increased pitta is known as Jalagardabha. (12)

Irivellika

पिडकामुत्तमाङ्गस्थां वृत्तामुग्ररुजाज्वराम् |
सर्वात्मिकां सर्वलिङ्गां जानीयादिरिवेल्लिकाम् ||१३||

A pidaka (papule) which occurs on the head, round, associated with severe pain, fever, caused by all the three doshas and having symptoms of increase of all the three doshas together, is known as Irivellika. (13)

Kaksha

बाहुपार्श्वांसकक्षेषु कृष्णस्फोटां सवेदनाम् |
पित्तप्रकोपसम्भूतां कक्षामित्यभिनिर्दिशेत् ||१४||
(सु. नि. अ. १३) |

Black coloured painful sphota (vesicle) appearing on arms, flanks, or sides of the arms, shoulders (shoulder blade, scapular region), or axillae, caused due to increase of pitta is known as Kaksa. (14)

Gandhamala

एकामेतादृशीं दृष्ट्वा पिडकां स्फोटसन्निभाम् |
त्वग्गतां पित्तकोपेन गन्धमालां प्रचक्षते ||१५||
(सु. नि. अ. १३) |

A single papule which is similar to the above-mentioned vesicle (which is similar to that explained in Kaksa – in the above context) manifesting superficially on the skin, which bursts out and is caused by increased pitta is called Gandhamala. (15)

Agnirohini

कक्षभागेषु ये स्फोटा जायन्ते मांसदारणाः |
अन्तर्दाहज्वरकरा दीप्तपावकसन्निभाः ||१६||
सप्ताहाद्वा दशाहाद्वा पक्षाद्वा हन्ति मानवम् |
तामग्निरोहिणीं विद्यादसाध्यां सर्वदोषजाम् ||१७||
(सु. नि. अ. १३) |

Sphotas (vesicles) developing in the axillae, which tears or bursts (burrow) deep into the muscles (and destroy them), associated with severe burning sensation inside the body and fever as if being enveloped by burning fire (being burnt by fire), which kills the patient within seven, ten or fifteen days is known as Agnirohini. It is caused by all the three doshas (aggravated together) and is said to be incurable. (16-17)

Chippa

नखमांसमधिष्ठाय वायुः पित्तः च देहिनाम् |
कुर्वते दाहपाकौ च तं व्याधिं चिप्पमादिशेत् ||१८||
तदेवाल्पतरैर्दोषैः परुषं कुनखं वदेत् ||१९||
(सु. नि. अ. १३) |

Vata and pitta which have undergone increase together get lodged in the muscles in and around the nails and produce burning sensation and suppuration (formation of pus) therein. This disease is called as Chippa. Kunakha is a similar condition caused by mild increase of doshas. (18-19)

Anusayi

गम्भीरामल्पसंरम्भां सवर्णामुपरिस्थिताम् |
पादस्यानुशयीं तां तु विद्यादन्तःप्रपाकिनीम् ||२०||
(सु. नि. अ. १३) |

A mild swelling which occurs on the upper portion of the foot and suppurates (produces pus) from deep inside and thus deep seated, has same colour of the skin (no discolouration), is known as Anusayi. (20)

Vidarika

विदारीकन्दवद्वृत्ता कक्षावङ्क्षणसन्धिषु |
विदारिका भवेद्रक्ता सर्वजा सर्वलक्षणा ||२१||
(सु. नि. अ. १३) |

A round papule resembling vidarikanda (tuber of Pueraria tuberosa), manifesting in the joints around axillae or groins, red in colour, caused by and presenting the symptoms of all the three doshas together is known as Vidarika. (21)

Sarkararbudam

प्राप्य मांससिरास्नायूः श्लेष्मा मेदस्तथाऽनिलः |
ग्रन्थिं करोत्यसौ भिन्नो मधुसर्पिर्वसानिभम् ||२२||

स्रवत्यास्रावमनिलस्तत्र वृद्धिं गतः पुनः |
मांसं संशोष्य ग्रथितां शर्करां जनयेत्ततः ||२३||
दुर्गन्धि क्लिन्नमत्यर्थं नानावर्णं ततः सिराः |
स्रवन्ति रक्तं सहसा तं विद्याच्छर्करार्बुदम् ||२४||
(सु. नि. अ. १३) |

Kapha, medas and vata undergoing increase invade the muscles, veins and ligaments (tendons, nerves), and produce a granthi (cystic swelling, tumour). When it bursts open discharges (exudates) resembling honey, ghee or muscle fat flow out of it. In due course of time, the vata aggravated (as an effect of destruction of tissues) dries up the muscles and produces small nodules which appear like sand particles in the muscles. Due to this, the veins instantly discharge excessive foul-smelling blood, containing watery content and of different colours. This condition is called as Sarkararbuda. (22-24)

Padadari

परिक्रमणशीलस्य वायुरत्यर्थरूक्षयोः |
पादयोः कुरुते दारीं पाददारीं तमादिशेत् ||२५||
(सु. नि. अ. १३) |

In persons who are in the habit of walking too much (on rough ground without footwear), the vata gets aggravated and produces fissures in the extremely dried (soles of the) feet. This condition is known as Padadari. (25)

Kadara

शर्करोन्मथिते पादे क्षते वा कण्टकादिभिः |
ग्रन्थिः कोलवदुत्सन्नो जायते कदरं हि तत् ||२६||
(सु. नि. अ. १३) |

When the foot gets pressed by (due to walking on) gravel or rough stones (without footwear) or gets injured (due to prick by) thorns etc, small (cystic) raised swelling of the size of a jujube fruit (Ziziphus jujuba) develop on (the sole) them. This condition is known as Kadara. (26)

Alasa

क्लिन्नाङ्गुल्यन्तरौ पादौ कण्डूदाहरुजान्वितौ |
दुष्टकर्दमसंस्पर्शादलसं तं विभावयेत् ||२७||

(सु. नि. अ. १३) |

Alasa is a disease characterized by ulcers formed between the toes from which discharges (exudation) occur (dampness between the toes), associated with itching, burning sensation and pain. This is caused by contact with contaminated slush. (27)

Indralupta

रोमकूपानुगं पित्तं वातेन सह मूर्छितम् |
प्रच्यावयति रोमाणि ततः श्लेष्मा सशोणितः ||२८||
रुणद्धि रोमकूपांस्तु ततोऽन्येषामसम्भवः |
तदिन्द्रलुप्तं खालित्यं रुह्येति च विभाव्यते ||२९||
(सु. नि. अ. १३) |

Increased pitta (Bhrajaka subtype) presents at the root of the body hairs, on getting association with (increased) vata, causes the hairs to fall off. Following this, increased kapha and blood together block the hair follicles (pores). This will not allow the new hairs to grow. This condition is known as Indralupta, Khalitya or Ruhya. (28-29)

Darunaka

दारुणा कण्डुरा रूक्षा केशभूमिः प्रपाट्यते |
कफमारुतकोपेन विद्याद्दारुणकं तु तम् ||३०||
(सु. नि. अ. १३) |

The skin on the scalp gets cracked, becomes hard (rough) and dry and will itch due to increase of kapha and vata together. This is known as Darunaka. (30)

Arumshika

अरूंषि बहुवक्त्राणि बहुक्लेदीनि मूर्ध्नि तु |
कफासृक्क्रिमिकोपेन नृणां विद्यादरूंषिकाम् ||३१||
(सु. नि. अ. १३) |

Small ulcers with many openings manifesting on the skin of the scalp, having discharges, caused due to aggravation of kapha, blood and worms (bacteria, infection) are called as Arumsika. (31)

Palita

क्रोधशोककश्रमकृतः शरीरोष्मा शिरोगतः |

पित्तं च केशान् पचति पलितं तेन जायते ||३२||
(सु. नि. अ. १३) |
The heat of the body produced by frequent bouts of anger, grief and physical strain (fatigue) reach the head along with increased pitta and make the hairs grey. This condition in which there is greying of hairs is known as palita. (32)

Yuvanapidaka

शाल्मलीकण्टकप्रख्याः कफमारुतरक्तजाः |
युवानपिडका यूनां विज्ञेया मुखदूषिकाः ||३३||
(सु. नि. अ. १३) |३४|
Papules resembling the sprouts (thorns, spikes) on the bark of salmali tree (Bombax malabaricum) appear on the face of adolescents caused by increase of kapha, vata and blood together is known as yuvanapidaka or mukhsdusika. (33)

Padminikantaka

कण्टकैराचितं वृत्तं मण्डलं पाण्डुकण्डुरम् |
पद्मिनीकण्टकप्रख्यैस्तदाख्यं कफवातजम् ||३४||
(सु. नि. अ. १३) |
Circular, pale (white) and itchy patches, studded with papules resembling thorn like projections of lotus flower, caused by increased kapha and vata together is called as Padminikantaka. (34)

Jatumani

सममुत्सन्नमरुजं मण्डलं कफरक्तजम् |
सहजं लक्ष्म चैकेषां लक्ष्यो जतुमणिस्तु सः ||३५||
(सु. नि. अ. १३) |
A congenital, even or slightly elevated, painless patch on the skin caused by increased kapha and rakta (blood) together is known as jatumani. According to the opinion of other experts it is called Laksma / Janmajata Lakshana. (35)

Masaka

अवेदनं स्थिरं चैव यस्मिन् गात्रे प्रदृश्यते |
माषवत्कृष्णमुत्सन्नमनिलान्मषकं तु तत् ||३६|| (सु. नि. अ. १३) |

Painless, fixed (immovable), elevated patches (nodules), black like a black-gram, appearing on the body and caused by increased vata are called as Masaka. (36)

Tilakalaka

कृष्णानि तिलमात्राणि नीरुजानि समानि च |
वातपित्तकफोच्छोषात्तान् विद्यात्तिलकालकान् ||३७||
(सु. नि. अ. १३) |

Black, painless, even (not raised above the level of the skin) spots resembling sesame seeds, is known as Tilakälaka. They are caused when kapha is dried by increased vata and pittta in the skin. (37)

Nyaccha

महद्वा यदि वा चाल्पं श्यावं वा यदि वाऽसितम् |
नीरुजं मण्डलं गात्रे न्यच्छमित्यभिधीयते ||३८||
(सु. नि. अ. १३) |

Broad (big) or small, blue or black, painless patches manifested on the skin is known as Nycha. (38)

Vyanga

क्रोधायासप्रकुपितो वायुः पित्तेन संयुतः |
मुखमागत्य सहसा मण्डलं विसृजत्यतः ||३९||
नीरुजं तनुकं श्यावं मुखे व्यङ्गं तमादिशेत् |
(सु. नि. अ. १३) |

Vata undergoes increase due to anger and physical exertion, associated with pitta gets localized in the face and would suddenly produce painless, thin, black (blackish blue) patches on the skin. This condition is known as Vyanga. (39)

Nilika

कृष्णमेवङ्गुणं गात्रे मुखे वा नीलिकां विदुः ||४०||

Similar black patches appearing on the face as well as on other parts of the body are known as Nilika. (40)

Parivartika

मर्दनात् पीडनाद्वाऽति तथैवाप्यभिघाततः |

मेढ्रचर्म यदा वायुर्भजते सर्वतश्चरन् ||४१||
तदा वातोपसृष्टत्वात्तच्चर्म परिवर्तते |
मणेरधस्तात् कोशश्च ग्रन्थिरूपेण लम्बते ||४२||
सरुजां वातसम्भूतां तां विद्यात् परिवर्तिकाम् |
सकण्डूः कठिना वापि सैव श्लेष्मसमुत्थिता ||४३||
(सु. नि. अ. १३) |

Due to too much indulgence in rubbing (hard friction) or squeezing (the penis) or by injury (to the penis or its skin), the vayu which is travelling throughout the body gets aggravated and reaches the skin on the penis and gets lodged therein. Being affected by the vitiated vata, the skin of the penis becomes upturned. The sac of the skin (prepuce) hangs under the glans penis in the form of a knot (appears like a cystic swelling). This condition is called parivartika. It causes pain if vata is predominant. If kapha is predominant in the same condition, it causes itching and hardness. (41-43)

Avapatika

अल्पीयःखां यदा हर्षाद्बलाद्गच्छेत् स्त्रियं नरः |
हस्ताभिघातादपि वा चर्मण्युद्वर्तिते बलात् ||४४||
यस्यावपाट्यते चर्म तां विद्यादवपाटिकाम् |
(सु. नि. अ. १३) |

When the man has forcible (aggressive, violent) coitus with a woman who has narrow vaginal opening due to extreme excitation or when he masturbates hard, forcibly with his hand, the skin of the glans penis forcibly gets upturned and eventually gets torn. This condition is known as Avapatika. (44-45)

Niruddhaprakasa

वातोपसृष्टे मेढ्रे वै चर्म संश्रयते मणिम् ||४५||
मणिश्चर्मोपनद्धस्तु मूत्रस्रोतो रुणद्धि च |
निरुद्धप्रकशे तस्मिन् मन्दधारमवेदनम् ||४६||
मूत्रं प्रवर्तते जन्तोर्मणिर्विव्रियते न च |
निरुद्धप्रकशं विद्यात् सरुजं वातसम्भवम् ||४७||
(सु. नि. अ. १३) |

Due to the effect of abnormally increased vata, the skin over the glans penis covers the glans tightly. The glans thus covered tightly by the skin will block the passage of urine. In this condition the urine flows out in slow streams and without any pain. The glans is always covered by the skin. This painful condition caused by increased vata is known as Niruddhaprakasa. (46-47)

Sanniruddhaguda

वेगसन्धारणाद्वायुर्विहतो गुदसंश्रितः |
निरुणद्धि महास्रोतः सूक्ष्मद्वारं करोति च ||४८||
मार्गस्य सौक्ष्म्यात् कृच्छ्रेण पुरीषं तस्य गच्छति |
सन्निरुद्धगुदं व्याधिमेतं विद्यात् सुदारुणम् ||४९||
(सु. नि. अ. १३) |

The vata which has got aggravated due to constant indulgence in suppression of the urge for defecation and fart (flatus) would reach the anal region (rectum) and causes blockage of the mahasrotas (rectal passage, colon) and causes narrowing of its opening (lumen). Due to the narrowing of the outlet (opening), the faeces is eliminated with difficulty. This highly distressing condition is known by the name sanniruddhaguda. (48-49)

Ahiputanaka

शकृन्मूत्रसमायुक्तेऽधौतेऽपाने शिशोर्भवेत् |
स्विन्ने वाऽस्नाप्यमाने वा कण्डू रक्तकफोद्भवा ||५०||
कण्डूयनात्ततः क्षिप्रं स्फोटः स्रावश्च जायते |
एकीभूतं व्रणैर्घोरं तं विद्यादहिपूतनम् ||५१||
(सु. नि. अ. १३) |

When the faeces and urine in and around the anal region of the infants are not cleansed (washed) properly or when the anal region is not washed in spite of sweating in that area there develops itching in that region caused due to increased blood and kapha. When scratched due to itching, it quickly produces pustules and discharges (exuding pustules). The ulcers of these pustules join together to form an intractable ulcer. This condition is known as Ahiputana. (50-51)

Vrushana kacchu

स्नानोत्सादनहीनस्य मलो वृषणसंस्थितः |
यदा प्रक्लिद्यते स्वेदात् कण्डूं जनयते तदा ||५२||
कण्डूयनात्ततः क्षिप्रं स्फोटः स्रावश्च जायते |
प्राहुर्वृषणकच्छूं तां श्लेष्मरक्तप्रकोपजाम् ||५३||

(सु. नि. अ. १३) |
In persons who do not take bath or oil massage regularly every day, the dirt accumulated on the skin of the scrotum gets wet on getting into contact (mixed with) with the sweat therein and produces itching. This condition is known as Vrsanakacchu. It is caused by simultaneous aggravation of kapha and rakta (blood). (52-53)

Gudabhramsa

प्रवाहणातीसाराभ्यां निर्गच्छति गुदं बहिः |
रूक्षदुर्बलदेहस्य गुदभ्रंशं तमादिशेत् ||५४||
(सु. नि. अ. १३) |
In persons who are dry (emaciated) and weak, the anus (muscles of anus) comes out due to (indulgence in) straining at defecation or due to (frequent episodes of) diarrhoea. This condition is known as Gudabhramsa. (54)

Varahadamstra / Sukaradamstra

सदाहो रक्तपर्यन्तस्त्वक्पाकी तीव्रवेदनः |
कण्डूमाञ्ज्वरकारी च स स्याच्छूकरदंष्ट्रकः ||५५||
The disease characterized by manifestation of skin ulcer with red edge, associated with severe burning sensation, suppuration, severe pain, itching and fever is known as Sakaradamstraka. (55)

इति श्रीमाधवकरविरचिते माधवनिदाने क्षुद्ररोगनिदानं समाप्तम् ||५५||
Thus ends the chapter on Kshudra Roga Nidanam in Madhava Nidana text written by Acharya Madhavakara.

56

Madhava Nidana Chapter 56 Mukha Roga Nidanam

Mukharoga Samanya Hetu

आनूपपिशितक्षीरदधिमत्स्यातिसेवनात् |
मुखमध्ये गदान् कुर्युः क्रुद्धा दोषाः कफोत्तराः ||१||

General Etiological Factors of 'Diseases of the Mouth'

Due to excessive indulgence in the foods prepared with meat of animals and birds of aquatic regions, milk, curds and fish, the doshas with the predominance of kapha would undergo abnormal increase and produce diseases of the mouth. (1)

Vataja Oshta Roga

कर्कशौ परुषौ स्तब्धौ सम्प्राप्तानिलवेदनौ |
दाल्येते परिपाट्यते ओष्ठौ मारुतकोपतः ||२||
(सु. नि. अ. १६) |

When vata gets increased in the lips, the lips become rough, hard, and immobile. There would be pain of vata nature (vata type of pain). Cracks and fissures appear on the lips. (2)

Pittaja Oshta Roga

चीयेते पिडकाभिश्च सरुजाभिः समन्ततः |
सदाहपाकपिडकौ पीताभासौ च पित्ततः ||३||

(सु. नि. अ. १६) |

In the disease of the lips caused by increase of pitta (in the lips), the lips are covered with painful papules along with burning sensation and suppuration. There is yellowish discoloration of the lips. (3)

Kaphaja Oshta Roga

सवर्णाभिश्च चीयेते पिडकाभिरवेदनौ |
भवतस्तु कफादोष्ठौ पिच्छिलौ शीतलौ गुरू ||४||
(सु. नि. अ. १६) |

When kapha gets abnormally increased in the lips, papules having colour of the skin (no discolouration) and are devoid of pain (slightly painful) develop on the lips. The lips are sticky, cold and heavy. (4)

Sannipataja Osta Roga

सकृत्कृष्णौ सकृत्पीतौ सकृच्छ्वेतौ तथैव च |
सन्निपातेन विज्ञेयावनेकपिडकाचितौ ||५||
(सु. नि. अ. १६) |

In the disease of the lips caused by simultaneous aggravation of all the three doshas the lips sometimes appear black, sometimes yellow and white at other times. Many types of pidakas (papules) will also appear on the lips. (5)

Raktaja Oshta Rog

खर्जूरफलवर्णाभिः पिडकाभिर्निपीडितौ |
रक्तोपसृष्टौ रुधिरं स्रवतः शोणितप्रभौ ||६||
(सु. नि. अ. १६) |

When the lips are affected by vitiated blood, papules resembling the fruits of date-palm (Phoenix sylvestris) in appearance, which discharge blood and are red in colour, develop on the lips. (6)

Mamsaja Oshta Rog

गुरू स्थूलौ मांसदुष्टौ मांसपिण्डवदुद्गतौ |
जन्तवश्चात्र मूर्छन्ति नरस्योभयतो मुखात् ||७||
(सु. नि. अ. १६) |

When the lips are contaminated by the muscles, they become heavy and thick and raised like lumps of muscles. Worms are formed on both sides of the mouth. (7)

Medoja Oshta Roga

सर्पिर्मण्डप्रतीकाशौ मेदसा कण्डुरौ गुरू |
अच्छं स्फटिकसङ्काशमास्रावं स्रवतो भृशम् ||८||
(सु. नि. अ. १६) |
तयोर्व्रणो न संरोहेन्मृदुत्वं च न गच्छति |९|

If the lips are contaminated by vitiated medas (fat), the lips appear like the fluid portion of the ghee, develop itching and heaviness, discharges fluids which are clear like spatika and are colourless in large quantities. The ulcers formed from this neither heal easily nor become soft. (8)

Abhighataja Oshta Roga

क्षतजाभौ विदीर्येते पाट्येते चाभिघाततः ||९||
ग्रथितौ च तथा स्यातामोष्ठौ कण्डूसमन्वितौ |१०|
(सु. नि. अ. १६) |

When the disease of the lips has occurred due to the injury (to the lips), the lips will be cut and become reddish as occurs in case of injury. They are cut or torn, will have lumps and will have itching. (9)

Dantamulagata Rogas (Diseases of the gums)

Sitada

शोणितं दन्तवेष्टेभ्यो यस्याकस्मात् प्रवर्तते |
दुर्गन्धीनि सकृष्णानि प्रक्लेदीनि मृदूनि च ||१०||
दन्तमांसानि शीर्यन्ते पचन्ति च परस्परम् |
शीतादो नाम स व्याधिः कफशोणितसम्भवः ||११||
(सु. नि. अ. १६) |

The disease in which bleeding occurs suddenly from the gums without any reason, the gums become foul smelling, black, wet (with discharges) and smooth, the muscles tear off (detach) and start suppurating each other, and is produced by abnormal increase of kapha and rakta (blood) is known as Sitada. (10-11)

Dantapupputaka

दन्तयोस्त्रिषु वा यस्य श्वयथुर्जायते महान् |

दन्तपुप्पुटको नाम स व्याधिः कफरक्तजः ||१२||
(सु. नि. अ. १६) |
When severe swelling occurs in the gums surrounding two or three gums, caused by abnormal increase of kapha and blood together is known by the name dantapupputaka. (12)

Dantavesta
स्रवन्ति पूयरुधिरं चला दन्ता भवन्ति च |
दन्तवेष्टः स विज्ञेयो दुष्टशोणितसम्भवः ||१३||
(सु. नि. अ. १६) |
The disease in which pus and blood (pus mixed blood) is discharged from the gums and the teeth begin to shake is known as dantavesta. This condition is caused by bad (contaminated) blood. (13)

Saushira
श्वयथुर्दन्तमूलेषु रुजावान् कफरक्तजः |
लालास्रावी स विज्ञेयः शौषिरो नाम नामतः ||१४||
(सु. नि. अ. १६)
A swelling which occurs at the root of the tooth caused by increased kapha and blood together is painful and causes free flow of saliva is known as sausira.

Mahasausira
दन्ताश्चलन्ति वेष्टेभ्यस्तालु चाप्यवदीर्यते |
यस्मिन् स सर्वजो व्याधिर्महाशौषिरसञ्ज्ञितः ||१५||
(सु. नि. अ. १६)
When in sausira (above explained condition), the teeth start getting loose from the gums and shaking, fissures occur in the palate (apart from the other symptoms of sausira), which is known as Mahasausira. This condition is caused by simultaneous increase of all the three doshas (together). (15)

Paridara
दन्तमांसानि शीर्यन्ते यस्मिन् ष्ठीवति चाप्यसृक् |
पितासृक्कफजो व्याधिर्ज्ञेयः परिदरो हि सः ||१६||
(सु. नि. अ. १६) |
The disease in which the gums undergo decomposition and causes frequent

spitting of blood is called paridara. It is caused by an increase of pitta, blood and kapha together. (16)

Upakusa

वेष्टेषु दाहः पाकश्च ताभ्यां दन्ताश्चलन्ति च |
यस्मिन् सोपकुशो नाम पित्तरक्तकृतो गदः ||१७||
(सु. नि. अ. १६) |

The disease in which there is burning sensation and suppuration in the gums and due to these the teeth become loose and shaking. This disease caused due to the abnormal increase in pitta and blood together is known by the name upakusa. (17)

Vaidarbha

घृष्टेषु दन्तमांसेषु संरम्भो जायते महान् |
चला भवन्ति दन्ताश्च स वैदर्भोऽभिघातजः ||१८||
(सु. नि. अ. १६) |

The disease in which the gums get frayed (grazed or rubbed) develop severe swelling, pain and burning sensation and the teeth become loose and shaky is called vaidarbha. This condition is caused due to trauma. (18)

Khalivardhana

मारुतेनाधिको दन्तो जायते तीव्रवेदनः |
खलिवर्धनसञ्ज्ञोऽसौ जाते रुक् च प्रशाम्यति ||१९||
(सु. नि. अ. १६) |

Due to the aggravation of vata an extra tooth erupts causing severe pain during its eruption. Once the extra tooth erupts, the pain subsides. This condition is known by the name khalivardhana. (19)

Karala

शनैः शनैः प्रकुरुते वायुर्दन्तसमाश्रितः |
करालान् विकटान् दन्तान् करालो न स सिध्यति ||२०||

The vata located in the teeth undergoes an increase and gradually (over a period of time) makes the teeth irregular and ugly. This condition is known as Karala. It is incurable and does not respond to any treatment. (20)

Adhimamsa

हानव्ये पश्चिमे दन्ते महाञ्छोथो महारुजः |

लालास्रावी कफकृतो विज्ञेयः सोऽधिमांसकः |२१|
(सु. नि. अ. १६) |
The condition in which a severe swelling appears in the gums surrounding the last molar tooth, which is highly painful and causes dribbling of saliva is known as adhimamsaka. It is caused by increased kapha. (21)

Dantanadi
दन्तमूलगता नाड्यः पञ्च ज्ञेया यथेरिताः ||२१||
(सु. नि. अ. १६) |
There are five kinds of nadis (sinus) which would manifest in the root of the teeth (gums). These are similar to those described previously (Nadivrana – sinus ulcers). (21)
Note - The five types of dantanadis are – vataja, pittaja, kaphaja, sannipataja and shalyaja.

Dantagata Rogas (Diseases of the teeth)

Dalana
दीर्यमाणेष्विव रुजा यस्य दन्तेषु जायते |
दालनो नाम स व्याधिः सदागतिनिमित्तजः ||२२||
(सु. नि. अ. १६) |
A condition of the teeth in which there is severe pain in the tooth as if they are breaking open or bursting is called Dalana. It is caused by increased vata. (22)

Krimidantaka
कृष्णच्छिद्रश्चलः स्रावी ससंरम्भो महारुजः |
अनिमित्तरुजो वाताद्विज्ञेयः क्रिमिदन्तकः ||२३||
(सु. नि. अ. १६) |
The condition in which the tooth which has black holes in them and are shaky (loose), which have discharges, swelling and severe pain which comes on without any apparent cause and caused by vitiated vata is called as krimidanta / krimidantaka. (23)

Bhanjanaka
वक्त्रं वक्रं भवेद्यस्य दन्तभङ्गश्च जायते |
कफवातकृतो व्याधिः स भञ्जनकसञ्ज्ञितः ||२४||

(सु. नि. अ. १६) |

A condition, in which the face assumes an irregular shape and the teeth get broken, is caused by increased kapha and vata together is called as Bhanjanaka. (24)

Dantaharsa

शीतरूक्षप्रवाताम्लस्पर्शानामसहा द्विजाः |
पित्तमारुतकोपेन दन्तहर्षः स नामतः ||२५||

A condition wherein due to the increased pitta and vata the teeth become incapable of tolerating the touch (contact of) of cold and dry foods, swift cold breeze and sour things (foods and drinks) is called by the name dantaharsa. (25)

Dantasarkara

मलो दन्तगतो यस्तु पित्तमारुतशोषितः |
शर्करेव खरस्पर्शा सा ज्ञेया दन्तशर्करा ||२६||

The dirt accumulated on the teeth gets dried up by the action of increased vata and pitta (together). This dried up dirt becomes hard, assumes the form of gravel and accumulates on the teeth. This condition is called as Dantasarkara. (26)

Kapalika

कपालेष्विव दीर्यत्सु दन्तानां सैव शर्करा |
कपालिकेति विज्ञेया सदा दन्तविनाशिनी ||२७||

Kapalika is a more complicated version of dantasarkara (discussed above). Here the pieces of teeth along with solidified and accumulated hard dirt (as in sarkara) on them, which appear like pieces of earthen vessel (big flakes of accretions) peel off along with parts of the tooth, and finally destroy the teeth. This condition is known as Kapalika. (27)

Syavadantaka

योऽसृङ्मिश्रेण पित्तेन दग्धो दन्तस्त्वशेषतः |
श्यावतां नीलतां वाऽपि गतः स श्यावदन्तकः ||२८||
(सु. नि. अ. १६) |

A condition in which the tooth becomes black of blue in colour, being burnt by the increased pitta combined with the vitiated blood is known as syavadantaka. (28)

Danta Vidradhi

दन्तमांसे मलैः सास्रैर्बाह्यान्तः श्वयथुर्गुरुः |
सदाहरुक् स्रवेद्भिन्नः पूयास्रं दन्तविद्रधिः ||२९||

A severe (big) swelling occurs inside and outside the gums caused by the vitiated blood and all the three increased doshas. It is associated with burning sensation and pain. On bursting open it discharges pus mixed with blood. This is called as Danta Vidradhi. (29)

Diseases of the tongue
Jihvagata Rogas

Jihvakantaka

जिह्वाऽनिलेन स्फुटिता प्रसुप्ता भवेच्च शाकच्छदनप्रकाशा |
पित्तेन दह्यत्युपचीयते च दीर्घैः सरक्तैरपि कण्टकैश्च |
कफेन गुर्वी बहुला चिता च मांसोच्छ्रयैः शाल्मलिकण्टकाभैः ||३०||
(सु. नि. अ. १६) |

Vataja Jihvakantaka – When increased vata affects the tongue it would become fissured, numb (loss of sensation) – loss of taste perception, and would resemble a leaf of a tree (rough, coarse).
Pittaja Jihvakantaka – When increased pitta affects the tongue there would be burning sensation in the tongue. The tongue would become studded with red coloured long thorny projections.
Kaphaja Jihvakantaka – When increased kapha affects the tongue, the tongue would become heavy, thick, and will be studded with muscular sprouts resembling those of Shalmali tree (Bombax malabaricum). (30)

Alasa

जिह्वातले यः श्वयथुः प्रगाढः सोऽलाससञ्ज्ञः कफरक्तमूर्तिः |
जिह्वां स तु स्तम्भयति प्रवृद्धो मूले च जिह्वा भृशमेति पाकम् ||३१||
(सु. नि. अ. १६) |

A condition in which a profound swelling occurs beneath the tongue caused by combined aggravation of kapha and rakta (blood) is called Alasa. This swelling would increase in size and cause stiffness (incapable of movement) of the tongue and also would cause severe suppuration at the root of the tongue. (31)

Upajihvika

जिह्वाग्ररूपः श्वयथुर्हि जिह्वामुन्नम्य जातः कफरक्तमूलः |
लालाकरः कण्डुयुतः सचोषः सा तूपजिह्वा पठिता भिषग्भिः ||३२||
(सु. नि. अ. १६) |

A condition in which a severe swelling caused by increased kapha and blood together, having the appearance of the tip of the tongue, is formed beneath the tongue and lifts up the tongue. This disease is called as upajihvika. This is associated with excessive salivation, itching and burning as if the tongue is in direct contact with the fire. (32)

Talugata Rogas (Diseases of the palate)

Kantasundi

श्लेष्मासृग्भ्यां तालुमूले प्रवृद्धो दीर्घः शोथो ध्मातबस्तिप्रकाशः |
तृष्णाकासश्वासकृत्तं वदन्ति व्याधिं वैद्याः कण्ठशुण्डीति नाम्ना ||३३||
(सु. नि. अ. १६) |

An elongated swelling resembling a bag inflated with air gets manifested at the root of the palate, caused by kapha and blood getting increased together, associated with thirst, cough and dyspnoea (breathing difficulty). This disease of the palate is called by the name Kanthasundi. (33)

Tundikeri

शोथः स्थूलस्तोददाहप्रपाकी प्रागुक्ताभ्यां तुण्डिकेरी मता तु |३४|
(सु. नि. अ. १६) |

The swelling which is caused by kapha and blood just like the condition explained above (kanthasundi) will be known as Tundikeri if it becomes thicker and is associated with pricking pain, burning sensation and suppuration. (34)

Adhrusa

मृदुः शोथो लोहितः शोणितोत्थो ज्ञेयोऽध्रुषः सज्वरस्तीव्ररुक् च ||३४||
(सु. नि. अ. १६) |

A condition, in which a soft, red swelling is caused by increased blood, is accompanied with fever and severe pain is known by the name adhrusa. (34)

Kacchapa

कूर्मोन्नतोऽवेदनोऽशीघ्रजन्मा रोगो ज्ञेयः कच्छपः श्लेष्मणा तु |३५|
(सु. नि. अ. १६) |

Kachchapa manifests in the form of a rounded big swelling resembling the upper surface of the shell of a tortoise. This condition is painless and develops slowly and is caused by increased kapha. (35)

Talvarbuda and Mamsa sanghata

पद्माकारं तालुमध्ये तु शोथं विद्याद्रक्तादर्बुदं प्रोक्तलिङ्गम् ||३५||
दुष्टं मांसं नीरुजं तालुमध्ये कफाच्छूनं मांससङ्घातमाहुः |
(सु. नि. अ. १६) |

It is a swelling which resembles a lotus flower and manifests at the center of the palate and has symptoms similar to that of raktarbuda.

It is a similar swelling (same as talvarbuda) manifesting at the centre of the palate involving mamsa – contaminated muscle tissue (it is a muscular swelling or lump at the centre of the palate), caused by increased kapha and is painless. (35)

Talupupputa

नीरुक् स्थायी कोलमात्रः कफात् स्यान्मेदोयुक्तात् पुप्पुटस्तालुदेशे ||३६||
शोषोऽत्यर्थं दीर्यते चापि तालुः श्वासश्चोग्रस्तालुशोषोऽनिलाच्च |
पित्तं कुर्यात् पाकमत्यर्थघोरं तालुन्येनं तालुपाकं वदन्ति ||३७||
(सु. नि. अ. १६) |

Talupupputa

A swelling (papule) of the size of a jujube fruit (Ziziphus jujuba) which is painless, fixed (immobile), caused by combination of abnormally increased kapha and medas (fat) together, developing in the palate is called by the name talupupputa.

Talusosa

Excessive dryness and fissures occurring in the palate, caused by aggravated vata and associated with severe dyspnoea (difficulty in breathing) is known as Talusosa.

Talupaka

Pitta aggravated in the palate causes severe and dreadful suppuration (in the palate). This is known as Talupaka. (36-37)

Galagata Rogas (Diseases of the throat:)

Rohini

गलेऽनिलः पित्तकफौ च मूर्च्छितौ प्रदूष्य मांसं च तथैव शोणितम् |
गलोपसंरोधकरैस्तथाऽङ्कुरैर्निहन्त्यसून् व्याधिरियं हि रोहिणी ||३८|| (सु. नि. अ. १६) |
जिह्वासमन्ताद्भृशवेदनास्तु मांसाङ्कुराः कण्ठनिरोधिनो ये |
सा रोहिणी वातकृता प्रदिष्टा वातात्मकोपद्रवगाढयुक्ता ||३९||
क्षिप्रोद्गमा क्षिप्रविदाहपाका तीव्रज्वरा पित्तनिमित्तजा तु |
स्रोतोविरोधिन्यचलोद्गता च स्थिराङ्कुरा या कफसम्भवा सा ||४०||
गम्भीरपाकिन्यनिवार्यवीर्या त्रिदोषलिङ्गा त्रितयोत्थिता च |
स्फोटैश्चिता पित्तसमानलिङ्गा साध्या प्रदिष्टा रुधिरात्मिका तु ||४१||
(सु. नि. अ. १६) |

Rohini and its types, symptoms

Vata, pitta and kapha getting increased in the throat (either individually or all together) would invade mamsa (muscle) and rakta (blood) and produce sprouts inside the throat subsequently causing obstruction of the throat passage and death. This disease is called Rohini.

Vataja Rohini – In vata predominant rohini there will be severe pain all over the tongue, muscular sprouts which cause obstruction to the throat, and severe complications (and other symptoms) of vata increase.

Pittaja Rohini – In pitta predominant rohini, there is quick appearance of sprouts, burning sensation and suppuration, and is associated with high fever.

Kaphaja Rohini – In kapha predominant rohini, the sprouts are immobile, big in size and fixed. They cause total obstruction of the throat.

Sannipataja Rohini – In Rohini caused by simultaneous aggravation of all the three doshas, suppuration occurs in the deeper tissues. It will not respond to any treatment (is incurable) and presents with symptoms of aggravation of all the three doshas.

Raktaja Rohini – In rohini caused by abnormally increased blood, there will be widespread red papules and will present with symptoms of pitta increase. This condition is curable. (39-41)

Kanthasaluka

कोलास्थिमात्रः कफसम्भवो यो ग्रन्थिर्गले कण्टकशूकभूतः |
खरः स्थिरः शस्त्रनिपातसाध्यस्तं कण्ठशालूकमिति ब्रुवन्ति ||४२||
(सु. नि. अ. १६) |

A cystic swelling (tumour) of the size of seed of jujube fruit, produced by increased kapha, occurring in the throat, appearing like thorns or spikes, rough, fixed (immobile), and curable only by surgical methods is called by the name Kanthasaluka. (42)

Adhijihva

जिह्वाग्ररूपः श्वयथुः कफात्तु जिह्वोपरिष्टादपि रक्तमिश्रात् |
ज्ञेयोऽधिजिह्वः खलु रोग एष विवर्जयेदागतपाकमेनम् ||४३||
(सु. नि. अ. १६) |

A swelling which occurs above the level of (top of) the root of the tongue, resembling the tip of the tongue, caused by kapha along with blood is known as adhijihva. If the swelling is found along with suppuration, it should be refused treatment (because it is incurable). (43)

Valaya

बलाश एवायतमुन्नतं च शोथं करोत्यन्नगतिं निवार्य |
तं सर्वथैवाप्रतिवार्यवीर्यं विवर्जनीयं वलयं वदन्ति ||४४||
(सु. नि. अ. १६) |

Kapha undergoing abnormal increase produces large sized swelling in the throat causing obstruction to the passage of food. This condition is called by the name valaya. It is an intractable disease which doesn't respond to any type of treatment and hence should be refused treatment. (44)

Balasa

गले तु शोथं कुरुतः प्रवृद्धौ श्लेष्मानिलौ श्वासरुजोपपन्नम् |
मर्मच्छिदं दुस्तरमेनमाहुर्बलाशसञ्ज्ञं निपुणा विकारम् ||४५||
(सु. नि. अ. १६) |

Kapha and vata having aggravated together produces a swelling in the throat which causes difficulty in breathing and pain, which tends to destroy (damage) the marmas (vital organs or spots in the body). This disease is identified as Balasa by the experts and is difficult to treat. (45)

Ekavrnda

वृत्तोन्नतोऽन्तः श्वयथुः सदाहः सकण्डुरोऽपाक्यमृदुर्गुरुश्च |
नाम्नैकवृन्दः परिकीर्तितोऽसौ व्याधिर्बलाशक्षतजप्रसूतः ||४६||
(सु. नि. अ. १६) |

A swelling developing inside the throat, which is round, elevated, accompanied with burning sensation, itching, not suppurating, not too smooth (little hard) and heavy is known as Ekavrnda. This condition is caused by kapha and blood together. (46)

Vrinda

समुन्नतं वृत्तममन्ददाहं तीव्रज्वरं वृन्दमुदाहरन्ति |
तच्चापि पित्तक्षतजप्रकोपाज्ज्ञेयं सतोदं पवनात्मकं तु ||४७||
(सु. नि. अ. १६) |

A condition in which an elevated and rounded swelling occurs in the throat being associated with severe burning sensation and high fever is called Vrnda. This is caused by combined vitiation of pitta and blood. If vata is involved in this condition there will also be pricking pain. (47)

Shataghni

वर्तिर्घना कण्ठनिरोधिनी या चिताऽतिमात्रं पिशितप्ररोहैः |
अनेकरुक् प्राणहरी त्रिदोषाज्ज्ञेया शतघ्नी च शतघ्निरूपा ||४८||
(सु. नि. अ. १६) |

A swelling obstructing the throat studded all over with multiple muscular sprouts resembling a Sataghni (a weapon in the form of an iron ball with sharp spikes), presenting with many kinds of pain and cause death is called as Sataghni. This condition is caused by simultaneous vitiation of all the three doshas together. (48)

Galayu

ग्रन्थिर्गले त्वामलकास्थिमात्रः स्थिरोऽतिरुग्यः कफरक्तमूर्तिः |
संलक्ष्यते सक्तमिवाशनं च स शस्त्रसाध्यस्तु गलायुसञ्ज्ञः ||४९||
(सु. नि. अ. १६) |

A cystic swelling occurring in the throat which is of the size of seed of Amalaka (Phyllanthus emblica), is immobile, very painful, and caused by combined aggravation of kapha and blood is known as Galayu. Due to this, the food remains obstructed in the throat (difficulty in swallowing the food) and can be treated by surgical methods (requires surgical treatment to cure this disease). (49)

Galavidradhi

सर्वं गलं व्याप्य समुत्थितो यः शोथो रुजः सन्ति च यत्र सर्वाः |
स सर्वदोषैर्गलविद्रधिस्तु तस्यैव तुल्यः खलु सर्वजस्य ||५०||
(सु. नि. अ. १६) |

The condition in which a swelling which involves all the areas of (entire) the throat develop, which presents with different kinds of pains caused by all the doshas, is called as galavidradhi. It is caused due to simultaneous aggravation of all the three doshas and is similar to tridoshaja vidradhi. (50)

Galaugha

शोथो महानन्नजलावरोधी तीव्रज्वरो वायुगतेर्निहन्ता |
कफेन जातो रुधिरान्वितेन गले गलौघः परिकीर्त्यते तु ||५१||
(सु. नि. अ. १६) |

A profound swelling in the throat, caused by increased kapha associated with vitiated blood, which causes obstruction to swallowing of food and water, associated with severe fever and causing the movements of vata (aeration, respiration) is called by the name Galaugha. (51)

Svaraghna

यस्ताम्यमानः श्वसिति प्रसक्तं भिन्नस्वरः शुष्कविमुक्तकण्ठः |
कफोपदिग्धेष्वनिलायनेषु ज्ञेयः स रोगः श्वसनात् स्वरघ्नः ||५२||
(सु. नि. अ. १६) |

A condition in which due to the coating and subsequent obstruction of the air passages by kapha (sputum, phlegm), the patient finds difficulty in breathing along with darkness before the eyes, has broken voice, dryness of the throat and loss of movement of the throat, is known as Svaraghna. This condition is caused by vitiated vata. (52)

Mamsatana

प्रतानवान् यः श्वयथुः सुकष्टो गलोपरोधं कुरुते क्रमेण |
स मांसतानः कथितोऽवलम्बी प्राणप्रणुत् सर्वकृतो विकारः ||५३||
(सु. नि. अ. १६) |

A broad swelling which has spread out in the throat, which is troublesome (with severe painful symptoms) and gradually obstructs the throat by hanging down and eventually causes death is known as Mamsatana. This condition is caused by simultaneous increase of all the three doshas together. (53)

Vidari

सदाहतोदं श्वयथुं सुताम्रमन्तर्गले पूतिविशीर्णमांसम् |
पित्तेन विद्याद्वदने विदारीं पार्श्वे विशेषात् स तु येन शेते ||५४||

(सु. नि. अ. १६) |

A swelling which occurs inside the throat and in the mouth, having burning sensation and pricking pain, has coppery colour, the muscles surrounding which has foul smell and fall off getting detached, is caused by predominant vitiation of pita is called by the name vidari. This occurs in the side of the face and throat on which the patient usually sleeps. (54)

Sarvasara Roga / Mukhapaka

स्फोटैः सतोदैर्वदनं समन्ताद्यस्याचितं सर्वसरः स वातात् |
रक्तैः सदाहैस्तनुभिः सपीतैर्यस्याचितं चापि स पित्तकोपात् |
अवेदनैः कण्डुयुतैः सवर्णैर्यस्याचितं चापि स वै कफेन ||५५||
(सु. नि. अ. १६) |

Vataja Sarvasara / Mukhapaka – In this condition the inside of the mouth is covered by papules (sores) having pricking pain.

Pittaja Sarvasara / Mukhapaka – In this condition the inside of the mouth is covered by papules which are red or yellow in colour, thin and have a burning sensation.

Kaphaja Sarvasara / Mukhapaka – In this condition the inside of the mouth is covered by papules which are painless, have itching and are of the same colour as that of the skin (surrounding area). (54-55)

Prognosis of Oshta kopa and other conditions

ओष्ठप्रकोपे वर्ज्याः स्युर्मांसरक्तत्रिदोषजाः |
दन्तमूलेषु वर्ज्यौ च त्रिलिङ्गगतिशौषिरौ ||५६||
दन्तेषु च न सिध्यन्ति श्यावदालनभञ्जनाः |
जिह्वारोगे बलाशस्तु तालव्येष्वर्बुदं तथा ||५७||
स्वरघ्नो वलयो वृन्दो बलाशश्च विदारिका |
गलौघो मांसतानश्च शतघ्नी रोहिणी गले ||५८||
असाध्याः कीर्तिता ह्येते रोगा नव दशैव तु |
तेषु चापि क्रियां वैद्यः प्रत्याख्याय समाचरेत् ||५९||
(सु. नि. अ. १६) |

Among the diseases of the lips – ostha prakopa produced by mamsa – muscle, rakta – blood, rakta – blood and all the three doshas should be rejected and should not be treated.

Among the diseases of the gums – tridoshaja nadivrana and saushira are considered as incurable and hence should be rejected.

Among the diseases of the teeth – Syavadanta, Dalana and Bhanjanaka are incurable.
Among the diseases of the tongue – Balasha is incurable.
Among the diseases of the palate – Arbuda is incurable.
Among the diseases of the throat – Svaraghna, Valaya, vrnda, Balasha, Vidarika, Galaudha, Mamsatana, Shataghni and Rohini are considered incurable.
These nineteen diseases are incurable and the physician should consider them as unfit for treatment and reject them. (56-59)

इति श्रीमाधवकरविरचिते माधवनिदाने मुखरोगनिदानं समाप्तम् ||५६||
Thus ends the chapter on Mukha Roga Nidanam in Madhava Nidana text written by Acharya Madhavakara.

57

Madhava Nidana Chapter 57 Karna Roga Nidanam

Karnashula

समीरणः श्रोत्रगतोऽन्यथाचरन् समन्ततः शूलमतीव कर्णयोः |
करोति दोषैश्च यथास्वमावृतः स कर्णशूलः कथितो दुराचरः ||१||
(सु. उ. तं. अ. २०) |

Vata which has been enveloped by the doshas (pitta and kapha) which have undergone abnormal increase due to their own etiological factors (etiological factors causing aggravation of pitta and kapha respectively) and has moved in upward direction (abnormal movement for vata) on reaching (and getting lodged in) the ears and produces pain in the ears. This condition is called Karnashula and is difficult to treat. (1)

Karnanada

कर्णस्रोतः स्थिते वाते शृणोति विविधान् स्वरान् |
भेरीमृदङ्गशङ्खानां कर्णनादः स उच्यते ||२||

When aggravated vata gets lodged in the canals of the ears the patient would hear many kinds of abnormal sounds similar to those produced by kettle drum, cymbal or conch etc. This condition is known as Karnanada. (2)

Badhirya

यदा शब्दवहं वायुः स्रोत आवृत्य तिष्ठति |

शुद्धः श्लेष्मान्वितो वाऽपि बाधिर्यं तेन जायते ||३||
When vata either alone or in association with kapha (vata enveloped by kapha) blocks the passages of sound, the patient develops deafness. This is known as Badhirya. (3)

Karna Kshveda
वायुः पित्तादिभिर्युक्तो वेणुघोषोपमं स्वनम् |
करोति कर्णयोः क्ष्वेडं कर्णक्ष्वेडः स उच्यते ||४||
A condition in which increased vata in association with pitta and other dosha (kapha) produces constant sound in the ear resembling the sound produced by a bamboo (when air is blown in hollow bamboo shoot) or flute. This is known as Karna Kshveda. (4)

Karnasrava
शिरोऽभिघातादथवा निमज्जतो जले प्रपाकादथवाऽपि विद्रधेः |
स्रवेद्धि पूयं श्रवणोऽनिलार्दितः स कर्णसंस्राव इति प्रकीर्तितः ||५||
(सु. उ. तं. अ. २०) |
Injury to the head, drowning in water (remaining underwater for long time) or ripening of an abscess in the ears causes discharge of pus from the ears. This is associated with pains and other symptoms of vata increase. This condition is known as Karnasrava. (5)

Karnakandu
मारुतः कफसंयुक्तः कर्णकण्डूं करोति च |
पित्तोष्मशोषितः श्लेष्मा कुरुते कर्णगूथकम् ||६||
Vata in association with kapha produces Karnakandu (itching inside the ears).

Karnaguthaka
स कर्णगूथो द्रवतां गतो यदा विलायितो घ्राणमुखं प्रपद्यते |
तदा स कर्णप्रतिनाहसञ्ज्ञितो भवेद्विकारः शिरसोऽर्धभेदकृत् ||७||
(सु. उ. तं. अ. २०) |
Kapha getting dried (and solidified) by the heat of pitta produces Karṇaguthaka (hardness of the wax). (6)

Karnapratinaha

यदा तु मूर्छन्त्यथवाऽपि जन्तवः सृजन्त्यपत्यान्यथवाऽपि मक्षिकाः |
तद्व्यञ्जनत्वाच्छ्रवणो निरुच्यते भिषग्भिराद्यैः क्रिमिकर्णको गदः ||८||
(सु. उ. तं. अ. २०) |

The condition in which this wax of the ears (explained above in karnaguthaka) gets liquefied (becoming watery), and reaches the nose and mouth (and gets discharged from there) is called Karnapratinaha. The patient also suffers from a headache in one half of the head. (7)

Krimikarnaka

पतङ्गाः शतपद्यश्च कर्णस्रोतः प्रविश्य हि |
अरतिं व्याकुलत्वं च भृशं कुर्वन्ति वेदनाम् ||९||
कर्णो निस्तुद्यते तस्य तथा फरफरायते |
कीटे चरति रुक् तीव्रा निष्पन्दे मन्दवेदना ||१०||

When insects or small worms forming (entering) in the ears (due to decaying of muscles and blood), or flies producing their larva inside the ears (in the decomposed or putrefied muscles of the ears), the physicians call this disease having symptoms similar to krimiroga (worm infestation disease) as krimikarnaka. (8)

If winged insects, centipedes or other insects have entered into the canals of the ears, they produce restlessness, a sense of fear or worry and severe pain. If these insects are alive and move around in the canals of the ear, they will produce pricking pain, sounds of movement of insects (movement of insects is felt), and severe pain. The pain will be mild if the insects are not moving inside the ear canals (if insects are dead). (9-10)

Karna Vidradhi

क्षताभिघातप्रभवस्तु विद्रधिर्भवेत्तथा दोषकृतोऽपरः पुनः |
सरक्तपीतारुणमस्रमास्रवेत् प्रतोदधूमायनदाहचोषवान् ||११||
(सु. उ. तं. अ. २०) |

One type of abscess develops due to injury or trauma to (inside) the ear and the other type develops due to aggravation of doshas inside the ear. This will cause discharge of fluids (pus) of red, yellow or crimson colour accompanied with pricking pain, feeling of hot fumes (smoke) being eliminated from the ears, burning sensation and feeling of sucking like pain. This disease is called as Karna Vidradhi. (11)

Karnapaka

कर्णपाकस्तु पित्तेन कोथविक्लेदकृद्भवेत् |
कर्णविद्रधिपाकाद्वा जायते चाम्बुपूरणात् ||१२||

Due to aggravation of pitta or due to ripening of ear abscess or due to water entering the ears a disease called karnapaka is produced. It causes putrefaction and foul discharges from the ears. (12)

Putikarnaka

पूयं स्रवति पूति वा स ज्ञेयः पूतिकर्णकः |१३|

A condition in which very foul-smelling pus is discharged from the ears is called Putikarnaka.

Karnashotha, Karnarbuda, Karnarsha

कर्णशोथार्बुदार्शांसि जानीयादुक्तलक्षणैः ||१३||

The symptoms of karnashotha, karnarbuda and karnarsha are similar to sotha (swelling, oedema), arbuda (tumour) and arsha (piles) which occur elsewhere in the body. (13)

Based on dosha predominance

नादोऽतिरुक् कर्णमलस्य शोषः स्रावस्तनुश्चाश्रवणं च वातात् |
शोथः सरागो दरणं विदाहः सपीतपूतिस्रवणं च पित्तात् ||१४||
वैश्रुत्यकण्डूस्थिरशोथशुक्लस्निग्धस्रुतिः स्वल्परुजः कफाच्च |
सर्वाणि रूपाणि च सन्निपातात् स्रावश्च तत्राधिकदोषवर्णः ||१५||
(च. चि. अ. २६) |

Karnarogas based on dosha predominance

Vataja Karnaroga – In the ear diseases caused due to predominant aggravation of vata, there will be noise in the ears, severe pain, drying (and hardening) of the dirt in the ears, less discharges (discharge of thin fluids), and loss of hearing (deafness).

Pittaja Karnaroga - In the ear diseases caused due to predominant aggravation of pitta, there will be reddish swelling, tearing / blasting pain, burning sensation, and yellowish offensive discharges from the ears.

Kaphaja Karnaroga – In the ear diseases caused due to predominant aggravation of kapha, there will be hearing of abnormal sounds, itching in the ears, hard and immobile (fixed) swelling, white and unctuous discharges and mild pain.

Sannipataja Karnaroga – In the ear diseases caused due to simultaneous aggravation of all the three doshas there will be symptoms of all the three doshas and the discharges will have the colour of the predominantly aggravated dosha. (14-15)

Paripotaka

सौकुमार्याच्चिरोत्सृष्टे सहसाऽतिप्रवर्धिते |
कर्णशोथो भवेत् पाल्यां सरुजः परिपोटवान् |
कृष्णारुणनिभः स्तब्धः स वातात् परिपोटकः ||१६||
(सु. चि. अ. २५) |

Due to the delicate / tender nature (of the child) if the hole punctured on the earlobe (as a part of childhood rituals) is left unattended for a long time and in later period if one tries to dilate the orifice all of a sudden, it would cause serious swelling along with pain in the ear (earlobe) which will have black or crimson colour. This hard swelling caused by increased vata is known as Paripotaka. (16)

Utpata

गुर्वाभरणसंयोगात्ताडनाद्घर्षणादपि |
शोथः पाल्यां भवेच्छ्यावो दाहपाकरुजान्वितः ||१७||
रक्तो वा रक्तपित्ताभ्यामुत्पातः स गदो मतः |
(सु. चि. अ. २५) |

Wearing of excessively heavy ornaments in the ears, blow (injury) or friction on the ears leads to the manifestation of swelling, black or red in colour, caused by aggravation of blood and pitta together, associated with burning sensation, suppuration and pain. This condition is known as Utpata. (17)

Unmanthaka

कर्णं बलाद्वर्धयतः पाल्यां वायुः प्रकुप्यति ||१८||
कफं सङ्गृह्य कुरुते शोथं स्तब्धमवेदनम् |
उन्मन्थकः सकण्डूको विकारः कफवातजः ||१९||

By forcibly attempting to pierce the pinna of the ears and trying to enhance the orifice, vata gets aggravated in the ears (earlobe). This vata getting associated with kapha produces stiff (hard) swelling without pain. This condition is called by the name Unmanthaka. It is caused by increased kapha and vata together and is associated with itching. (18-19)

Dukhavardhana

संवर्ध्यमाने दुर्विद्धे कण्डूपाकरुजान्वितः |
शोथो भवति पाकश्च त्रिदोषो दुःखवर्धनः ||२०||
(सु. चि. अ. २५) |

When the pinna of the ear is pierced at the wrong place and when that orifice becomes bigger, it leads to the development of swelling and ripening accompanied with itching, suppuration and pain. This condition is called Dukhavardhana and is caused by increase of all the three doshas together. (20)

Parilehina

कफासृक्क्रिमयः क्रुद्धाः सर्षपाभा विसर्पिणः |
कुर्वन्ति पाल्यां पिडकाः कण्डूदाहरुजान्विताः ||२१||
कफासृक्क्रिमिसम्भूतः स विसर्पन्नितस्ततः |
लिहेत् सशष्कुलीं पालीं परिलेहीति स स्मृतः ||२२||
(सु. चि. अ. २५)

Increase of kapha and blood and presence of bacteria together produce pustules on the pinna of the ear, of the size of mustard seeds, spreading in nature, accompanied with itching, burning sensation, pain causing a disease called as Parilehi. This disease caused by increased kapha, blood and worms (bacteria) will spread all through the ears and eat off (destroy) the entire pinna and lobes. (21-22)

इति श्रीमाधवकरविरचिते माधवनिदाने कर्णरोगनिदानं समाप्तम् ||५७||

Thus ends the chapter on Karna Roga Nidanam in Madhava Nidana text written by Acharya Madhavakara.

58

Madhava Nidana Chapter 58 Nasa Roga Nidanam

Apinasa

आनह्यते यस्य विशुष्यते च प्रक्लिद्यते धूप्यति चापि नासा |
न वेत्ति यो गन्धरसांश्च जन्तुर्जुष्टं व्यवस्येदिह पीनसेन |
तं चानिलश्लेष्मभवं विकारं ब्रूयात् प्रतिश्यायसमानलिङ्गम् ||१||
(सु. उ. तं. अ. २२) |

The condition in which the nasal passage of the person is obstructed (being stuffed with kapha dried by vata), dried up or moist and feeling of raised warmth (feeling of smoke being eliminated from the nose) and the person not understand (appreciate) the smell or taste of materials shall be considered as suffering from the disease Apinasa. It will have symptoms similar to that of pratisyaya and is caused by the increase of vata and kapha together. (1)

Putinasya

दोषैर्विदग्धैर्गलतालुमूले सम्मूर्छितो यस्य समीरणस्तु |
निरेति पूतिर्मुखनासिकाभ्यां तं पूतिनस्यं प्रवदन्ति रोगम् ||२||
(सु. उ. तं. अ. २२) |

Vāta getting associated with the other (pitta and kapha) morbid (severely increased, burnt and accumulated) doshas localized at the roots of the throat and palate gets eliminated producing foul smell from the mouth and nose. This disease is called as putinasya. (2)

Nasikapaka

घ्राणाश्रितं पित्तमरूंषि कुर्याद्यस्मिन् विकारे बलवांश्च पाकः |
तं नासिकापाकमिति व्यवस्येद्विक्लेदकोथावथवाऽपि यत्र ||३||
(सु. उ. तं. अ. २२) |

The disease in which the pitta located in the nose undergoing abnormal increase produce ulcerations inside the nose or causes severe suppuration or produces moistness and putrefaction inside the nose is known as Nasikapaka. (3)

Puyarakta

दोषैर्विदग्धैरथवाऽपि जन्तोर्ललाटदेशेऽभिहतस्य तैस्तैः |
नासा स्रवेत् पूयमसृग्विमिश्रं तं पूयरक्तं प्रवदन्ति रोगम् ||४||
(सु. उ. तं. अ. २२) |

A condition in which due to abnormal increase of doshas or different kinds of injuries occurring on the forehead, there is continuous discharge of blood mixed pus from the nose is known as Puyarakta. (4)

Kshavathu

घ्राणाश्रिते मर्मणि सम्प्रदुष्टो यस्यानिलो नासिकया निरेति |
कफानुजातो बहुशोऽतिशब्दस्तं रोगमाहुः क्षवथुं विधिज्ञाः ||५||
(सु. उ. तं. अ. २२) |

The disease in which vata getting aggravated in the vital spots located inside the nose comes out of the nose frequently getting associated with kapha, with great force, making great (loud) sounds is named as Kshavathu by the learned people. (5)

Agantuja Kshavathu

तीक्ष्णोपयोगादभिजिघ्रतो वा भावान् कटूनर्कनिरीक्षणाद्वा |
सूत्रादिभिर्वा तरुणास्थिमर्मण्युद्घाटितेऽन्यः क्षवथुर्निरेति ||६||
(सु. उ. तं. अ. २२) |

Kshavathu (sneezing) may also arise from various other external causes like - the ingestion of pungent (deep penetrating) food substances or use of similar substances, smelling of spicy materials (irritants), looking up at the sun, or injury to the cartilage and vital spots inside the nose due to introduction of thread, grass etc things into the nose. (Such kshavathu is called as agantuja kshavathu.) (6)

Bramshathu

प्रभ्रश्यते नासिकया तु यस्य सान्द्रो विदग्धो लवणः कफस्तु |
प्राक्सञ्चितो मूर्धनि सूर्यतप्तस्तं भ्रंशथुं रोगमुदाहरन्ति ||७||
(सु. उ. तं. अ. २२) |

The thick, burnt (improperly formed) and salty kapha which had been previously accumulated inside the head melts and undergoes liquefaction by the heat of the sun and falls (comes) out of the nose. Such a condition is described as the disease Bhramsathu. (7)

Dipta Roga

घ्राणे भृशं दाहसमन्विते तु विनिःसरेद्धूम इवेह वायुः |
नासा प्रदीप्तेव च यस्य जन्तोर्व्याधिं तु तं दीप्तमुदाहरन्ति ||८||
(सु. उ. तं. अ. २२) |

The disease of the nose in which the air comes out just like smoke (hot air) from the nose wherein severe burning sensation is already present and the person feels as if his nose is being burnt by the fire is known by the name Dipta Roga. (8)

Pratinaha

उच्छ्वासमार्गं तु कफः सवातो रुन्ध्यात् प्रतीनाहमुदाहरेत्तम् |९|
(च. चि. अ. २६) |

Kapha along with Vata causes blockage of the passage of respiration. This condition is called Pratinaha.

Nasasrava

घ्राणाद्घनः पीतसितस्तनुर्वा दोषः स्रवेत् स्रावमुदाहरेत्तम् ||९||
(च. चि. अ. २६) |

Discharge of thick or thin, yellow or white coloured dosha (kapha) from the nose is known as Nasasrava. (9)

Nasashosha, Nasa parishosha

घ्राणाश्रिते स्रोतसि मारुतेन गाढं प्रतप्ते परिशोषिते च |
कृच्छ्राच्छ्वसेदूर्ध्वमधश्च जन्तुर्यस्मिन् स नासापरिशोष उक्तः ||१०||
(सु. उ. तं. अ. २२) |

The disease in which the nasal passages become dry by the action of vata and warm due to the action of pitta and the person experiences difficulty in inspiration and expiration (breathing) is known as Nasasosa or Nasaparisosa. (10)

Pinasa

शिरोगुरुत्वमरुचिर्नासास्रावस्तनुः स्वरः |
क्षामः ष्ठीवत्यथाभीक्ष्णमामपीनसलक्षणम् ||११||
आमलिङ्गान्वितः श्लेष्मा घनः खेषु निमज्जति |
स्वरवर्णविशुद्धिश्च परिपक्वस्य लक्षणम् ||१२||

Symptoms of Ama (unripe, early stage) Pinasa – include feeling of heaviness of the head, loss of taste / appetite, discharge of thin fluid from the nose, feeble voice and frequent expectoration of the sputum.

Symptoms of Pakva (ripened stage) Pinasa – include decrease of symptoms of ama pinasa, discharges becoming thick and adhering to the inside of nasal passages, restoration of normal voice (clarity of voice) and restoration of normal colour. (11-12)

Pratishyaya

सन्धारणाजीर्णरजोतिभाष्यक्रोधर्तुवैषम्यशिरोभितापैः |
प्रजागरातिस्वपनाम्बुशीतैरवश्यया मैथुनबाष्पधूमैः |
संस्त्यानदोषे शिरसि प्रवृद्धो वायुः प्रतिश्यायमुदीरयेत्तु ||१३||
(च. चि. अ. २६) |
चयं गता मूर्धनि मारुतादयः पृथक् समस्ताश्च तथैव शोणितम् |
प्रकुप्यमाणा विविधैः प्रकोपणैस्ततः प्रतिश्यायकरा भवन्ति हि ||१४||
(सु. उ. तं. अ. २४) |

Causative factors of Pratishyaya include - suppression of the natural urges of the body, having indigestion (ingestion of uncooked foods), exposure to excessive dust (frequently), excessive talking, excessive anger, seasonal abnormalities, injury to head or exposure to etiological factors which cause headache (dust, fumes, smoke etc which enter the head through the nose and cause headache), habit of keeping awake at night, excessive sleep or excessive day-sleep, excessive consumption of cold water, excessive exposure to snowfall (thin rain, frost, mist, dew), excessive indulgence in sexual act and excessive exposure to steam (vapours) and smoke.

Pathogenesis of Pratishyaya – The above-mentioned etiological factors (and similar others) lead to aggravation of vata in the head in which kapha has

already solidified which in turn causes the disease pratishyaya.
Vata and the other doshas i.e., pitta and kapha and rakta (blood) accumulate in the head, suddenly get excited (and aggravated) either individually or in combination by their respective exciting causes (etiological factors) and produce pratishyaya. (13-14)

Pratishyaya Purvarupa

क्षवप्रवृत्तिः शिरसोऽतिपूर्णता स्तम्भोऽङ्गमर्दः परिहृष्टरोमता ।
उपद्रवाश्चाप्यपरे पृथग्विधा नृणां प्रतिश्यायपुरःसराः स्मृताः ॥१५॥
(सु. उ. तं. अ. २४) ।

Premonitory Symptoms of Pratishyaya

The symptoms seen in the premonitory stage of pratishyaya include – frequent bouts of sneezing, feeling of fullness of the head, stiffness / inactivity, pain all over the body, horripilation and many other complications. (15)

Symptoms of Vataja, Pittaja and Kaphaja Pratishyaya

Symptoms of Vataja Pratishyaya

आनद्धा पिहिता नासा तनुस्रावप्रसेकिनी ।
गलताल्वोष्ठशोषश्च निस्तोदः शङ्खयोस्तथा ॥१६॥
(सु. उ. तं. अ. २४) ।
क्षवप्रवृत्तिरत्यर्थं वक्त्रवैरस्यमेव च ।
भवेत् स्वरोपघातश्च प्रतिश्यायेऽनिलात्मके ॥१७॥

– In this condition there is obstruction or covering inside the nose (full or partial blockage of nose), dripping out of thin fluid from the nose, dryness of the throat, palate and lips, pricking pain in the temples, excessive sneezing, distaste in the mouth and destruction of voice (broken voice). (16-17)

Symptoms of Pittaja Pratishyaya

उष्णः सपीतकः स्रावो घ्राणात् स्रवति पैत्तिके ।
कृशोऽतिपाण्डुः सन्तप्तो भवेदुष्णाभिपीडितः ॥१८॥
सधूममग्निं सहसा वमतीव स मानवः ।

In this condition there will be feeling of warmth inside the nose, yellowish discharges from the nose, emaciation, severe pallor, raised temperature (worried, restless), and exhaustion by heat (of pittta). The person feels as if he is vomiting fire along with the smoke (excessive hot air is eliminated from the mouth). (18)

Symptoms of Kaphaja Pratishyaya

घ्राणात् कफः कफकृते शीतः पाण्डुः स्रवेद्बहुः |
शुक्लावभासः शुक्लाक्षो भवेद्गुरुशिरा नरः ||१९||
कण्ठताल्वोष्ठशिरसां कण्डूभिरभिपीडितः |
(सु. उ. तं. अ. २४) |

In this condition there will be excessive discharge of cold, pale (whitish yellow), thick mucus (phlegm) from the nose, the body and eyes would become (appear) white in colour. The person would also experience heaviness of the head, and excessive itching in the throat, palate, lips and head. (19-20)

Sannipataja Pratishyaya

भूत्वा भूत्वा प्रतिश्यायो यस्याकस्मान्निवर्तते ||२०||
सम्पक्वो वाऽप्यपक्वो वा स सर्वप्रभवः स्मृतः |
(सु. उ. तं. अ. २४) |

Symptoms of Sannipataja Pratishyaya - Partisyaya appearing and disappearing frequently without any apparent reason and is either in ripened or unripe state should be understood as being caused by all the three doshas together i.e., sannipataja pratishyaya. (20)

Dushta Pratishyaya

प्रक्लिद्यते पुनर्नासा पुनश्च परिशुष्यति ||२१||
पुनरानह्यते वाऽपि पुनर्विव्रियते तथा |
निःश्वासो वाऽतिदुर्गन्धो नरो गन्धान् न वेत्ति च ||२२||
एवं दुष्टप्रतिश्यायं जानीयात् कृच्छ्रसाधनम् |
(सु. उ. तं. अ. २४) |

In this condition, the inside of the nose will become too wet (due to too much fluid) or too dry alternatively (and repeatedly). Similarly, the nose gets blocked and gets cleared (of blockage) on its own accord (repeatedly). There will be foul smell in the breath and the person would not appreciate smell (loss of sense of smell). This condition is called Dusta Pratishyaya and is difficult to treat. (21-22)

Raktaja Pratishyaya

रक्तजे तु प्रतिश्याये रक्तस्रावः प्रवर्तते ||२३||
ताम्राक्षश्च भवेज्जन्तुरुरोघातप्रपीडितः |
दुर्गन्धोच्छ्वासवदनो गन्धानपि न वेत्ति सः ||२४||
(सु. उ. तं. अ. २४) |

In pratishyaya caused due to increase of rakta (blood) there will be bleeding from the nose, coppery colour of the eyes, and severe pain in the chest, foul smell in the breath and mouth and the person will not appreciate smell (loss of sense of smell). (23-24)

Transformation of all Pratishyayas into Dusta Pratishyaya

सर्व एव प्रतिश्याया नरस्याप्रतिकारिणः |
दुष्टतां यान्ति कालेन तदाऽसाध्या भवन्ति हि ||२५||
मूर्छन्ति चात्र क्रिमयः श्वेताः स्निग्धास्तथाऽणवः |
क्रिमितो यः शिरोरोगस्तुल्यं तेनास्य लक्षणम् ||२६||
(सु. उ. तं. अ. २४) |

If not treated properly at proper time, all kinds of pratishyaya would ultimately get converted into dusta pratishyaya and become incurable in due course of time. Following this, there will be the appearance of worms which are white, unctuous (oily) and minute and the patient will develop symptoms similar to those of krimija siroroga (headache caused due to worms, bacteria). (25-26)

Pratishyaya Upadrava

बाधिर्यमान्ध्यमघ्रत्वं घोरांश्च नयनामयान् |
शोथाग्निसादकासांश्च वृद्धाः कुर्वन्ति पीनसाः ||२७||
(सु. उ. तं. अ. २४) |

Complications of Pratishyaya

All varieties of peenasa when become progressive (neglected) will, in due course of time, produce deafness, blindness, loss of sense of smell, severe kinds of eye diseases, swelling of the body, poor digestion and cough. (27)

Other diseases manifesting in the nose

अर्बुदं सप्तधा शोथाश्चत्वारोऽर्शश्चतुर्विधम् |
चतुर्विधं रक्तपित्तमुक्तं घ्राणेऽपि तद्विदुः ||२८||

The seven kinds of abruda, four kinds of sotha, four kinds of arsas and four kinds of raktapitta described previously might also manifest in the nose (or these may also develop as complications / sequelae of diseases of the nose).

इति श्रीमाधवकरविरचिते माधवनिदाने नासारोगनिदानं समाप्तम् ||५८||
Thus ends the chapter on Nasa Roga Nidanam in Madhava Nidana text written by Acharya Madhavakara.

59

Madhava Nidana Chapter 59 Netra Roga Nidanam

Netra Roga Samanya Hetu

उष्णाभितप्तस्य जले प्रवेशाद्दूरेक्षणात् स्वप्नविपर्ययाच्च |
स्वेदाद्रजोधूमनिषेवणाच्च छर्देर्विघाताद्वमनातियोगात् ||१||
द्रवात्तथाऽन्नान्निशि सेविताच्च विण्मूत्रवातक्रमनिग्रहाच्च |
प्रसक्तसंरोदनकोपशोकाच्छिरोऽभिघातादतिमद्यपानात् ||२||
तथा ऋतूनां च विपर्ययेण क्लेशाभिघातादतिमैथुनाच्च |
बाष्पग्रहात् सूक्ष्मनिरीक्षणाच्च नेत्रे विकाराञ्जनयन्ति दोषाः ||३||
(सु. उ. तं. अ. १) |

General Causes of Eye Diseases

Entering into the water (taking bath in cold water) immediately after exposure to heat, seeing objects which are far away (by straining one's eyes), abnormal sleeping habits (like not sleeping at proper time, keeping awake during night time, sleeping in excess during day time etc), sudation or fumigation to the eyes, excessive contact / exposure of the eyes to dust and smoke, forcibly withholding the urge for vomiting or vomiting in excess (too much vomiting, too much of emesis therapy), taking watery foods (liquid foods) at night in excess, habitually suppressing the natural urges of faeces, urine and flatus, constantly weeping, getting angry and grieving, injury to the head, excessive consumption of alcoholic drinks, abnormal seasonal changes, physical and mental exhaustion, excessive indulgence in sexual act, controlling tears, seeing minute objects (microscopic objects) for prolonged periods of time, etc are the etiological factors of eye disorders. The above-mentioned etiological factors cause abnormal increase of doshas which in turn produce various diseases of the eyes. (1-3)

Types of Abhisyanda

वातात् पित्तात् कफाद्रक्तादभिष्यन्दश्चतुर्विधः |
प्रायेण जायते घोरः सर्वनेत्रामयाकरः ||४||

Abhsyanda is of four types - vātaja, pittaja, kaphaja and raktaja. It is a very dreadful disease which probably is the main cause for all other (almost) eye diseases. (4)

Vataja Abisyanda

निस्तोदनस्तम्भनरोमहर्षसङ्घर्षपारुष्यशिरोऽभितापाः |
विशुष्कभावः शिशिराश्रुता च वाताभिपन्ने नयने भवन्ति ||५||
(सु. उ. तं. अ. ६) |

Symptoms of Abisyanda caused by increased vata include pricking pain, stiffness (loss of movements or restricted movements), horripilation, irritation and roughness (friction) in the eyes, headache, absence of excretions in the eyes (dryness of eyes) and cold tears flowing out of the eyes. (5)

Pittaja Abhishyanda

दाहप्रपाकौ शिशिराभिनन्दा धूमायनं बाष्पसमुच्छ्रयश्च |
उष्णाश्रुता पीतकनेत्रता च पित्ताभिपन्ने नयने भवन्ति ||६||
(सु. उ. तं. अ. ६) |

Symptoms of Abisyanda caused by increased pitta include feeling of burning sensation, suppuration, desire for cold things and comforts, feeling as if hot smoke is being eliminated from the eyes, excessive flow of tears, hot tears coming from the eyes and yellowish discolouration of the eyes. (6)

Kaphaja Abhisyanda

उष्णाभिनन्दा गुरुताऽक्षिशोथः कण्डूपदेहावतिशीतता च |
स्रावो मुहुः पिच्छिल एव चापि कफाभिपन्ने नयने भवन्ति ||७||
(सु. उ. तं. अ. ६) |

Symptoms of Abhisyanda caused by increased kapha include desire for warm things and comforts, feeling of heaviness in the eyes, swelling, itching, accumulation of dirty excretions, excessive coldness, excessive and frequent discharge of sticky secretions (discharges, tears) from the eyes. (7)

Raktaja Abhishyanda

ताम्राश्रुता लोहितनेत्रता च नाड्यः समन्तादतिलोहिताश्च |
पित्तस्य लिङ्गानि च यानि तानि रक्ताभिपन्ने नयने भवन्ति ||८||
(सु. उ. तं. अ. ६) |

Symptoms of Abhisyanda caused by increased rakta (blood) include discharge of copper-coloured tears, redness of the eyes, redness of the capillaries in all corners of the eyes and presence of other symptoms of pittaja abhisyanda (explained above). (8)

Adhimantha

वृद्धैरेतैरभिष्यन्दैर्नराणामक्रियावताम् |
तावन्तस्त्वधिमन्थाः स्युर्नयने तीव्रवेदनाः ||९||
(सु. उ. तं. अ. ६) |

Any of the above types of abhiṣyanda, if not treated at the proper time, will undergo abnormal increase and lead to another condition called as adhimantha which causes severe pain in the eyes. (9)

Adhimantha Samanya Lakshana

उत्पाट्यत इवात्यर्थं नेत्रं निर्मथ्यते तथा |
शिरसोऽर्धं च तं विद्यादधिमन्थं स्वलक्षणैः ||१०||
(सु. उ. तं. अ. ६) |

General symptoms of Adhimantha

A condition of the eye in which the person feels as though someone is pulling out or churning (squeezing) his eyes and half portion of his head with force is known as adhimantha. In addition to this the other symptoms of predominant doshas (as explained in dosha types of abhisyanda above) are also seen in this condition. (10)

Effect of Adhimantha

हन्याद्दृष्टिं श्लैष्मिकः सप्तरात्राद‍धिमन्थो रक्तजः पञ्चरात्रात् |
षड्रात्राद्वातिको वै निहन्यान्मिथ्याचारात् पैत्तिकः सद्य एव ||११||
(सु. उ. तं. अ. ६) |

When improperly managed and not treated properly at proper time –

Kaphaja Adhimantha will destroy the vision within seven days.
Raktaja Adhimantha will destroy the vision within five days.
Vataja Adhimantha will destroy the vision within six days.
Pittaja Adhimantha will destroy the vision immediately / very soon (within three days). (11)

Sama Lakshanas of Netra Roga

उदीर्णवेदनं नेत्रं रागशोथसमन्वितम् |
घर्षनिस्तोदशूलाश्रुयुक्तमामान्वितं विदुः ||१२||

Symptoms of eye diseases associated with ama (unripe stage)
The symptoms of ama (unripe) stage of eye diseases include progressively increasing severe pain, redness, swelling and rubbing pain (friction, irritation), pricking pain, pain, and discharges (excessive flow of tears) from the eyes. (12)

Pakva Lakshanas of Netra Roga

मन्दवेदनता कण्डूः संरम्भाश्रुप्रशान्तता |
प्रशस्तवर्णता चाक्ष्णोः सम्पक्वदोषमादिशेत् ||१३||

Symptoms of eye diseases devoid of ama association (ripe stage)
The symptoms of pakva (ripe) stage of eye diseases include mild pain (reduction in severity of pain) in the eyes, itching, swelling, reduction of discharges (tears) from the eyes, colour of the eyes (discolouration) returning to normal. (13)

Shothaja and Ashothaja Netrapaka

कण्डूपदेहाश्रुयुतः पक्वोदुम्बरसन्निभः |
संरम्भी पच्यते यस्तु नेत्रपाकः स शोथजः |
शोथहीनानि लिङ्गानि नेत्रपाके त्वशोथजे ||१४||
(सु. उ. तं. अ. ६) |

Shothaja Netrapaka

In this condition the eyes will have itching, accumulation of excretion / dirt (in the eyes), excessive tearing, and will resemble the ripe Udumbara fruit. Suppuration will occur following the appearance of swelling.

Ashothaja Netrapaka

In this condition all symptoms mentioned above (in sothaja netrapaka) will be found except the appearance of swelling (suppuration of eyes occur even without the appearance of swelling). (14)

Hatadimantha

उपेक्षणादक्षि यदाऽधिमन्थो वातात्मकः सादयति प्रसह्य |
रुजाभिरुग्राभिरसाध्य एष हताधिमन्थः खलु नाम रोगः ||१५||
(सु. उ. तं. अ. ६) |

When neglected (not properly treated at proper time), the Vataja Adhimantha forcefully causes severe pain in the eyes and leads to destruction of vision. This incurable disease is known as Hatadhimantha. (15)

Vataparyaya

वारंवारं च पर्येति भ्रुवौ नेत्रे च मारुतः |
रुजश्च विविधास्तीव्राः स ज्ञेयो वातपर्ययः ||१६|

A condition in which vata which has abnormally increased repeatedly causes different kinds of pain in the eyebrows and eyes (areas surrounding the eyes) is called as Vataparyaya. (16)

Sushka akshipaka

यत् कूणितं दारुणरूक्षवर्त्म सन्दह्यते चाविलदर्शनं यत् |
सुदारुणं यत् प्रतिबोधने च शुष्काक्षिपाकोपहतं तदक्षि ||१७||
(सु. उ. तं. अ. ६) |

The condition in which the eyelids become closed, hard and dry to touch, has burning sensation, is cloudy and unclear vision, and it becomes difficult to open the eyelids and on opening the eyes look dry is known as Suska Akshipaka. (17)

Anyatovata

यस्यावटुकर्णशिरोहनुस्थो मन्यागतो वाऽप्यनिलोऽन्यतो वा |
कुर्याद्रुजं वै भ्रुवि लोचने च तमन्यतोवातमुदाहरन्ति ||१८||
(सु. उ. तं. अ. ६) |

A condition in which vata aggravating in the posterior part of the neck, ears, head, jaw (lower) and sides of the neck causes severe pain in the eyebrows and eye is known as Anyatovata. (18)

Amladhyusita

श्यावं लोहितपर्यन्तं सर्वं चाक्षि प्रपच्यते |

सदाहशोथं सास्रावमम्लाध्युषितमम्लतः ||१९||

The condition in which the pitta undergoing abnormal increase due to excessive consumption of sour foods would cause bluish discolouration of the eyes with reddish borders and suppuration in the entire eye is known as Amladhyusita. This condition is also associated with burning sensation, swelling and discharges (excessive flow of tears) from the eyes. (19)

Sirotpata

अवेदना वाऽपि सवेदना वा यस्याक्षिराज्यो हि भवन्ति ताम्राः |
मुहुर्विरज्यन्ति च याः स ताद्दग्व्याधिः सिरोत्पात इति प्रदिष्टः ||२०||
(सु. उ. तं. अ. ६) |

The disease in which the network of blood vessels in the eye become coppery or red in colour, is associated or not associated with pain and the eye becomes angry red repeatedly is known by the name Sirotpata. (20)

Sirapraharsha

मोहात् सिरोत्पात उपेक्षितस्तु जायेत रोगस्तु [२] सिराप्रहर्षः |
ताम्राभमस्रं स्रवति प्रगाढं तथा न शक्नोत्यभिवीक्षितुं च ||२१||
(सु. उ. तं. अ. ६) |

When sirotpata disease (explained above) is neglected (not treated promptly) due to ignorance, yet another disease known as Sirapraharsha gets manifested. In this condition the person would discharge thick coppery / red coloured fluids in large quantities and will be unable to see anything. (21)

Savrana Shukla

निमग्नरूपं तु भवेद्धि कृष्णे सूच्येव विद्धं प्रतिभाति यद्वै |
स्रावं स्रवेदुष्णमतीव यच्च तत् सव्रणं शुक्ल(क्र)मुदाहरन्ति ||२२||
(सु. उ. तं. अ. ५) |

A deep-seated spot which is difficult to identify, which appears as if pierced by a sharp needle, located in the black of the eye (cornea) is known as Savrana Shukla or Savrana Shukra. In this condition, very hot tears discharge (tears) flow out of the eyes. (22)

Savrana Shukla

दृष्टेः समीपे न भवेत्तु यच्च न चावगाढं न च संस्रवेद्धि |
अवेदनं वा न युग्मशुक्लं तत् सिद्धिमायाति कदाचिदेव ||२३||

(सु. उ. तं. अ. ५) |

An ulcer which is not very near to the pupil, which is not deep rooted, not having too much of discharge, is painless (has mild pain) and which doesn't have two ulcers (not affecting both eyes together) and is sometimes curable (sometimes responds to treatment and sometimes will not, especially if both eyes are afflicted with ulcers) is known as Savrana Shukla or Savrana Shukra. (23)

Symptoms of Curability of Avrana Shukla

स्यन्दात्मकं कृष्णगतं सचोषं शङ्खेन्दुकुन्दप्रतिमावभासम् |
वैहायसाभ्रप्रतनुप्रकाशमथाव्रणं साध्यतमं वदन्ति ||२४||
(सु. उ. तं. अ. ५) |

Due to the effect of Abhisyanda there appears a white coloured scar resembling the colour of conch, moon or lily flower on the cornea or the cornea appears cloudy, as if it is covered by thin (waterless) cloud, and is associated with burning sensation. This condition is known as Avrana Shukla which is easily curable. (24)

Prognosis of Avrana Shukla

गम्भीरजातं बहुलं च शुक्लं चिरोत्थितं चापि वदन्ति कृच्छ्रम् |
विच्छिन्नमध्यं पिशितावृतं वा चलं [१] सिरासूक्ष्ममदृष्टिकृच्च |
द्वित्वग्गतं लोहितमन्ततश्च चिरोत्थितं चापि विवर्जनीयम् ||२५||
(सु. उ. तं. अ. ५) |
उष्णाश्रुपातः पिडका च नेत्रे यस्मिन् भवेन्मुद्गनिभं च शुक्लम् |
तदप्यसाध्यं प्रवदन्ति केचिदन्यच्च यत्तित्तिरिपक्षतुल्यम् ||२६||
(सु. उ. तं. अ. ५) |

Avranashukla developing from deep inside (second or third layer / tunic), is thick, and has been for a long time (has become chronic) is difficult to cure.

Avrana Shukla in which there is a tear in the middle or is covered by muscle, movable, and is minute / invisible (interferes with vision) because of being enveloped with a thin network of veins should be refused treatment since it is incurable.

Avrana Shukla occurring (involving) in the second layer, having reddish edges and has become chronic is also incurable.

Similarly, avrana shukla in which warm tears are eliminated from the eyes, there is appearance of white coloured nodules of the size of green gram and that which assumes the colour of feather of tittira bird (grey partridge) should also be considered as incurable. (25-26)

Akshipakatyaya

श्वेतः समाक्रामति सर्वतो हि दोषेण यस्यासितमण्डलं च |
तमक्षिपाकात्ययमक्षिरोगं सर्वात्मकं वर्जयितव्यमाहुः ||२७||
(सु. उ. तं. अ. ५) |

The eye disease in which the entire cornea becomes white (in colour) by the action of all the three abnormally increased doshas, caused by all three aggravated doshas should be rejected treatment (because it is incurable). (27)

Ajakajata

अजापुरीषप्रतिमो रुजावान् सलोहितो लोहितपिच्छिलास्रः |
विगृह्य कृष्णं प्रचयोऽभ्युपैति तच्चाजकाजातमिति व्यवस्येत् ||२८||
(इति कृष्णजाः) | (सु. उ. तं. अ. ५) |

A growth (projection) resembling a dried pellet of goat excreta, which is painful, red in colour, discharges red sticky fluid, and projects out piercing the cornea is called as Ajakajata. (28)

Pratama Patalagata Timira

प्रथमे पटले दोषा यस्य दृष्ट्यां व्यवस्थिताः |
अव्यक्तानि स रूपाणि कदाचिदथ पश्यति ||२९||
(सु. उ. तं. अ. ५) |

When timira manifests due to the increased doshas localized in the first patala (layer) of the drsti (lens), the person sees things in an indistinct or unclear way (does not see the objects clearly). (29)

Dwitiya Patalagata Timira

दृष्टिर्भृशं विह्वलति द्वितीयं पटलं गते |
मक्षिकामशकांश्चापि जालकानि च पश्यति ||३०||
मण्डलानि पताकांश्च मरीचिं कुण्डलानि च |
परिप्लवांश्च विविधान् वर्षमभ्रं तमांसि च ||३१||
दूरस्थानि च रूपाणि मन्यते स समीपतः |
समीपस्थानि दूरे च दृष्टेर्गोचरविभ्रमात् ||३२||
यत्नवानपि चात्यर्थं सूचीपाशं न पश्यति |

(सु. उ. तं. अ. ७) |

When the timira manifests due to the increased doshas getting localized (invade the) in the second patala (layer), his vision becomes distorted. He sees flies, mosquitoes, spider webs, round things (circular objects), flags, various types of shining things like rays of light etc, rings, jumping frogs etc, rain, clouds, and darkness. He sees distant objects to be very near to him and nearby things to be very far away due to distortion and perversion of vision and visual objects. In spite of making all efforts the person will not be able to see the eye of the needle and its thread (will not be able to put the thread into the eye of the needle). (31-32)

Trtiya Patalagata Timira

ऊर्ध्वं पश्यति नाधस्तात्तृतीयं पटलं गते ||३३||
महान्त्यपि च रूपाणि छादितानीव चाम्बरैः |
कर्णनासाक्षिहीनानि विकृतानीव पश्यति ||३४||
यथादोषं च रज्येत दृष्टिर्दोषे बलीयसि |
(सु. उ. तं. अ. ७) |
अधःस्थिते समीपस्थं दूरस्थं चोपरिस्थिते ||३५||
पार्श्वस्थिते तथा दोषे पार्श्वस्थं नैव पश्यति |
समन्ततः स्थिते दोषे सङ्कुलानीव पश्यति ||३६||
दृष्टिमध्यस्थिते दोषे महद्ध्रस्वं च पश्यति |
द्विधा स्थिते द्विधा पश्येद्बहुधा चानवस्थिते ||३७||
(सु. उ. तं. अ. ७) |

When the timira manifests due to the increased doshas getting localized (invade the) in the third patala (layer), the person will be able to see objects which are at the top but cannot see the objects placed at the bottom. Even the larger objects appear to him as though covered by cloth. He sees the other people as being devoid of ears, nose and eyes or sees them (ears, nose and eyes) as abnormal and distorted. Depending on the doshas which become predominant in the disease, the colour corresponding to that particular predominant dosha will manifest in the drsti – lens.

When the doshas get localized in the lower portion of the drsti (lens) one cannot see the objects which are nearby. If the doshas are located in the upper portion, one cannot see the objects which are far away. When the doshas are localized at the sides, one cannot see the objects which are on the sides.

If doshas are spread all over, in all directions, the objects will be seen as mixed up in different ways. On the other hand, if the doshas are located at the centre, the big objects are seen as small by the patient. If the doshas are located in two places, all the objects appear double. If the doshas are located in many places, all objects appear to be of many types. If the doshas are located obliquely in the drsti, the person sees one object as two. (33-37)

Chaturtha Patalagata Timira
तिमिराख्यः स वै दोषश्चतुर्थं पटलं गतः ||३८||
रुणद्धि सर्वतो दृष्टिं लिङ्गनाशमतः परम् |
अस्मिन्नपि तमोभूते नातिरूढे महागदे ||३९||
चन्द्रादित्यौ सनक्षत्रावन्तरीक्षे च विद्युतः |
निर्मलानि च तेजांसि भ्राजिष्णून्यथ पश्यति ||४०||
(सु. उ. तं. अ. ७) |
स एव लिङ्गनाशस्तु नीलिका काचसञ्ज्ञितः |४१|
(सु. उ. तं. अ. ७) |
When the same increased doshas of (having the form of) timira located in the third patala (layer) reaches to invade the fourth patala (layer), they cause complete loss of vision. This condition is called Linganasha (loss of capacity to see and perceive the objects – total loss of vision).
If this dreadful disease which is in the form of darkness is not deep rooted or if it has not run a long course and become chronic (much time has not lapsed since the onset of blindness), the person will be able to see very bright objects such as the moon, sun, stars and lightning in the sky and also other clear bright objects elsewhere. This linganasha is also known as Nilika or Kacha. (38-40)

Timira Symptoms based on 'predominant dosha' involved
वातेन चापि रूपाणि भ्रमन्तीव च पश्यति ||४१||
आविलान्यरुणाभानि व्याविद्धानीव मानवः |
पित्तेनादित्यखद्योतशक्रचापतडिद्गुणान् ||४२||
नृत्यतश्चैव शिखिनः सर्वं नीलं च पश्यति |
कफेन पश्येद्रूपाणि स्निग्धानि च सितानि च ||४३||
(गौरचामरगौराणि श्वेताभ्रप्रतिमानि च |
पश्येदसूक्ष्माण्यत्यर्थं व्यभ्रे चैवाभ्रसम्प्लवम्) |
सलिलप्लावितानीव परिजाड्यानि मानवः |
पश्येद्रक्तेन रक्तानि तमांसि विविधानि च ||४४||

स सितान्यपि कृष्णानि पीतान्यपि च मानवः |
सन्निपातेन चित्राणि विप्लुतानीव पश्यति ||४५||
बहुधा च द्विधा चापि सर्वाण्येव समन्ततः |
हीनाधिकाङ्गान्यपि तु ज्योतींष्यपि च भूयसा ||४६||
(सु. उ. तं. अ. ७) |

Vataja Timira – In timira, when vata is predominant, the patient sees the objects constantly moving in front of his eyes. The objects are perceived as being dirty, of slightly red (reddish yellow) in colour and crooked (irregular or broken).

Pittaja Timira – In timira, when pitta is predominant, the patient sees the (shapes, forms of) sun, glow-worm, rainbow, and sparks of fire and dancing peacocks – all objects blue in colour.

Kaphaja Timira – In timira, when kapha is predominant, the patient sees all objects as being unctuous and white in colour and very big in size. He sees a clear sky as if covered by clouds. He sees all the objects being drowned in the water and devoid of any movement (still and stagnant).

Raktaja Timira – In timira, when rakta (vitiated blood) is predominant, the person sees all the objects red in colour. He also would see different types of darkness (darkness of varying intensity). Even the white coloured objects are seen as being black or yellow coloured.

Sannipataja Timira – In timira caused by predominance of all the three doshas, the person sees different objects and also strange objects and in different forms (not in their actual form) with many colours and irregularities. He sees one object as many (all objects everywhere) or one object as two or many (many mingled into one). He sees people etc with absence of some body parts or with extra parts. He also sees the stars as being deformed. (41-46)

Parimlayi Kacha

पित्तं कुर्यात् परिम्लायि मूर्छितं पित्ततेजसा |
पीता दिशस्तु खद्योतान् भास्करं चापि पश्यति ||४७||
विकीर्यमाणान् खद्योतैर्वृक्षांस्तेजोभिरेव वा |
(सु. उ. तं. अ. ७) |

Pitta in association with blood produces another condition known as Parimlayi. In this condition, the patient sees yellow in everything and everywhere. He also sees glow worms and sun here and there (at any time). He sees trees surrounded by glow worms, fire or any other shining things.

(47)

Types of Linganasha

वक्ष्यामि षड्विधं रागैर्लिङ्गनाशमतः परम् ||४८||

Further on, I will describe six types of **Linganashas** pertaining to (based on) colours.

Manifestation of different colours in different types of doshaja Linganasha

रागोऽरुणो मारुतजः प्रदिष्टो म्लायी च नीलश्च तथैव पित्तात् |
कफात् सितः शोणितजः सरक्तः समस्तदोषप्रभवो विचित्रः ||४९||
(सु. उ. तं. अ. ७) |
अरुणं मण्डलं दृष्ट्यां स्थूलकाचारुणप्रभम् |५०|

In timira / linganasha caused by increased vata, all objects will appear crimson red in colour.

In linganasha caused by increased pitta, all the objects will appear yellowish blue or blue in colour.

In linganasha caused by increased kapha, all the objects will appear white in colour.

In linganasha caused by increased blood, all objects will appear red in colour.

In linganasha caused by all the three doshas increased together, all objects will appear to have strangely mixed colours. (49)

The crimson red colour described (for vātaja linganasha) will be like bright circular rings as seen coming out of a thick lens. (50)

Specific features of Parimlayi

परिम्लायिनि रोगे स्यान्म्लायि नीलं च मण्डलम् ||५०||
दोषक्षयात् स्वयं तत्र कदाचित् स्यात्तु दर्शनम् |
(सु. उ. तं. अ. ७) |

In parimlaayi, lens becomes dirty and blue coloured. Sometimes when the doshas decrease on their own accord in due course of time, the person regains sight even without any treatment. (50)

Symptoms of coloured lens in accordance to dosha predominance

अरुणं मण्डलं वाताच्चञ्चलं परुषं तथा ||५१||
पित्तान्मण्डलमानीलं कांस्याभं पीतमेव च |
श्लेष्मणा बहुलं पीतं शङ्खकुन्देन्दुपाण्डुरम् ||५२||

चलत्पद्मपलाशस्थः शुक्लो बिन्दुरिवाम्भसः |
मृज्यमाने च नयने मण्डलं तद्विसर्पति ||५३||
प्रवालपद्मपत्राभं मण्डलं शोणितात्मकम् |
दृष्टिरागो भवेच्चित्रो लिङ्गनाशे त्रिदोषजे |
यथास्वं दोषलिङ्गानि सर्वेष्वेव भवन्ति हि ||५४||
(सु. उ. तं. अ. ७) |

In case of increase of vata, the vision / lens become crimson in colour, unsteady and rough (irregular).

In case of increase of pitta, the lens becomes blue, whitish yellow like bronze and yellow in colour.

In case of increase of kapha, the lens becomes thick, yellow or of the colour (resemblance) of conch, jasmine flower or moon, whitish yellow in colour or white in colour resembles a drop of water on a moving lotus leaf. The lens moves here and there while rubbing the eyes.

In case of increase of rakta – blood, the rings (lens) will resemble coral or leaf of red coloured lotus.

In case of increase of all the three doshas together, the rings (lens) will be of mixed colours. The other symptoms in this condition will be in accordance to the predominance of particular dosha in the combined vitiation. (51-54)

To sum up

षड् लिङ्गनाशाः षडिमे च रोगा दृष्ट्याश्रयाः षट् च षडेव वाच्याः |५५|
(सु. उ. तं. अ. ७) |

Six types of linganashas occur in the eye as explained above. Six other diseases affecting the lens (vision) will be detailed further on. (55)

Pitta Vidagdha Dristi

पित्तेन दुष्टेन सदा तु दृष्टिः पीता भवेद्यस्य नरस्य किञ्चित् ||५५||
पीतानि रूपाणि च तेन पश्येत् स वै नरः पित्तविदग्धदृष्टिः |
प्राप्ते तृतीयं पटलं तु दोषे दिवा न पश्येन्निशि चेक्षते सः ||५६||
रात्रौ च शीतानुगृहीतदृष्टिः पित्ताल्पभावादपि तानि पश्येत् |
(सु. उ. तं. अ. ७) |

If the drsti (lens, vision) due to the influence of vitiated pitta always remains slight yellowish in color, the person starts seeing everything in his surrounding as being yellow in colour. This condition is called as pitta vidagdha drsti (also called divandhya – day blindness). If pitta gets localized in the third patala (layer) of drsti mandala (eye, lens) the person cannot see any objects during day time. He can only see things during night time. Due to the influence of coldness prevailing at night, the pitta gets subsided and hence he can see things during night time. (55-56)

Kapha Vidagdha Drushti

तथा नरः श्लेष्मविदग्धदृष्टिस्तान्येव शुक्लानि तु मन्यते सः ||५७||
त्रिषु स्थितोऽल्पः पटलेषु दोषो नक्तान्ध्यमापादयति प्रसह्य |
दिवा स सूर्यानुगृहीतदृष्टिः पश्येत्तु रूपाणि कफाल्पभावात् ||५८||
(सु. उ. तं. अ. ७) |

Similarly, when the drsti (lens, vision) of the person is afflicted by vitiated kapha, the person sees everything (all objects) as white (in colour). When the doshas get lodged in all the three patalas (layers), the person would suffer from a condition called naktandhya (night blindness). In the day time, due to less quantity of kapha and due to the influence of (heat of) the Sun, he can see the objects properly. This condition is called as Kaphavidagdha Drsti or Naktandya which means night blindness. (57-58)

Dhumadarsi

शोकज्वरायासशिरोऽभितापैरभ्याहता यस्य नरस्य दृष्टिः |
धूम्रांस्तथा पश्यति सर्वभावान् स धूमदर्शीति नरः प्रदिष्टः ||५९||
(सु. उ. तं. अ. ७) |

Drsti (lens, vision) getting affected by causes such as grief, fever, excessive exertion and headache etc leads to the manifestation of a disease called Dhumadarsi in which the person sees all objects as if covered by smoke. (59)

Hrisvajadya

यो ह्रस्वजाड्यो दिवसेषु कृच्छ्राद्ध्रस्वानि रूपाणि च तेन पश्येत् |६०|
(सु. उ. तं. अ. ७) |

The disease in which the person finds it very difficult to see the objects during daytime and also sees big objects as small is known as Hrisvajādya. (60)

Nakulandhya

विद्योतते यस्य नरस्य दृष्टिर्दोषाभिपन्ना नकुलस्य यद्वत् ||६०||
चित्राणि रूपाणि दिवा स पश्येत् स वै विकारो नकुलान्ध्यसञ्ज्ञः |

(सु. उ. तं. अ. ७) |

When all the three vitiated doshas affect the drsti (vision, lens) the eyes of the person shine like the eyes of mongoose. Such a person sees objects in different (mixed) shapes and colours. This condition is known as Nakulandhya. (60)

Gambhirika

दृष्टिर्विरूपा श्वसनोपसृष्टा सङ्कोचमभ्यन्तरतस्तु याति ||६१||
रुजावगाढा च तमक्षिरोगं गम्भीरिकेति प्रवदन्ति तज्ज्ञाः |
(सु. उ. तं. अ. ७) |

The drsti (lens, vision, eyes) affected by vitiated vata makes the eye deformed (sees things in unnatural state) and the eyeball sinks deep inside the socket of the eye. In this condition there is severe pain in the eye. This disease is called Gambhirika by experts. (61)

Agantuja Linganasha

बाह्यौ पुनर्द्वाविह सम्प्रदिष्टौ निमित्ततश्चाप्यनिमित्ततश्च ||६२||
निमित्ततस्तत्र शिरोऽभितापाज्ज्ञेयस्त्वभिष्यन्दनिदर्शनः सः |
सुरर्षिगन्धर्वमहोरगाणां सन्दर्शनेनापि च भास्करस्य ||६३||
हन्येत दृष्टिर्मनुजस्य यस्य स लिङ्गनाशस्त्वनिमित्तसञ्ज्ञः |
तत्राक्षि विस्पृष्टमिवावभाति वैदूर्यवर्णा विमला च दृष्टिः ||६४||
(इति दृष्टिगताः) | (सु. उ. तं. अ. ७) |

Agantuja Linganasha (that caused by external agents) is of two types. They are – Nimittaja Linganasha and Animittaja Linganasha.

Nimittaja Linganasha– Linganasha caused due to headache (caused by etiological factors like poisons, smell of flowers, exposure to severe winds etc) is called as Nimittaja Linganasa. This will have symptoms similar to those of Abhisyanda (conjunctivitis).

Animittaja Linganasha – Loss of vision caused due to unusual (sudden) sight of gods, sages, gandharvas, divine serpents, or the Sun is known as Animittaja Linganasha . In this condition the eyes are quite normal and not deformed. The lens too will be bright and will have the colour and glitter of vaidurya (Cat's Eye) and clear (but they would have lost the capacity to see and perceive). (62-64)

Prastaryarma (Prastari Arma)

प्रस्तार्यर्म तनु स्तीर्णं श्यावं रक्तनिभं सिते |६५|

A thin, broad, black or blackish blue or red coloured mass of tissue (fleshy growth) formed on the white of the eye (sclera – sita mandala) is known as Prastaryarma. (65)

Shuklarma

सश्वेतं मृदु शुक्लार्म शुक्ले तद्वर्धते चिरात् ||६५||

A white soft mass (fleshy strip), developing slowly (over many days) on the white portion of the eye (sclera) is known as Shuklarma (Sukla Arma). (65)

Rakta Arma

पद्माभं मृदु रक्तार्म यन्मांसं चीयते सिते |६६|
पृथु मृद्वधिमांसार्म बहुलं च यकृन्निभम् |६६|

A soft muscular tissue / strip resembling a red lotus petal developing on the white of the eye (sclera) is known as Raktarma (Rakta Arma).
A muscular strip / fleshy strip which is soft, thick and resembling a piece of liver, developing on the white of the eye (sclera) is known as Adhimāṁsārma (Adhimamsa Arma). (66)

Snayu Arma

स्थिरं प्रस्तारि मांसाढ्यं शुक्लं स्नाय्वर्म पञ्चमम् ||६६||

Immovable, widespread, dry, muscular (or tendinous) tissue is the fifth kind of arma. It is known as Snayvarma (Snayu Arma). (66)

Shuktika, Arjuna

श्यावाः स्युः पिशितनिभाश्च बिन्दवो ये शुक्त्याभाः सितनियताः स शुक्तिसञ्ज्ञः |६७|
(सु. उ. तं. अ. ७) |
एको यः शशरुधिरोपमश्च बिन्दुः शुक्लस्थो भवति तमर्जुनं वदन्ति ||६७||
(सु. उ. तं. अ. ४) |

A spot (papule) which is blackish blue in colour, which resembles muscle tissue and oyster shell developing on the white of the eye (sclera) is known as Shuktika.
Arjuna – A single spot (papule) resembling the blood of a rabbit (deep / dark red in colour) which occurs on the white of the eye (sclera) is known as Arjuna. (67)

Pistaka

श्लेष्ममारुतकोपेन शुक्ले पिष्टं समुन्नतम् |

पिष्टवत् पिष्टकं विद्धि मलाक्तादर्शसन्निभम् ||६८||

Kapha and vata getting increased causes a raised papule resembling ground rice flour or of the colour of a dirty mirror (dust laden mirror) on the white of the eye (sclera). This condition is called as Pistaka. (68)

Sirajala

जालाभः कठिनसिरो महान् सरक्तः सन्तानः स्मृत इह जालसञ्ज्ञितस्तु |६९|

(सु. उ. तं. अ. ४) |

A big and red coloured covering having a network of hard veins developing over the white of the eye (sclera) is known as Sirajala. (68)

Siraja Pidaka

शुक्लस्थाः सितपिडकाः सिरावृता यास्ता ब्रूयादसितसमीपजाः सिराजाः |६९|

(सु. उ. तं. अ. ४) |

White papules covered with veins, developing on the white of the eye (sclera), very near to the black of the eye (cornea, iris) is known as Siraja Pidaka.

Balasa Grathita

कांस्याभोऽमृदुरथ वारिबिन्दुकल्पो विज्ञेयो नयनसिते बलाससञ्ज्ञः ||६९||

(सु. उ. तं. अ. ४) |

A papule (cyst) developing on the white of the eye (sclera), having the colour of bronze, raised – resembling water bubble and hard to touch is known as Balasa or Balasagrathita. (69)

Puyalasaka

पक्वः शोथः सन्धिजो यः सतोदः स्रवेत् पूयं पूति पूयालसाख्यः |७०|

(सु. उ. तं. अ. २) |

A well-formed (matured) swelling (vesicle), which occurs at the inner angle (corner) of the eye, along with pain and discharge of foul-smelling pus is known as Puyalasaka.

Upanaha

ग्रन्थिर्नाल्पो दृष्टिसन्धावपाकी कण्डूप्रायो नीरुजस्तूपनाहः ||७०||

(सु. उ. तं. अ. २) |

A big sized cyst (tumour) occurring at the junction of cornea and pupil, not suppurating (not forming pus) having itching and devoid of pain is known as Upanaha. (70)

Chaturvidha Srava

गत्वा सन्धीनश्रुमार्गेण दोषाः कुर्युः स्रावान् लक्षणैः स्वैरुपेतान् |
तं हि स्रावं नेत्रनाडीति चैके तस्या लिङ्गं कीर्तयिष्ये चतुर्धा ||७१||
(सु. उ. तं. अ. २) |

Four types of discharges

The aggravated doshas reach the joints of the eyes through the asruvahi nadis i.e., channels which carry tears and cause discharges associated with their corresponding features (symptoms). This is called Netrasrava. Some experts also call it Netranadi. Four types of symptoms of these nadis shall be enumerated ahead. (71)

Symptoms of 4 kinds of Srava

पाकात् सन्धौ संस्रवेद्यस्तु पूयं पूयास्रावोऽसौ गदः सर्वजस्तु |७२|
(सु. उ. तं. अ. २) |
श्वेतं सान्द्रं पिच्छिलं यः स्रवेत्तु श्लेष्मास्रावोऽसौ विकारो मतस्तु ||७२||
(सु. उ. तं. अ. २) |
रक्तस्रावः शोणितोत्थो विकारः स्रवेद्दुष्टं तत्र रक्तं प्रभूतम् |७३|
(सु. उ. तं. अ. २) |
हरिद्राभं पीतमुष्णं जलाभं पित्तात् स्रावः संस्रवेत् सन्धिमध्यात् ||७३||
(सु. उ. तं. अ. २) |

Puyasraava – Due to suppuration (formation of pus) in the angles (corners) of the eye, there will be discharge of pus caused due to simultaneous increase of all the three doshas. This condition is called Puyasrava.

Shlesmasrava – The disease in which there is white, thick and sticky discharge is called Kaphaja Puyasrava or Shlesmasrava.

Raktasrava – The disease caused by vitiated rakta (blood) in which there is excessive bleeding from the corner (inner angle) of the eye is called Raktaja Puyasrava or Raktasrava.

Pittasrava – Discharges which resemble turmeric colour, yellow, hot and watery in nature which occurs from the inner angle of the eye caused by aggravated pitta is called as Pittaja Puyasrava or Pittasrava. (72-73)

Parvani and Alaji

ताम्रा तन्वी दाहशूलोपपन्ना रक्ताज्ज्ञेया पर्वणी वृत्तशोथा |

जाता सन्धौ कृष्णशुक्ले ऽलजी स्यात् तस्मिन्नेव ख्यापिता पूर्वलिङ्गै ||७४||
(सु. उ. तं. अ. २) |

Parvani - A rounded swelling of coppery (red) colour, thin (small), associated with burning sensation and pain, caused by aggravated blood, developing at the junction of sclera and cornea is known as Parvani.
Alaji – Another identical disease known as Alaji occurs at the same place i.e. at the junction of sclera and cornea, will have the symptoms of the disease alaji which has already been described (under Prameha Pidaka). (74)

Krimigranthi

क्रिमिग्रन्थिर्वर्त्मनः पक्ष्मणश्च कण्डूं कुर्युः क्रिमयः सन्धिजाताः |
नानारूपा वर्त्मशुक्लान्तसन्धौ चरन्त्यन्तर्लोचनं दूषयन्तः ||७५||
(सु. उ. तं. अ. २) |

The micro-organisms which are produced at the corners of the eyes (inner and outer angles of the eye) on reaching the eyelids and eyelashes produce itching therein. These organisms are of different kinds. They move around and on reaching the junction between eyelids and the white of the eye (sclera), they also gain entry into and contaminate the inside of the eye. This disease is known as Krimigranthi. (75)

Utsangini / Utsanga Pidaka

अभ्यन्तरमुखी ताम्रा बाह्यतो वर्त्मनश्च या |
सोत्सङ्गोत्सङ्गपिडका सर्वजा स्थूलकण्डुरा ||७६||
(सु. उ. तं. अ. २) |

A cyst is formed on the outer side of the eyelid with its opening pointed inwards into the eye, is coppery (red) in colour, covered by many small cysts (papules), elevated (big in size), with severe itching and caused by increase of all three doshas together is called as Utsangini or Utsanga Pidaka. (76)

Kumbhika

वर्त्मान्ते पिडका ध्माता भिद्यन्ते च स्रवन्ति च |
कुम्भीकाबीजप्रतिमाः कुम्भीकाः सन्निपातजाः ||७७||
(सु. उ. तं. अ. ३) |

Multiple papules of the size of seeds of kumbhika formed on the margins of the eyelids, which get swollen and burst open repeatedly and produce discharges, caused by increase of all the three doshas together is known as

Kumbika. (77)

Pothaki
स्राविण्यः कण्डुरा गुर्व्यो रक्तसर्षपसन्निभाः |
रुजावत्यश्च पिडकाः पोथक्य इति कीर्तिताः ||७८||
(सु. उ. तं. अ. ३) |
A disease in which many papules are formed inside the eyelids, which has discharges, itching, is heavy (hard), resembling (size of) red mustard seeds, and has pain is known as Pothaki. (78)

Vartmasharkara
पिडका या खरा स्थूला सूक्ष्माभिरभिसंवृता |
वर्त्मस्था शर्करा नाम स रोगो वर्त्मदूषकः ||७९||
(सु. उ. तं. अ. ३) |
A rough and hard papule, surrounded by many smaller ones inside the lids, is known as Vartmasharkara. This disease causes distortion of eyelids. (79)

Arsovartma
एर्वारुबीजप्रतिमाः पिडका मन्दवेदनाः |
श्लक्ष्णाः खराश्च वर्त्मस्थास्तदर्शोवर्त्म कीर्त्यते ||८०||
(सु. उ. तं. अ. ३) |
A papule which resembles a seed of a melon, is slightly painful, unctuous (smooth), rough and is caused either inside or outside or obth sides of the eyelid is known as Arshovartma. (80)

Shushka Arshas
दीर्घाङ्कुरः खरः स्तब्धो दारुणोऽभ्यन्तरोद्भवः |
व्याधिरेषोऽभिविख्यातः शुष्कार्शो नाम नामतः ||८१||
(सु. उ. तं. अ. ३) |
A papule comprising of long sprouts, rough, stiff (hard), immovable, very troublesome (painful) and arising from deep inside the eyelid is known as Shushka Arshas. (81)

Anjana Namika
दाहतोदवती ताम्रा पिडका वर्त्मसम्भवा |
मृद्वी मन्दरुजा सूक्ष्मा ज्ञेया साऽञ्जननामिका ||८२||

(सु. उ. तं. अ. ३) |

A papule associated with burning sensation, pricking pain, coppery (red) coloured, occurring inside the eyelid, is soft, with mild pain, and small in size is known as Anjana Namika. (82)

Bahala Vartma

वर्त्मोपचीयते यस्य पिडकाभिः समन्ततः |
सवर्णाभिः स्थिराभिश्च विद्याद्बहुलवर्त्म तत् ||८३||
(सु. उ. तं. अ. ३) |

The disease in which the eyelid becomes with numerous hard papules which are of the same colour of the surrounding skin (not discoloured) developing inside the eyelid is known as Bahulavartma or Bahalavartma. (83)

Vartma Bandhaka

कण्डूमताऽल्पतोदेन वर्त्मशोथेन यो नरः |
न स सञ्च्छादयेदक्षि यत्रासौ वर्त्मबन्धकः ||८४||
(सु. उ. तं. अ. ३) |

The disease in which eyelids get swollen being associated with itching and mild pricking pain and the person is unable to cover the eye (with the lids) i.e., unable to close the eyes properly is known as Vartma Bandhaka. (84)

Klista Vartma

मृद्वल्पवेदनं ताम्रं यद्वर्त्म सममेव च |
अकस्माच्च भवेद्रक्तं क्लिष्टवर्त्मेति तद्विदुः ||८५||
(सु. उ. तं. अ. ३) |

The disease in which the eyelids become soft, slightly painful, and coppery red in colour and even and the eyelids suddenly become angry red without any apparent reason is known as Klista Vartma. (35)

Vartmakardama

क्लिष्टं पुनः पित्तयुतं शोणितं विदहेद्यदा |
ततः क्लिन्नत्वमापन्नमुच्यते वर्त्मकर्दमः ||८६||
(सु. उ. तं. अ. ३) |

In the same Klista Vartma disease (mentioned above) when increased pitta associated with rakta (blood) causes burning sensation, the lids become moist. This condition is called as Vartmakardama. (86)

Syava Vartma

यद्वर्त्म बाह्यतोऽन्तश्च श्यावं शूलं सवेदनम् |
तदाहुः श्याववर्त्मेति वर्त्मरोगविशारदाः ||८७||
(सु. उ. तं. अ. ३) |

The disease in which the eyelids become blackish blue both inside and outside, gets swollen and becomes painful is called as Syavavartma by experts. (87)

Praklinna Vartma

अरुजं बाह्यतः शूनं वर्त्म यस्य नरस्य हि |
प्रक्लिन्नवर्त्म तद्विद्यात् क्लिन्नमत्यर्थमन्ततः ||८८||
(सु. उ. तं. अ. ३) |

The disease in which the eyelids are swollen and painless from outside (externally) but the inside of the lids is moist with discharges is known as Praklinna Vartma. (88)

Aklinna Vartma

यस्य धौतान्यधौतानि सम्बध्यन्ते पुनः पुनः |
वर्त्मान्यपरिपक्वानि विद्यादक्लिन्नवर्त्म तत् ||८९||
(सु. उ. तं. अ. ३) |

A disease in which the lids stick (together) to each other often whether they are washed with water or not and suppuration of the eyelids do not take place (lids show signs of unripe state – pus not being formed) is known as Aklinna Vartma. (89)

Vatahara Vartma

विमुक्तसन्धि निश्चेष्टं वर्त्म यस्य न मील्यते |
एतद्वातहतं वर्त्म जानीयादक्षिचिन्तकः ||९०||
(सु. उ. तं. अ. ३) |

The disease in which the lids get displaced from their joints (junction between the eyelids and the white of the eyes – sclera) and becomes motionless and the person unable to close or open his eyelids is known by the experts as Vatahata Vartma. (90)

Vartma Arbuda

वर्त्मान्तरस्थं विषमं ग्रन्थिभूतमवेदनम् |
आचक्षीतार्बुदमिति सरक्तमविलम्बितम् ||९१||
(सु. उ. तं. अ. ३) |

A cystic swelling (tumour) developing from inside the eyelids, irregular in shape, having mild pain (or painless), red coloured and quickly increasing in size is known as Vartmarbuda. (91)

Nimesha

निमेषिणीः सिरा वायुः प्रविष्टः सन्धिसंश्रयाः |
प्रचालयति वर्त्मानि निमेषं नाम तद्विदुः ||९२||
(सु. उ. तं. अ. ३) |

A disease in which the vata which has got increased gets lodged in the siras (veins, blood vessels) responsible for winking the eyes located in the junction of the eyelid and white of the eye (sclera) and causes too much of winking (blinking) of the eyelids is known as Nimesha. (92)

Shonitarshas (Raktarshas)

यः स्थितो वर्त्ममध्ये तु लोहितो मृदुरङ्कुरः |
तद्रक्तजं शोणितार्शश्छिन्नं छिन्नं प्रवर्धते ||९३||
(सु. उ. तं. अ. ३) |

A disease in which red coloured soft sprouts develop at the centre of the inside of the eyelid, caused by increased rakta (blood) is known as Shonitarsha or Raktarsha. Thes sprouts continuously (again and again) keep growing even after they are excised. (93)

Lagana

अपाकी कठिनः स्थूलो ग्रन्थिर्वर्त्मभवोऽरुजः,
लगणो नाम स व्याधिर्लिङ्गतः परिकीर्तितः ||९४|| (सु. उ. तं. अ. ३) |

A disease in which a non-suppurating, hard, big, painless cystic swelling (tumour) develops inside the eyelid is known as Lagana. (94)

Bisa Vartma

त्रयो दोषा बहिःशोथं कुर्युश्छिद्राणि वर्त्मनोः |
प्रस्रवन्त्यन्तरुदकं बिसवद्बिसवर्त्म तत् ||९५||
(वा. उ. अ. ८) |

A disease caused by all the three doshas increased together, wherein a swelling is produced on the exterior (outside) of the eyelid, having many small openings through which watery discharges come out from inside the lids, just like from the stalk of a lotus flower is called by the name Bisa Vartma. (95)

Kunchana

वाताद्या वर्त्मसङ्कोचं जनयन्ति मला यदा |
तदा द्रष्टुं न शक्नोति कुञ्चनं नाम तद्विदुः ||९६||

A disease in which when vata and other doshas (pitta, kapha) undergo increase together and cause contractures of the eyelids leading to inability (of the person) to see things (due to inability to open the eyelids) is known as Kunchana. (96)

Pakshmakopa

प्रचालितानि वातेन पक्ष्माण्यक्षि विशन्ति हि |
घृष्यन्त्यक्षि मुहुस्तानि संरम्भं जनयन्ति च ||९७||
असिते सितभागे च मूलकोषात् पतन्त्यपि |
पक्ष्मकोपः स विज्ञेयो व्याधिः परमदारुणः ||९८||

When the aggravated vata causes the eyelashes turned inwards into the eye, and causes friction on the eyeball repeatedly, and swelling of both white and black portions of the eye, and the hairs may also get dislodged from their roots and fall off. This dreadful disease is known as Pakshmakopa. (97-98)

Pakshmashata

वर्त्मपक्ष्माशयगतं पित्तं रोमाणि शातयेत् |
कण्डूं दाहं च कुरुते पक्ष्मशातं तमादिशेत् ||९९||

A disease in which increased pitta located in the eyelids and lashes (junction of eyelids and eyelashes) makes the eyelashes to fall off from their roots (eyelids) and is associated with itching and burning sensation is known as Pakshmashata. (99)

Compilation of all the eye diseases

नव सन्ध्याश्रयास्तेषु वर्त्मजास्त्वेकविंशतिः |
शुक्लभागे दशैकश्च चत्वारः कृष्णभागजाः ||१००||
सर्वाश्रयाः सप्तदश दृष्टिजा द्वादशैव तु |
बाह्यजौ द्वौ समाख्यातौ रोगौ परमदारुणौ ||१०१||

भूय एतान् प्रवक्ष्यामि सङ्ख्यारूपचिकित्सितैः ||१०२||
(इति वर्त्मगताः) |
(सु. उ. तं. अ. १) |

(So far have been described nine diseases of joints of the eye, twenty-one diseases of the eyelids, eleven diseases of the white of the eye i.e. sclera, four diseases of the black portion of the eye, seventeen diseases occurring in the entire eye, twelve diseases of the vision and two external diseases of the lashes which are dreadful in nature).

इति श्रीमाधवकरविरचिते माधवनिदाने नेत्ररोगनिदानं समाप्तम् ||५९||

Thus ends the chapter on Netra Roga Nidanam in Madhava Nidana text written by Acharya Madhavakara.

60

Madhava Nidana Chapter 60 Shiro Roga Nidanam

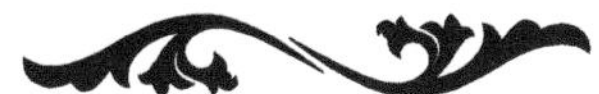

Shiroroga Bheda

शिरोरोगास्तु जायन्ते वातपित्तकफैस्त्रिभिः |
सन्निपातेन रक्तेन क्षयेण क्रिमिभिस्तथा |
सूर्यावर्तानन्तवातार्धावभेदकशङ्खकैः ||१||
(सु. उ. तं. अ. २५) |

Types of Shiroroga based on the causes

The diseases of the head (headache) are caused by individual doshas i.e. aggravated vata, pitta and kapha or by simultaneous vitiation of all three doshas together (sannipataja). They are also caused by rakta (vitiated blood), ksaya (loss, decrease of the tissues) or by krimis (infection from microorganisms). They also manifest by the names Suryavarta, Anantavata, Ardhavabheda and Sankhaka. (1)

Notes - Shiroroga is of 11 kinds. They are –

Vataja Shiroroga, Pittaja Shiroroga, Kaphaja Shiroroga, Sannipataja Shiroroga

Raktaja Shiroroga, Kshayaja Shiroroga , Krimija Shiroroga

Suryavarta, Anantavata, Ardhavabhedaka, Shankhaka

Vataja Shiroroga

यस्यानिमित्तं शिरसो रुजश्च भवन्ति तीव्रा निशि चातिमात्रम् |

बन्धोपतापैः प्रशमश्च यत्र शिरोऽभितापः स समीरणेन ||२||
(सु. उ. तं. अ. २५) |
The symptoms of headache caused by increased vata are –
sudden appearance of severe headache without any apparent cause,
headache being more severe at night (gets worse at night)
gets reduced (relieved) by applying tight bandage and fomentation (warm comforts) (2)

Pittaja Shiroroga
यस्योष्णमङ्गारचितं यथैव भवेच्छिरो धूप्यति चाक्षिनासम् |
शीतेन रात्रौ च भवेच्छमश्च शिरोभितापः स तु पित्तकोपात् ||३||
(सु. उ. तं. अ. २५) |
The symptoms of headache caused by increased pitta are –
the head of the patient feels hot as if his head is enveloped by burning charcoal
feeling as if smoke is coming out of the eyes and nose
gets relieved with cold comforts and at night time (3)

Kaphaja Shiroroga
शिरो भवेद्यस्य कफोपदिग्धं गुरु प्रतिष्टब्धमतो हिमं च |
शूनाक्षिकूटं वदनं च यस्य शिरोऽभितापः स कफप्रकोपात् ||४||
(सु. उ. तं. अ. २५) |
The symptoms of headache caused by increased kapha are –
the head becomes coated with kapha (feeling as if the head is full or is coated with kapha)
heaviness of the head
tightness of the head
coldness of the head
swelling of the face and orbits (region around the eyes) (4)

Sannipataja Shirorog
शिरोऽभितापे त्रितयप्रवृत्ते सर्वाणि लिङ्गानि समुद्भवन्ति |५|
(सु. उ. तं. अ. २५) |
In the headache caused by all the three doshas increased together, there will be presence of the symptoms of (aggravation of) all the three doshas at the same time.

Raktaja Shiroroga

रक्तात्मकः पित्तसमानलिङ्गः स्पर्शासहत्वं शिरसो भवेच्च ||५||

(सु. उ. तं. अ. २५) |

In the headache caused by (abnormally) increased blood the symptoms will be similar to those of pittaja Shiroroga. In addition there will be intolerance to touch / tenderness of the head (the person cannot tolerate if his head is touched / will not allow the head to be touched). (5)

Ksayaja Shiroroga

असृग्वसाश्लेष्मसमीरणानां शिरोगतानामिह सङ्क्षयेण |
क्षयप्रवृत्तः शिरसोऽभितापः कष्टो भवेदुग्ररुजोऽतिमात्रम् |
संस्वेदनच्छर्दनधूमनस्यैरसृग्विमोक्षैश्च विवृद्धिमेति ||६||

(सु. उ. तं. अ. २५) |

When there is loss or abnormal decrease of blood, muscle-fat, kapha and vata residing normally in the head a severe form of headache which is difficult to cure manifests with severe pain in the head. This type of headache is called Ksayaja Shiroroga. The headache increases by administering of therapies like sudation, emesis, herbal (medicated) smoking, instillation of nasal drops and bloodletting. (6)

Krimija Shiroroga

निस्तुद्यते यस्य शिरोऽतिमात्रं सम्भक्ष्यमाणं स्फुरतीव चान्तः |
घ्राणाच्च गच्छेत् सलिलं सपूयं शिरोभितापः क्रिमिभिः स घोरः ||७||

(सु. उ. तं. अ. २५) |

The symptoms of headache caused by krimis (infection by microorganisms) are –

excessive and constant pricking pain in the head,
a feeling as if the head is being eaten away from inside
feeling of pulsations or movements within the head
watery discharges mixed with pus flowing out of the nose
This headache is said to be dreadful in nature. (7)

Suryavarta

सूर्योदयं या प्रति मन्दमन्दमक्षिभ्रुवं रुक् समुपैति गाढा |
विवर्धते चांशुमता सहैव सूर्यापवृत्तौ विनिवर्तते च |
सर्वात्मकं कष्टतमं विकारं सूर्यापवर्तं तमुदाहरन्ति ||८||

(सु. उ. तं. अ. २५) |

The headache which starts at sunrise and the pain gradually increases and spreads to involve the eyes and eyebrows, which gradually increases in severity as the sun reaches its peak (ascent - upward movement of the sun, towards noon) and gradually decreases with the descent of the sun i.e. sunset is called as Suryavarta or Suryapavarta. It is a troublesome (dreadful) disease and is caused by all the three doshas (undergoing increase together). (8)

Anantavata

दोषास्तु दुष्टास्त्रय एव मन्यां सम्पीड्य घाटासु रुजां सुतीव्राम् |
कुर्वन्ति योऽक्षिभ्रुवि शङ्खदेशे स्थितिं करोत्याशु विशेषतस्तु ||९||
गण्डस्य पार्श्वे तु करोति कम्पं हनुग्रहं लोचनजांश्च रोगान् |
अनन्तवातं तमुदाहरन्ति दोषत्रयोत्थं शिरसो विकारम् ||१०||
(सु. उ. तं. अ. २५) |

All the three doshas (vata, pitta and kapha) which have undergone excessive increase together get lodged (invade) and troubles (pain) in the nape of the neck and produce severe pain at the back of the neck. This pain quickly spreads to the eyes, eyebrows and temples and gets localized therein. This will lead to throbbing (pulsation) on the sides of the cheek bones, stiffness of the lower jaw and many diseases of the eyes. This disease of the head caused by simultaneous vitiation of all the three doshas is known as Anantavata. (9-10)

Ardhavabheda

रूक्षाशनात्यध्यशनप्राग्वातावश्यमैथुनैः |
वेगसन्धारणायासव्यायामैः कुपितोऽनिलः ||११||
केवलः सकफो वाऽर्धं गृहीत्वा शिरसो बली |
मन्याभ्रूशङ्खकर्णाक्षिललाटार्धेऽतिवेदनाम् ||१२||
शस्त्रारणिनिभां कुर्यात्तीव्रां सोऽर्धावभेदकः |
नयनं वाऽथवा श्रोत्रमतिवृद्धो विनाशयेत् ||१३||

Causes of Ardhavabheda – Excessive indulgence in (eating) dry foods, too much food frequently, habit of eating food before the previously consumed food is properly digested (eating in presence of indigestion), exposure to heavy breeze coming from the east direction, excessive exposure to snowfall, excessive indulgence in sexual intercourse, habit of suppressing the natural urges, excessive physical exertion and excessive indulgence in physical exercises are the causative factors which cause increase of vata and subsequent manifestation of Ardhavabhedaka.

Pathogenesis – The above said etiological factors would cause abnormal increase of vata. This vata, either alone or gaining strength due to its association with kapha, would invade half the portion of the head and cause the disease Ardhavabhedaka.

Symptoms of Ardhavabhedaka – Ardhavabhedaka is marked by severe pain in the sides of the neck, eyebrows, temples, ears, eyes and forehead of any one side i.e. left or right side. The pain of Ardhavabhedaka is very severe. The person feels as if his head is being cut by a sharp weapon or being burnt by fire or being churned by a churner. If the disease progresses, it will also cause destruction of the functions of eyes or ears.

This disease is called as Ardhavabhedaka. (11-13)

Sankhaka

रक्तपित्तानिला दुष्टाः शङ्खदेशे विमूर्च्छिताः |
तीव्ररुग्दाहरागं हि शोथं कुर्वन्ति दारुणम् ||१४||
स शिरो विषवद्वेगी निरुन्ध्याशु गलं तथा |
त्रिरात्राज्जीवितं हन्ति शङ्खको नामतः परम् |
त्र्यहाज्जीवति भैषज्यं प्रत्याख्याय समाचरेत् ||१५||

Abnormally increased rakta (blood), pitta and vata get lodged and mixed with each other in the temples and would cause severe pain, burning sensation and reddish swelling therein (in the temples). This swelling having the intensity and velocity (as powerful as) of a life threatening poison quickly causes obstruction in the head and neck and takes away the life of the person within three days. This disease is known as Sankhaka.

By chance if the patient survives even after three days (many times the patient will not survive after three days), it should be treated by considering (announcing) that it is incurable (treating in refusal). According to Master Videha, the treatment of Sankhaka should be done in refusal (announcing that it is difficult to cure or incurable) within three days. After three days this disease becomes incurable. (14-15)

इति श्रीमाधवकरविचिते माधवनिदाने शिरोरोगनिदानं समाप्तम् ||६०||

Thus ends the chapter on Shiro Roga Nidanam in Madhava Nidana text written by Acharya Madhavakara.

61

Madhava Nidana Chapter 61 Asrigdara Nidanam

Asrigdara Nidana, Bheda

विरुद्धमद्याध्यशनादजीर्णाद्गर्भप्रपातादतिमैथुनाच्च |
यानाध्वशोकादतिकर्षणाच्च भाराभिघाताच्छयनाद्दिवा च |
तं श्लेष्मपित्तानिलसन्निपातैश्चतुष्प्रकारं प्रदरं वदन्ति ||१||

Causative factors –

excessive indulgence (by the woman) in incompatible foods (foods mutually opposite / antagonistic in nature), alcoholic beverages and over-eating,
eating (in excess) uncooked foods / having indigestion
frequent abortions
indulgence in excessive sexual intercourse
excessive riding on animals
walking long distances
excessive grief
emaciation – excessive loss of tissues due to excessive starvation / fasting and similar other causes
carrying heavy loads
trauma
excessive sleeping during day time

Types of Pradara / Asrigdara – The above-mentioned etiological factors lead to manifestation of four kinds of pradara (excessive menstruation). The four types of pradara are – kaphaja, pittaja, vataja and sannipataja (caused by all doshas together. (1)

Asrigdhara Samanya Lakshana

असृग्दरं भवेत् सर्वं साङ्गमर्दं सवेदनम् |२|

(सु. शा. अ. २) |

General symptoms of Asrigdhara

Aches all over the body and abdominal pain during menstrual periods.

Complications of excessive menstrual bleeding

तस्यातिवृत्तौ दौर्बल्यं भ्रमो मूर्छा मदस्तृषा |

दाहः प्रलापः पाण्डुत्वं तन्द्रा रोगाश्च वातजाः ||२||

(सु. शा. अ. २) |

Excessive bleeding during menstruation leads to many complications like debility, giddiness, fainting, intoxication, excessive thirst, burning sensation, delirium, pallor, stupor and some diseases of vata origin. (2)

Symptoms of types of Asrigdara

आमं सपिच्छाप्रतिमं सपाण्डु पुलाकतोयप्रतिमं कफात्तु |

सपीतनीलासितरक्तमुष्णं पित्तार्तियुक्तं भृशवेगि पित्तात् ||३||

रूक्षारुणं फेनिलमल्पमल्पं वातार्ति वातात् पिशितोदकाभम् |

सक्षौद्रसर्पिर्हरितालवर्णं मज्जप्रकाशं कुणपं त्रिदोषात् ||४||

Kaphaja Asrigdara – In this type of pradara caused by increased kapha, the menstrual discharge will be ill-processed (ama), is sticky (mixed with mucus), is pale (yellowish-white) coloured, resembles ground sesamum (or some bad grain) or meat or mallow plant washed water.

Pittaja Asrigdara – In this type of pradara caused by increased pitta, the menstrual discharge will be yellow, blue, black or red in colour, hot (warm), will have pitta type of pains and comes out with great force (in gushes).

Vataja Asrigdara – In this type of pradara caused by increased vata, the menstrual blood will be dry (viscid), of crimson colour, frothy, scanty, will have vata type of pains, and resembles meat (mutton) washed water.

Tridoshaja / Sannipataja Asrigdara – In this type of pradara caused by all the three doshas together, the flow / discharges will appear like honey, ghee, orpiment or bone marrow in colour, and will emit cadaveric smell.

Asrigdhara Asadhyata

चाप्यसाध्यं प्रवदन्ति तज्ज्ञा, न तत्र कुर्वीत भिषक् चिकित्साम् |
शश्वत् स्रवन्तीमास्रावं तृष्णादाहज्वरान्विताम् |
क्षीणरक्तां दुर्बलां च तामसाध्यां विनिर्दिशेत् ||५||

Prognosis of Asrigdara

The expert physicians consider tridoshaja type of asrigdara as incurable and hence shall not be treated.

Similarly, the asrigdara in which there is continuous menstrual bleeding for long time, and the woman develops thirst, burning sensation, fever, severe loss of blood and debility should also be considered as incurable. (3-5)

Vishuddha Artava Lakshana

मासान्निष्पिच्छदाहार्ति पञ्चरात्रानुबन्धि च |
नैवातिबहुलात्यल्पमार्तवं शुद्धमादिशेत् ||६||
शशासृक्प्रतिमं यच्च यद्वा लाक्षारसोपमम् |
तदार्तवं प्रशंसन्ति यच्चाप्सु न विरज्यते ||७||
(सु. शा. अ. २) |

Signs / symptoms of normal or clean (un-contaminated) menstrual blood

Menstrual blood (Menstruation) is considered to be normal if it occurs regularly every month, for a period of five days, the fluid not being sticky (not having mucus), and not associated with burning sensation and pain and the flow being neither too much in quantity or too less.

The menstrual fluid (blood) which resembles the blood of a rabbit or a solution of lac and the cloth soaked in such fluid when washed in water does not retain any blood stains (can be washed off easily) is considered to be healthy. (6-7)

इति श्रीमाधवकरविरचिते माधवनिदाने असृग्दरनिदानं समाप्तम् ||६१||

Thus ends the chapter on Asrigdara Nidanam in Madhava Nidana text written by Acharya Madhavakara.

62

Madhava Nidana Chapter 62 Yonivyapat Nidanam

Yonivyapat Sankhya, Samanya Nidana

विंशतिर्व्यापदो योनौ निर्दिष्टा रोगसङ्ग्रहे |
मिथ्याचारेण ताः स्त्रीणां प्रदुष्टेनार्तवेन च ||१||
जायन्ते बीजदोषाच्च दैवाच्च शृणु ताः पृथक् |
(च. चि. अ. ३०) |

Number of Yonivyapat -

Twenty diseases of the vaginal tract have been enumerated in the rogasangraha (Ashtodariya chapter – chapter 19 of sutrasthana section of Charaka Samhita).

Etiological Factors of Yonivyapat - These diseases occur in women who indulge in unhealthy foods and habits, due to contamination of menstrual blood or disorders of menstruation, due to bijadosha (disease of the ovary and ovum) and by influence of gods. (1)

Vataja Yoni Vyapad (5 in number)

सा फेनिलमुदावर्ता रजः कृच्छ्रेण मुञ्चति ||२||
वन्ध्यां नष्टार्तवां विद्याद्विप्लुतां नित्यवेदनाम् |
परिप्लुतायां भवति ग्राम्यधर्मेण रुग्भृशम् ||३||
वातला कर्कशा स्तब्धा शूलनिस्तोदपीडिता |
चतसृष्वपि चाद्यासु भवन्त्यनिलवेदनाः ||४||

(सु. उ. तं. अ. ३८) |

Caused due to predominance of vata – Udavarta, Vandhya, Vipluta, Paripluta, Vatala yoni

Udavarta Yonivyapat – In this condition the woman discharges frothy menstrual blood with difficulty (pain).

Vandhya Yonivyapat - the woman in whom the menstrual blood has been destroyed (who has stopped menstruating and is sterile) is known as Vandhyā. Such a condition is known as Vandhya Yonivyapat.

Vipluta Yonivyapat – In this condition the woman always has pain (constant pain).

Paripluta Yonivyapat – In this condition the woman experiences severe pain during sexual intercourse.

Vatala Yonivyapat – It is a condition in which the vagina afflicted by aggravated vata is rough and stiff and is associated with pain and pricking pain.

In the first four conditions (explained above) also there will be vataja types of pains (and other symptoms of vata increase). (2-4)

Pittaja Yoni Vyapad (5 in number)

क्षीयते रक्तं यस्यां सा लोहितक्षया |
सवातमुद्गिरेद्बीजं वामिनी रजसा युतम् ||५||
प्रस्रंसिनी स्रंसते च क्षोभिता दुष्प्रजायिनी |
स्थितं स्थितं हन्ति गर्भं पुत्रघ्नी रक्तसङ्क्षयात् ||६||
अत्यर्थं पित्तला योनिर्दाहपाकज्वरान्विता |
चतसृष्वपि चाद्यासु पित्तलिङ्गोच्छ्रयो भवेत् ||७||
(सु. उ. तं. अ. ३८) |

Caused due to predominance of pitta – Lohitaksaya, Vamini, Prasramsini, Putraghni, Pittala yoni

Lohitaksaya Yonivyapat – It is a condition in which the woman has large quantities of menstrual flow along with burning sensation. There is severe loss of blood and hence this condition is known as Lohitaksaya.

Vamini Yonivyapat – In this condition both the ovum and menstrual fluid (blood) are expelled out from the vagina along with vata.

Prasramsini Yonivyapat – It is a condition in which the vagina is displaced from its place repeatedly due to irritation. This woman gives birth to a child with great difficulty.

Putraghni Yonivyapat – The woman who repeatedly undergoes abortion after having conceived the embryo due to severe loss of blood is said to be suffering from Putraghni Yonivyapat.

Pittala Yonivyapat – In this condition there will be severe burning sensation and suppuration in the vaginal tract and is accompanied with fever.

In the first four conditions (explained above) also there will be pittaja types of pains (and other symptoms of pitta increase). (5-7)

Kaphaja Yoni Vyapad (5 in number)

न सन्तोषं ग्राम्यधर्मेण गच्छति |
कर्णिन्यां कर्णिका योनौ श्लेष्मासृग्भ्यां [१] प्रजायते ||८||
मैथुनेऽचरणा पूर्वं पुरुषादतिरिच्यते |
बहुशश्चातिचरणा तयोर्बीजं न विन्दति ||९||
श्लेष्मला पिच्छिला योनिः कण्डूग्रस्ताऽतिशीतला |
चतसृष्वपि चाद्यासु श्लेष्मलिङ्गोच्छ्रयो भवेत् ||१०||
(सु. उ. तं. अ. ३८) |

Caused due to predominance of kapha – Atyananda, Karnini, Acarana, Aticarana, Shleshmala yoni

Atyananda Yonivyapat – In this condition the woman does not experience pleasure during coitus.

Karnini Yonivyapat – In this condition a ring-like muscular mass is produced by vitiated kapha and blood inside the vaginal passage.

Acarana Yonivyapat – In this condition the woman (uterus) discharges much earlier than the man (ejaculates the semen) during coitus.

Aticarana Yonivyapat – In this condition the woman (uterus) discharges only after excessive and prolonged coitus. Both these conditions (acarana and aticarana) will not retain the seed / sperm (i.e., women having these two conditions do not conceive).

Shlesmala Yonivyapat – In this condition the vaginal passage of the woman will be sticky; will have severe itching and coldness.

In the first four conditions (explained above) also there will be kaphaja types of pains / symptoms (and other symptoms of kapha increase). (8-10)

Sannipataja Yoni Vyapad (5 in number)

अनार्तवाऽस्तनी षण्डी खरस्पर्शा च मैथुने |
अतिकायगृहीतायास्तरुण्यास्त्वण्डली भवेत् ||११||
विवृता च महायोनिः सूचीवक्त्राऽतिसंवृता |

सर्वलिङ्गसमुत्थाना सर्वदोषप्रकोपजा ||१२||
चतसृष्वपि चाद्यासु सर्वलिङ्गोच्छ्रयो भवेत् |
पञ्चासाध्या भवन्तीह योनयः सर्वदोषजाः ||१३||
(सु. उ. तं. अ. ३८) |

Caused due to predominance of all three doshas – Sandi, Andali, Vivrta, Sucimukhi, Tridoshaja yoni

Sandi Yonivyapat – It is a condition in which the woman would not menstruate (not menstruating), not have breasts or have small and under-developed breasts and will have roughness of the vagina during coitus.

Andali Yonivyapat – In this condition the young woman would have a prolapsed vagina (uterus) caused due to coitus with a person having a big or stout penis.

Vivrta Yonivyapat – In this condition the vaginal passage (opening) of the woman would be very wide.

Sucivaktra / Sucimukhi Yonivyapat – It is a condition in which the woman would have a very narrow vaginal (uterine) passage.

Tridoshaja Yonivyapat – In this condition caused due to simultaneous vitiation of all three doshas, the causative factors and symptoms of all the three doshas will be found together.

In the first four conditions (explained above) also there will be tridoshaja types of pains / symptoms (and other symptoms of tridosha increase).

All these five kinds of tridoshaja yonivyapat are said to be incurable.(11-13)

इति श्रीमाधवकरविरचिते माधवनिदाने योनिव्यापन्निदानं समाप्तम् ||६२||

Thus ends the chapter on Yoni vyapat in Madhava Nidana text written by Acharya Madhavakara.

63

Madhava Nidana Chapter 63 Yoni Kanda Nidanam

Yonikanda Hetu

दिवास्वप्नादतिक्रोधाद्व्यायामादतिमैथुनात् |
क्षताच्च नखदन्ताद्यैर्वाताद्याः कुपिता यदा ||१||
पूयशोणितसङ्काशं निकुचाकृतिसन्निभम् |
जनयन्ति यदा योनौ नाम्ना कन्दः स योनिजः ||२||
दिवास्वप्नादतिक्रोधाद्व्यायामादतिमैथुनात् |
क्षताच्च नखदन्ताद्यैर्वाताद्याः कुपिता यदा ||१||
पूयशोणितसङ्काशं निकुचाकृतिसन्निभम् |
जनयन्ति यदा योनौ नाम्ना कन्दः स योनिजः ||२||

Etiological factors - excessive sleeping during the daytime, excessive (frequent episodes) of anger, indulgence in excessive exercises (physical strain) and sexual intercourse, injury (to the vagina) by nails, teeth and other foreign bodies

Pathogenesis, nature and form of yonikanda – the above-mentioned etiological factors cause excessive (abnormal) increase of vata and other doshas (pitta and kapha). These doshas produce a mass in the vagina which has the size and shape of a jujube fruit, round, having the colour of pus mixed blood. This is known as Yonikanda. (1-2)

Yonikanda Bheda, Lakshana

रूक्षं विवर्णं स्फुटितं वातिकं तं विनिर्दिशेत् |
दाहरागज्वरयुतं विद्यात् पित्तात्मकं तु तम् ||३||
नीलपुष्पप्रतीकाशं कण्डूमन्तं कफात्मकम् |
सर्वलिङ्गसमायुक्तं सन्निपातात्मकं विदुः ||४||
रूक्षं विवर्णं स्फुटितं वातिकं तं विनिर्दिशेत् |
दाहरागज्वरयुतं विद्यात् पित्तात्मकं तु तम् ||३||
नीलपुष्पप्रतीकाशं कण्डूमन्तं कफात्मकम् |
सर्वलिङ्गसमायुक्तं सन्निपातात्मकं विदुः ||४||

Types and symptoms of Yonikanda

Vataja Yonikanda – Yonikanda caused by increased vata is dry, discoloured and fissured.

Pittaja Yonikanda – Yonikanda caused by increased pitta presents with burning sensation, redness and fever.

Kaphaja Yonikanda – Yonikanda caused by increased kapha has colour of nilapuspa i.e. flower of atasi (linseed) and has itching.

Sannipataja Yonikanda – In Yonikanda caused by the increase of all the three doshas together, the symptoms of all the three doshas are seen together. (3-4)

इति श्रीमाधवकरविरचिते माधवनिदाने योनिकन्दनिदानं समाप्तम् ||६३||

Thus ends the chapter on Yoni Kanda Nidanam in Madhava Nidana text written by Acharya Madhavakara.

64

Madhava Nidana Chapter 64 Mudhagarba Nidanam

Definition

सर्वावयवसम्पूर्णो मनोबुद्ध्यादिसंयुतः ।
विगुणापानसंमूढो मूढगर्भोऽभिधीयते ॥ 1॥

Mudha Garbha -The condition in which the foetus whose body parts have been properly and completely formed (matured), and has been endowed (associated) with mind, intellect etc, gets obstructed in the birth passage due to the influence of aggravated apana vata is called as mudhagarbha.

Garbhapata

भयाभिघातात्तीक्ष्णोष्णपानाशननिषेवणात् |
गर्भे पतति रक्तस्य सशूलं दर्शनं भवेत् ||१||

Sudden fear, injury (assault), excessive consumption of foods and drinks which are sharp and hot in nature causes falling off (abortion) of the embryo accompanied with pain and heavy bleeding. (This condition is known as garbhapata – miscarriage or abortion). (1)

Types of Garbhapata

आचतुर्थात्ततो मासात् प्रस्रवेद्गर्भविद्रवः |
ततः स्थिरशरीरस्य पातः पञ्चमषष्ठयोः ||२||
(सु. नि. अ. ८) |

Garbhasrava - If this (premature falling off of the embryo) happens within the first four months of pregnancy when the uterine contents are still in fluid state (embryo is in fluid state) it is known as Garbhasrava (abortion).
Garbhapata - If the premature embryo is expelled from the uterus in the fifth or sixth month when the embryo has been developed and the body parts are stable (hard parts), it is known as Garbhapata (miscarriage). (2)

Garbhapata hetu
गर्भोऽभिघातविषमाशनपीडनाद्यैः पक्वं द्रुमादिव फलं पतति क्षणेन |३|
Causative factors for miscarriage
Just as a ripe fruit fall from a tree, the embryo too falls off suddenly (garbhpat takes place) by trauma on the abdomen, consumption of unhealthy foods, and unnecessary massage or pressure over abdomen.

Nature and symptoms of Mudhagarbha
मूढः करोति पवनः खलु मूढगर्भं शूलं च योनिजठरादिषु मूत्रसङ्गम् ||३||
If vata (apana vata) gets increased (goes out of balance), it causes difficulty in delivery. This condition is accompanied with pain in the vagina (uterine passages), abdomen etc and urinary obstruction. (3)

Mudhagarbha Ashta Vidha
भुग्नोऽनिलेन विगुणेन ततः स गर्भः सङ्ख्यामतीत्य बहुधा समुपैति योनिम् |
द्वारं निरुध्य शिरसा जठरेण कश्चित् कश्चिच्छरीरपरिवर्तितकुब्जदेहः ||४||
एकेन कश्चिदपरस्तु भुजद्वयेन तिर्यग्गतो भवति कश्चिदवाङ्मुखोऽन्यः |
पार्श्वापवृत्तगतिरेति तथैव कश्चिदित्यष्टधा गतिरियं ह्यपरा चतुर्धा ||५||
Eight kinds of Mudhagarbha
Väta undergoing increase affects the foetus and creates many kinds of abnormal presentations of the foetus inside the vagina (in the vaginal tract). Among such abnormal presentations of the foetus, eight main presentations are mentioned here. They are –

- obstruction of the mouth (opening) of the uterus by the face of the foetus
- obstruction of the opening of the uterus by the abdomen of the foetus
- obstruction of the mouth of the uterus by the back of the foetus, curved and shortened
- obstruction of the mouth of the uterus by one shoulder of the foetus

- obstruction of the mouth of the uterus by both the shoulders of the foetus
- obstruction of the mouth of the uterus by the body of the foetus placed in transverse position
- obstruction of the mouth of the uterus by the face of the foetus bent down (foetus faces downwards)
- obstruction of the mouth of the uterus by the flanks of the foetus (3-5)

Four special types of presentations of the foetus

सङ्कीलकः प्रतिखुरः परिघोऽथ बीजस्तेषूर्ध्वबाहुचरणैः शिरसा च योनिम् |
सङ्गी च यो भवति कीलकवत् स कीलो दृश्यैः खुरैः प्रतिखुरं स हि कायसङ्गी |
गच्छेद्भुजद्वयशिराः स च बीजकाख्यो योनौ स्थितः स परिघः परिघेण तुल्यः ||६||

Some other authorities enumerate four other kinds of presentations of foetus. They are named as Kilaka, Pratikhura, Parigha and Bijaka.

Kilaka / sankilaka – It is the presentation in which the foetus blocks the mouth of the uterus / vagina, like a wedge, by raising its hands, feet and head upwards.

Pratikhura – In this presentation we can see the bending of the body of the foetus like a horse's hoof with hands, feet and head of the foetus obstructing the opening of the uterus / vagina. Even in this, the body becomes obstructed.

Bijaka – It is a presentation in which both the shoulders (hands) and head cause obstruction to the opening of the uterus (which may prolapse).

Parigha – Here we can see the transverse position of the foetus, like the bolt of a door inside the uterus (obstructing the vaginal passage / uterus). (6)

Prognosis of Mudha Garbha

अपविद्धशिरा या तु शीताङ्गी निरपत्रपा |
नीलोद्गतसिरा हन्ति सा गर्भं स च तां तथा ||७||
(सु. नि. अ. ८) |

The woman in labour who is unable to keep / hold her head straight (in position) i.e., the head keeps falling to one or the other side, whose body has become cold, who is devoid of (natural) shyness and on whose abdomen has blue prominent veins would kill the child and that child would kill her (mother). (7)

Mruta Garbha

गर्भास्पन्दनमावीनां प्रणाशः श्यावपाण्डुता |
भवेदुच्छ्वासपूतित्वं शूनताऽन्तर्मृते शिशौ ||८||
(सु. नि. अ. ८) |

Absence of movements of the foetus and cessation of labour pains, blackish yellow or bluish yellow discolouration of the skin, bad smell in her breath and swelling (abnormally swollen abdomen) are the symptoms of the woman whose foetus is dead inside (the womb). (8)

Reason for the death of the foetus

मानसागन्तुभिर्मातुरुपतापैः प्रपीडितः |
गर्भो व्यापद्यते कुक्षौ व्याधिभिश्च निपीडितः ||९||
(सु. नि. अ. ८) |

Due to mental disorders, external injury, excessive physical strain for the mother and as an effect of many diseases, the foetus would die inside the womb (uterus). (9)

Prognosis of Mudhagarbha

योनिसंवरणं सङ्गः कुक्षौ मक्कल्ल एव च |
हन्युः स्त्रियं मूढगर्भां यथोक्ताश्चाप्युपद्रवाः ||१०||

Yonisamvaraṇa (total obstruction of the uterus), kukṣisanga (obstruction of the foetus inside the abdomen / womb or dead foetus staying in the uterus for long time) and makkalla (pain after delivery) developing as complications of mūḍhagarbha and other complications are going to kill the woman. (10)

Makkalla

वायुः प्रकुपितः कुर्यात् संरुध्य रुधिरं स्रुतम् |
सूताया हृच्छिरोबस्तिशूलं मक्कल्लसञ्ज्ञकम् ||११||

(A condition in which abnormally increased vata causes obstruction of the blood being discharged after delivery and causes pain in the region of the heart, head and urinary bladder is called Makkalla.) Thus ends the chapter on Mudha Garbha.

इति श्रीमाधवकरविरचिते माधवनिदाने मूढगर्भनिदानं समाप्तम् ||६४||

Thus ends the chapter on Mudhagarba Nidanam in Madhava Nidana text written by Acharya Madhavakara.

65

Madhava Nidana Chapter 65 Sutikaroga Nidanam

Sutikaroga Lakshana

अङ्गमर्दो ज्वरः कम्पः पिपासा गुरुगात्रता |
शोथः शूलातिसारौ च सूतिकारोगलक्षणम् ||१||

Symptoms of disease of puerperium

The symptoms of Sutikaroga (puerperal disorders) are – pain in the body parts / general malaise, fever, tremors, thirst, feeling of heaviness of the body, swelling, pain in the abdomen and diarrhoea. (1)

Sutikaroga Hetu

मिथ्योपचारात् सङ्क्लेशाद्विषमाजीर्णभोजनत् |
सूतिकायाश्च ये रोगा जायन्ते दारुणास्तु ते ||२||

Etiological factors of Sutikaroga

Improper management of puerperium i.e., woman indulging in unhealthy foods and activities soon after delivery, consumption of foods which would increase the doshas or mental strain, consumption of improper foods and drinks and uncooked foods (consumption of foods in the presence of indigestion) lead to the manifestation of many kinds of diseases in the woman in puerperium, which are dreadful (difficult to cure). These diseases are called as sutikaroga – puerperal diseases. (2)

Sutikaroga

ज्वरातीसारशोथाश्च शूलानाहबलक्षयाः |
तन्द्रारुचिप्रसेकाद्याः कफवातामयोद्भवाः ||३||

Puerperal disorders

Fever, diarrhoea, oedema, pain in the abdomen (colic) and flatulence (distension of the abdomen), debility, stupor, loss of taste / appetite, excessive salivation and other disorders caused by increase of kapha and vāta manifest in the puerperal period.

Prognosis

कृच्छ्रसाध्या हि ते रोगाः क्षीणमांसबलाग्नितः |
ते सर्वे सूतिकानाम्ना रोगास्ते चाप्युपद्रवाः ||४||

The above-mentioned diseases become difficult to treat in those who have weak muscles, strength and digestive strength (activity). These diseases are called sutika rogas – puerperal diseases. There may also occur many complications of these diseases. These diseases will also be called by the name sutikarogas. (2-7)

इति श्रीमाधवकरविरचिते माधवनिदाने सूतिकारोगनिदानं समाप्तम् ||६५||

Thus ends the chapter on Sutikaroga Nidanam in Madhava Nidana text written by Acharya Madhavakara.

66

Madhava Nidana Chapter 66 Stanaroga Nidanam

Stana Roga Samprapti

सक्षीरौ वाऽप्यदुग्धौ वा प्राप्य दोषः स्तनौ स्त्रियाः |
प्रदूष्य मांसरुधिरं स्तनरोगाय कल्पते ||१||

Pathogenesis of diseases of the breast

The doshas which have undergone abnormal increase (vitiation) get localized in the breasts filled with milk (during the period of lactation) or without milk (other than lactation period – when mother is not feeding the child), contaminate the muscles and blood therein and produce many diseases of the breasts. (1)

Stanaroga Bheda, Lakshana

पञ्चानामपि तेषां हि रक्तजं विद्रधिं विना |
लक्षणानि समानानि बाह्यविद्रधिलक्षणैः ||२||

Types and symptoms of breast diseases

The five kinds of diseases of the breasts (produced by the increase of vata, pitta, kapha and all the three doshas together and that caused due to external agents) will have similar symptoms as those of five types of bahya vidradhi i.e. abscesses occurring outside (on the exterior) the body i.e. the symptoms of vataja, pittaja, kaphaja, sannipataja and agantuja vidradhi respectively, while excluding the raktaja vidradhi (abscess caused by the vitiated blood) i.e. there will be no raktaja stana roga as in raktaja vidradhi. (2)

इति श्रीमाधवकरविरचिते माधवनिदाने स्तनरोगनिदानं समाप्तम् ||६६||

Thus ends the chapter on Stana Roga Nidanam in Madhava Nidana text written by Acharya Madhavakara.

67

Madhava Nidana Chapter 67 Stanya dushti Nidanam

Similarities between discharge of sukra (semen) in men and stanya (breast milk) in women

विशंस्तेष्वपि गात्रेषु यथा शुक्रं न दृश्यते |
सर्वदेहाश्रितत्वाच्च शुक्रलक्षणमुच्यते ||१||
तदेव चेष्टयुवतेर्दर्शनात् स्मरणादपि |
शब्दसंश्रवणात् स्पर्शात् संहर्षाच्च प्रवर्तते ||२||
सुप्रसन्नं मनस्तत्र हर्षणे हेतुरुच्यते |
आहाररसयोनित्वादेवं स्तन्यमपि स्त्रियाः ||३||
तदेवापत्यसंस्पर्शाद्दर्शनात् स्मरणादपि |
ग्रहणाच्च शरीरस्य शुक्रवत् सम्प्रवर्तते |
स्नेहो निरन्तरस्तत्र प्रस्रवे हेतुरुच्यते ||४||

Just as sukra (semen, reproductive element of the male) though (described as) present all over the body cannot be seen even if any part of the body is cut open but comes out of the body on its own (ejaculated) by the sight, remembrance, hearing or excitement caused due to touch of the beloved woman. Sheer pleasantness (pleasure) of the mind is the cause for sexual excitation (and consequent discharge of semen).

Similar is the case with stanya (breast milk). Since stanya is the product of (produced by) the food that we consume (ahara rasa – essence or juice of the digested food) it is also (like sukra – semen) spread out all through the body. This breast milk will also flow freely out of the breasts by the touch, sight, and remembrance and fondling of the baby, just like the semen (as explained above).

The cause of continuous lactation (flow of breast milk) is the love of the mother towards her child. (3-4)

Stanya Dushti Hetu

गुरुभिर्विविधैरन्नैर्दुष्टैर्दोषैः प्रदूषितम् |
क्षीरं मातुः कुमारस्य नानारोगाय कल्पते ||५||

Etiological factors for contamination of breast milk

The doshas which undergo vitiation due to indulgence in different kinds of heavy (to digest) foods and similar other types of foods contaminate the breast milk of the mother which eventually becomes the cause for manifestation of many diseases in the child (which would consume such contaminated milk). (5)

Dushta Stanya Lakshana

कषायं सलिलप्लावि स्तन्यं मारुतदूषितम् |
कट्वम्ललवणं पीतराजीमत् पित्तसञ्ज्ञितम् ||६||
कफदुष्टं घनं तोये निमज्जति सपिच्छलम् |
द्विलिङ्गं द्वन्द्वजं विद्यात् सर्वलिङ्गं त्रिदोषजम् ||७||

Symptoms of milk contaminated by the doshas

Vata Dusta Stanya – The breast milk vitiated by increased vata will be astringent in taste and float on the water.

Pitta Dusta Stanya – The breast milk vitiated by increased pitta will be pungent, sour or salty in taste and appears with yellowish threads (milk appears to have yellow thread like suspensions). **Kapha Dusta Stanya** – The breast milk vitiated by increased kapha is thick, sinks in water and is sticky.

Dwidosha and Tridosha Dusta Stanya – The breast milk vitiated by two or all three doshas which have simultaneously undergone vitiation will produce symptoms of two or three doshas together respectively. (6-7)

Shuddha Dugdha Swarupa

अदुष्टं चाम्बुनिक्षिप्तमेकीभवति पाण्डुरम् |
मधुरं चाविवर्णं च प्रसन्नं तत् प्रशस्यते ||८||

Features of normal / pure (not contaminated by doshas) breast milk

Breast milk is said to be normal or pure (not contaminated with doshas) when it is found to mix evenly with water when put into water, is pale / slightly yellowish white in colour, is sweet in taste, doesn't have abnormal colours and is clear. (8)

इति श्रीमाधवकरविरचिते माधवनिदाने स्तन्यदुष्टिनिदानं समाप्तम् ||६७||

Thus ends the chapter called 'Stanya Dusti Nidana' in the book Madhava Nidana, written by Acharya Madhavakara.

68

Madhava Nidana Chapter 68 Bala Roga Nidanam

Balarogas caused by milk vitiated by Vata

वातदुष्टं शिशुः स्तन्यं पिबन् वातगदातुरः |
क्षामस्वरः कृशाङ्गः स्याद्बद्धविण्मूत्रमारुतः ||१||

When the child drinks milk which is vitiated by increased vata (in the lactating mother) it will become afflicted with diseases of vata origin. As a result, the child's voice becomes feeble and the child gets emaciated. The faeces, urine and flatus will not get eliminated. (1)

Balarogas caused by milk vitiated by Pitta

स्विन्नो भिन्नमलो बालः कामलापित्तरोगवान् |
तृष्णालुरुष्णसर्वाङ्गः पित्तदुष्टं पयः पिबन् ||२||

Drinking milk which is vitiated by pitta will make the child get afflicted with excessive sweating, diarrhea, jaundice or other diseases of pitta origin. The child will suffer from severe thirst and the body will become extremely hot (increased body temperature). (2)

Balarogas caused by milk vitiated by Kapha

कफदुष्टं पिबन् क्षीरं लालालुः श्लेष्मरोगवान् |
निद्रान्वितो जडः शूनवक्त्राक्षश्छर्दनः शिशुः ||३||

Drinking milk which is vitiated by increased kapha, will cause excessive salivation in the child. The child would be afflicted by many diseases of kapha origin. Apart from this excessive sleep, inactiveness, swelling of the face and eyes and vomiting are also present. (3)

Balarogas caused by simultaneous vitiation of milk by two or three doshas together

द्वन्द्वजे द्वन्द्वजं रूपं सर्वजे सर्वलक्षणम् |४|

Milk vitiated by the increase of two doshas would produce symptoms of two doshas together and the milk vitiated by the increase of all three doshas together would produce symptoms of all three doshas together.

Antargata Vedana Jnana Upaya

शिशोस्तीव्रामतीव्रां च रोदनाल्लक्षयेद्रुजम् ||४||
स यं स्पृशेद्भृशं देशं यत्र च स्पर्शनाक्षमः |
तत्र विद्याद्रुजं मूर्ध्नि रुजं चाक्षिनिमीलनात् ||५||
हृदि जिह्वौष्ठदशनश्वासमुष्टिनिपीडनैः |
कोष्ठे विबन्धवमथुस्तनदंशान्त्रकूजनैः |
आध्मानपृष्ठनमनजठरोन्नमनैरपि ||६||
बस्तौ गुह्ये च विण्मूत्रसङ्गत्रासदिगीक्षणैः |
स्रोतांस्यङ्गानि सन्धींश्च पश्येद्यत्नान्मुहुर्मुहुः ||७||

Methods of knowing (diagnosing) different types of pains in the child

Recognizing the nature and intensity of pain - The nature of pain (or discomfort) in the child i.e., whether the pain is severe or less severe shall be recognized by the nature of crying, i.e., if the child is crying loudly, it indicates that the pain is severe and if the child is crying mildly it means to tell that the intensity of the pain is less severe.

Knowing the seat of pain - The part of the body which the child touches by its hands repeatedly or the part of the body which the child does not allow anyone to touch shall be recognized as the painful part (part affected by the disease).

Recognizing Headache or other diseases of the head – When the child keeps his eyes closed, it should be understood that the child is suffering from headache.

Recognizing pain or diseases of the abdomen – It should be inferred (understood) that the child is suffering from pain (or diseases) in the abdomen when the child has constipation, vomiting, biting of breast (of mother), gurgling noises in the intestines, distension of abdomen, bending

(backward or forward) of back or abdomen.
Recognizing pain or diseases of urinary bladder and genitals / groins – Obstruction to the passage of faeces and urine, fear and unsteady vision (seeing in either directions and getting scared / terrified) indicate pain or disease in urinary bladder / genitals in children.
This is the reason that the physician should carefully observe the channels (orifices), body parts, joints and other places of the body of the child frequently. (4-7)

Kukunaka

कुकूणकः क्षीरदोषाच्छिशूनामेव वर्त्मनि |
जायते तेन तन्नेत्रं कण्डूरं च स्रवेन्मुहुः ||८||
शिशुः कुर्याल्ललाटाक्षिकूटनासावघर्षणम् |
शक्तो नार्कप्रभां द्रष्टुं न वर्त्मोन्मीलनक्षमः ||९||

Kukūṇaka is a disease which occurs in the eyelids of the children. It is caused due to the effect of the child (infant) drinking the vitiated breast milk.
In this condition there will be itching and repeated discharges (exudates) from the eye / eyes. The child will repeatedly rub its forehead, region around the eye (orbit) and nose. The child will be incapable of seeing the sunlight and also in making movements of the eyelids (opening, closing). (8-9)

Parigarbhika

मातुः कुमारो गर्भिण्याः स्तन्यं प्रायः पिबन्नपि |
कासाग्निसादवमथुतन्द्राकार्श्यारुचिभ्रमैः ||१०||
युज्यते कोष्ठवृद्ध्या च तमाहुः पारिगर्भिकम् |
रोगं परिभवाख्यं च युञ्ज्यात्तत्राग्निदीपनम् ||११||

Children drinking milk of the pregnant mother (i.e., mother of the child whom she is feeding, who has concurrently become pregnant) will develop cough, loss of digestion capacity (poor digestive capacity), vomiting, stupor, emaciation, loss of taste / appetite, giddiness and enlargement of abdomen. This disease is known by the name Parigarbhika or Paribhava. This condition shall be treated with herbs / medicines which increases digestion (power of digestion). (10-11)

Talukantaka

तालुमांसे कफः क्रुद्धः कुरुते तालुकण्टकम् |
तेन तालुप्रदेशस्य निम्नता मूर्ध्नि जायते ||१२||
तालुपातः स्तनद्वेषः कृच्छ्रात् पानं शकृद्द्रवम् |
तृडक्षिकण्ठास्यरुजा ग्रीवादुर्धरता वमिः ||१३||

Kapha undergoing increase in the muscles of the palate of the child produces a disease known as Talukaṇṭaka. In this condition, a depression appears in the upper part of the palate. The palate hangs down; the child will have aversion towards breasts and the child drinks breast milk with difficulty. The child will also have watery stools (diarrhoea), thirst, pain in the eyes, throat (neck) and mouth, instability of neck (inability to hold the neck / head upright) and vomiting. (12-13)

Mahapadma

विसर्पस्तु शिशोः प्राणनाशनो बस्तिशीर्षजः |
पद्मवर्णो महापद्मनामा दोषत्रयोद्भवः ||१४||
शङ्खाभ्यां हृदयं याति हृदयाद्वा गुदं व्रजेत् |१५|

Visarpa (erysipelas) developing in the urinary bladder and on the head in children is dreadful and life threatening. This condition caused by all the three doshas increased together will be red in colour resembling that of petals of red coloured lotus flower and hence called by the name Mahapadma. This disease may spread from temples to the region of the heart (chest) or from the chest to the anal / rectal region. (14)

Ajagallika, Ahiputana

क्षुद्ररोगे च कथिते त्वजगल्ल्यहिपूतने ||१५||

The two diseases Ajagallika and Ahipūtana which have been described under ksudrarogas will also occur commonly in children. (15)

Jwara (fever) & other diseases occurring in children

ज्वराद्या व्याधयः सर्वे महतां ये पुरेरिताः |
बालदेहेऽपि ते तद्वद्विज्ञेयाः कुशलैः सदा ||१६||

Jwara (fever) and all other major diseases which are explained earlier (which manifest in adults) will also affect the children. They should be recognized by the learned physicians in the same way (as they would recognize and diagnose them in adults) by their specific symptoms. (16)

Grahajusta Laksanas

क्षणादुद्विजते बालः क्षणात्त्रस्यति रोदिति |
नखैर्दन्तैर्दारयति धात्रीमात्मानमेव वा ||१७||
ऊर्ध्वं निरीक्षते दन्तान् खादेत् कूजति जृम्भते |
भ्रुवौ क्षिपति दन्तौष्ठं फेनं वमति चासकृत् ||१८||
क्षामोऽति निशि जागर्ति शूनाक्षो भिन्नविट्स्वरः |
मांसशोणितगन्धिश्च न चाश्नाति यथा पुरा ||१९||
सामान्यं ग्रहजुष्टानां लक्षणं समुदाहृतम् |२०|

Symptoms of child affected by grahas (spirits)

(When the child is affected by grahas – spirits) the child suddenly becomes agitated (perturbed, frightened, terrified, irritable), frightened and begins to cry without any apparent cause. The child scratches / injures self and also the wet-nurse (mother) by his nails and teeth, would stare upwards, bites/ grinds his own teeth, moans / makes indistinct sounds of helplessness and yawns frequently. He moves (throws, scatters) the brows (frown), teeth and lips here and there, vomits froth frequently. The child becomes excessively emaciated, does not sleep at night, has swelling around his eyes, diarrhoea and broken voice. The child's body emits the smell of flesh and blood and he would not take the food like before.

These are the general symptoms seen when the child is possessed by the Grahas i.e., evil spirits. (17-19)

Symptoms of child possessed by Skandagraha

एकनेत्रस्य गात्रस्य स्रावः स्पन्दनकम्पनम् ||२०||
ऊर्ध्वं दृष्ट्या निरीक्षेत वक्रास्यो रक्तगन्धिकः |
दन्तान् खादति वित्रस्तः स्तन्यं नैवाभिनन्दति ||२१||
स्कन्दग्रहगृहीतानां रोदनं चाल्पमेव च |२२|

Below mentioned are the symptoms of child possessed by Skandagraha –
Tearing from one eye (left or right eye)
Excessive sweating from one side (half) of the body
Pulsations / shivering in one side of the body
Convulsions / tremors on one side of the body
Gaze of the child is fixed upwards
Deviation of one side of the face
Smell of blood emitted from the face / skin
Biting / grinding of the teeth
Fretfulness
Does not like (relish) drinking breast milk

Crying less (crying mildly) (20-21)

Symptoms of child possessed by Skandapasmara

नष्टसञ्ज्ञो वमेत् फेनं सञ्ज्ञावानतिरोदिति ।
पूयशोणितगन्धित्वं स्कन्दापस्मारलक्षणम् ॥२२॥

Below mentioned are the symptoms of child possessed by Skandapasmara –
Fainting along with frothy vomiting
Too much crying after gaining consciousness
Smell of pus and blood emitted from the body of the child (22)

Symptoms of child possessed by Sakunigraha

स्रस्ताङ्गो भयचकितो विहङ्गगन्धिः सास्रावव्रणपरिपीडितः समन्तात् ।
स्फोटैश्च प्रचिततनुः सदाहपाकैर्विज्ञेयो भवति शिशुः क्षतः शकुन्या ॥२३॥
(सु. उ. तं. अ. २७) ।

Below mentioned are the symptoms of child possessed by Sakunigraha –
Drooping of the limbs / body parts
Fretfulness
Alarmed / shocked
Smell resembling that of the aquatic birds emitted from the body of the child,
Many ulcers / papules along with discharges spread out all over the body
Many blisters spread out all over the body along with burning sensation and suppuration (23)

Symptoms of child possessed by Revatigraha

व्रणैः स्फोटैश्चितं गात्रं पङ्कगन्धं स्रवेदसृक् ।
भिन्नवर्चा ज्वरी दाही रेवतीग्रहलक्षणम् ॥२४॥

Below mentioned are the symptoms of child possessed by Revatigraha –
Ulcers and boils spread out all through the body
Blood having the smell of silt is discharged from the ulcers
Watery stools (diarrhoea)
Fever
Burning sensation in the body (24)

Symptoms of child possessed by Putanagraha

अतीसारो ज्वरस्तृष्णा तिर्यक्प्रेक्षणरोदनम् ।
नष्टनिद्रस्तथोद्विग्नो ग्रस्तः पूतनया शिशुः ॥२५॥

Below mentioned are the symptoms of child possessed by Putanagraha –

- Diarrhoea
- Fever
- Thirst
- Looking side-wards
- Crying
- Loss of sleep
- Irritability (25)

Symptoms of child possessed by Andhaputana

छर्दिः कासो ज्वरस्तृष्णा वसागन्धोऽतिरोदनम् |
स्तन्यद्वेषोऽतिसारश्च अन्धपूतनया भवेत् ||२६||

Below mentioned are the symptoms of child possessed by Andhaputana graha –

- Vomiting
- Cough
- Fever
- Thirst
- Body emitting smell of muscle fat
- Excessive crying
- Aversion to breast milk
- Diarrhoea (26)

Symptoms of child possessed by Shitaputana

वेपते कासते क्षीणो नेत्ररोगो विगन्धिता |
छर्द्यतीसारयुक्तश्च शीतपूतनया शिशुः ||२७||

Below mentioned are the symptoms of child possessed by Shitaputana graha –

- Tremors / abnormal movements in the body parts
- Cough
- Emaciation
- Eye disorders

- Abnormal smell emitted from the body
- Vomiting
- Diarrhoea (27)

Symptoms of child possessed by Mukhamandika Graha

प्रसन्नवर्णवदनः सिराभिरभिसंवृतः |
मूत्रगन्धी च बह्वाशी मुखमण्डिकया भवेत् ||२८||

Below mentioned are the symptoms of child possessed by Mukhamandika graha –

- Pleasantness of body colour
- Pleasantness / brightness of the face,
- Presence of prominent veins all over the body
- Smell of urine emitted from the body
- Eating too much food (28)

Symptoms of child possessed by Naigamesa Graha

छर्दिस्प(स्य)न्दनकण्ठास्यशोषमूर्छाविगन्धिताः |
ऊर्ध्वं पश्येद्दशेद्दन्तान् नैगमेयग्रहं वदेत् ||२९||

Below mentioned are the symptoms of child possessed by Naigamesa graha –

- Vomiting,
- Visible pulsations
- Dryness of the throat and mouth
- Fainting
- Bad / foul smell emitted from the body
- Gaze fixed upwards
- Biting / grinding of teeth (29)

Prognosis of possession by evil spirits

प्रस्तब्धाक्षः स्तनद्वेषी मुह्यते चानिशं मुहुः |
तं बालमचिराद्धन्ति ग्रहः सम्पूर्णलक्षणः |
विपरीततमं साध्यं चिकित्सेदचिरार्दितम् ||३०||

The grahas (possession by evil spirits) will kill the child in quick time in the presence of the below mentioned symptoms (symptoms of bad prognosis) –

Loss of movements in the eyes (and other sense organs)
Aversion towards breast / breast milk
Frequent fainting
Appearance of all the symptoms of grahas (30)

इति श्रीमाधवकरविरचिते माधवनिदाने बालरोगनिदानं समाप्तम् ||६८||

Thus ends the chapter on BalaRoga Nidanam in Madhava Nidana text written by Acharya Madhavakara.

69

Madhava Nidana Chapter 69 Visha Roga Nidanam

Visha Bheda

स्थावरं जङ्गमं चैव द्विविधं विषमुच्यते |
मूलाद्यात्मकमाद्यं स्यात् परं सर्पादिसम्भवम् ||१||

Types of Poisons

Poisons are of two kinds - Sthavara Visha and Jangama Visha.

Poisons obtained from roots and other parts of the plants (leaves, flowers etc) are known as Sthavara Visa.

Poisons of animals like snakes are called Jangama Visa. (1)

General symptoms caused by the effect of Jangama Visha

निद्रां तन्द्रां क्लमं दाहमपाकं लोमहर्षणम् |
शोथं चैवातिसारं च जङ्गमं कुरुते विषम् ||२||
(च. चि. अ. २३) |३|

Sleep, stupor, exhaustion, burning sensation, indigestion, horripilations, swelling and diarrhoea are the general symptoms caused by (the effect of) Jangama Visha (animal poison).(2)

General symptoms caused by the effect of Sthavara Visha

स्थावरं च ज्वरं हिक्कां दन्तहर्षं गलग्रहम् |
फेनच्छर्द्यरुचिश्वासं मूर्छां च कुरुते भृशम् ||३||

(च. चि. अ. २३) |४|

The general symptoms caused (by the effect of) Sthavara Visha include - fever, hiccough, tingling sensation in the teeth (gums), catch / stiffness / choking in the throat, vomiting of froth, loss of taste (appetite), difficulty in breathing and fainting. (3)

Visha Datara

इङ्गितज्ञो मनुष्याणां वाक्चेष्टामुखवैकृतैः |
जानीयाद्विषदातारमेभिर्लिङ्गैश्च बुद्धिमान् ||४||
न ददात्युत्तरं पृष्टो विवक्षुर्मोहमेति च |
अपार्थं बहु सङ्कीर्णं भाषते चापि मूढवत् ||५||
हसत्यकस्मात् स्फोटयत्यङ्गुलीर्विलिखेन्महीम् |
वेपथुश्चास्य भवति त्रस्तश्चान्योन्यमीक्षते ||६||
विवर्णवक्त्रो ध्यामश्च नखैः किञ्चिच्छिनत्त्यपि |
आलभेतासनं दीनं करेण व शिरोरुहम् ||७||
वर्तते विपरीतं च विषदाता विचेतनः |
(सु. क. अ. १) |

Signs of person who is habituated to administer poisons to others

An intelligent person (physician) who can identify the signs and expressions of anyone should also find out the characteristic features of a Vishadata (person who is habituated to administer poisons to others) by his talks, actions and facial expressions and also with the help of below mentioned signs –

When asked about anything the person (who has poisoned) will either not reply or even if he tries to reply he fumbles or gets confused (scared), acts ignorant

Gives wrong replies, speaks too much or gives irrelevant replies (in an unclear way) just like a fool / idiot

Laughs suddenly without any reason

Cracks his knuckles (makes sounds from his fingers)

Scratches the ground (earth) with his toes / fingers

Keeps shivering, gets scared and looks at others (for help or support),

Face becomes discoloured and unclean (bad expressions)

Keeps cutting something or the other (grass etc) with his nails,

Takes seat (sits) with timidity and hesitation,

Repeatedly touches (pulls) the hairs on his head with his hands

Keeps changing his seat and position every now and then

Will not be in his senses (behaves in an unusual manner) (4-7)

General symptoms produced by poisons derived from roots etc.

उद्वेष्टनं मूलविषैः प्रलापो मोह एव च ||८||
जृम्भणं वेपनं श्वासो मोहः पत्रविषेण तु |
मुष्कशोथः फलविषैर्दाहोऽन्नद्वेष एव च ||९||
भवेत् पुष्पविषैश्छर्दिराध्मानं श्वास एव च |
त्वक्सारनिर्यासविषैरुपयुक्तैर्भवन्ति हि ||१०||
आस्यदौर्गन्ध्यपारुष्यशिरोरुक्कफसंस्रवाः |
फेनागमः क्षीरविषैर्विड्भेदो गुरुगात्रता ||११||
हृत्पीडनं धातुविषैर्मूर्छा दाहश्च तालुनि |
प्रायेण कालघातीनि विषाण्येतानि निर्दिशेत् ||१२||
(सु. क. अ. २) |

Mula Visha/ Poisonous roots – when consumed will produce pain all over the body as though hit by a stick, delirium and delusion.
Patra Visha/ Poisonous leaves – when consumed will produce excess yawning, tremors, difficulty in breathing and delusion.
Phala Visha/ Poisonous fruits – when consumed will cause swelling in the scrotum, burning sensation and aversion towards food.
Puspa Visha/ Poisonous flowers – when consumed will produce vomiting, distension of the abdomen and difficulty in breathing.
Twaksara & Niryasa Visha / Poisonous bark and resin (gum) – when consumed will produce foul smell in the mouth, roughness of the body, headache and discharge of kapha from mouth.
Ksira Visha / Poisonous latex – when consumed will cause frothy discharges from the mouth, diarrhoea and feeling of heaviness in the body.
Dhatu Visha / Poisonous minerals (ores) etc – when consumed will produce pain in the region of the heart (cardiac region), fainting / loss of consciousness and burning sensation in the palate.
Probably all the above kinds of poisons are considered to be kalaghatini i.e., would kill the person in due course of time. (8-12)

Digdahata Lakshana

सद्यःक्षतं पच्यते यस्य जन्तोः स्रवेद्रक्तं पच्यते चाप्यभीक्ष्णम् |
कृष्णीभूतं क्लिन्नमत्यर्थपूति क्षतान्मांसं शीर्यते चापि यस्य ||१३||
तृष्णा मूर्छा ज्वरदाहौ च यस्य दिग्धाहतं तं पुरुषं व्यवस्येत् |

लिङ्गान्येतान्येव कुर्यादमित्रैर्व्रणे विषं यस्य दत्तं प्रमादात् ||१४||
सपीतं गृहधूमाभं पुरीषं योऽतिसार्यते |
फेनमुद्वमते चापि विषपीतं तमादिशेत् ||१५||
(सु. क. अ. ३) |

Digdahata (wounds caused by poison smeared weapons) - The person in whom the fresh wound undergoes immediate suppuration, discharges plenty of blood and suppuration becomes progressive (occurs repeatedly), the wound becomes black in colour, has too much of discharge, is foul smelling and the muscles surrounding the wound fall off all by themselves (after getting decomposed) are the signs of wounds caused by weapons smeared with poison. The person will also suffer from thirst, fainting, fever and burning sensation.

Vishadigdha Lakshana

Vishadigdha (wounds poisoned by poison) – Sometimes when a person is not cautious, some enemies will poison their wounds (or even make the wounded person drink poison forcefully). Even in these conditions the signs and symptoms mentioned above (digdahata) will be found. This is called Visadigda.

Vishapita Lakshana

Vishapita (one who has drunk poison) – A person should be considered to have consumed (administered) poison when he repeatedly eliminates stools (diarrhoea) which are yellow in colour or a colour resembling soot of chimney (black), and has frothy vomiting. (13-15)

1.It is more appropriate to read 'Mukha' instead of Muska in this stanza.

Sarpa and Sarpavisha

वातपित्तकफात्मानो भोगिमण्डलिराजिलाः |
यथाक्रमं समाख्याता द्व्यन्तरा द्वन्द्वरूपिणः ||१६||

Snakes and snake poison

Bhogi - snakes with a hood, Mandala – snakes with patches and Rajila – snakes with stripes are predominant in vata, pitta and kapha doshas respectively (tend to vitiate these doshas respectively). The hybrid snakes will have mixed qualities of two or more doshas. (16)

Symptoms of bites of different kinds of snakes

दंशो भोगिकृतः कृष्णः सर्ववातविकारकृत् |
पीतो मण्डलिजः शोथो मृदुः पित्तविकारवान् ||१७||

राजिलोत्थो भवेद्दंशः स्थिरशोथश्च पिच्छिलः |
पाण्डुः स्निग्धोऽतिसान्द्रसृक् सर्वश्लेष्मविकारकृत् ||१८||

Bhogi Sarpa - The site of the bite by a hooded snake will become black. It causes all the symptoms (diseases) of vata increase.

Mandala Sarpa – The bite of the mandala snake (snake with patches) will become yellow in colour. The swelling which occurs is soft and it causes all the symptoms (diseases) of pitta to increase.

Rajila Sarpa – The site of the bite of rajila snake (striped snakes) will have an immobile (hard) swelling, is sticky, of yellowish white (pale) colour and discharges very thick blood. It causes all the symptoms (diseases) of kapha to increase. (17-18)

Prognosis of snake bite

अश्वत्थदेवायतनश्मशानवल्मीकसन्ध्यासु चतुष्पथेषु |
याम्ये च दष्टाः परिवर्जनीया ऋक्षे सिरामर्मसु ये च दष्टाः ||१९||
(सु. क. अ. ३) |

Snake bite happening in the below mentioned places should be rejected treatment (because they are incurable) –

- Near / Below Aswattha tree (Ficus religiosa)
- In a temple
- In a crematorium
- In / near an anthill
- In the evening time
- At crossroads
- In Bharani constellation
- If the bite is on veins and vital spots of the body (or vital spots of the body wherein there is predominance of veins) (19)

Effect of snake bite on life

दर्वीकराणां विषमाशुघाति सर्वाणि चोष्णे द्विगुणीभवन्ति |२०|
(सु. क. अ. ३) |

The poison of darvikara sarpa i.e., hooded snakes kill the person immediately (quickly). The effect of the other poisons becomes twice powerful in hot season (or when associated with heat – as in exposure to sunlight, fire, hot objects, fomentation etc). (20)

Other conditions in which the effect of poisons becomes powerful

अजीर्णपित्तातपपीडितेषु बालेषु वृद्धेषु बुभुक्षितेषु ||२०||
क्षीणक्षते मेहिनि कुष्ठयुक्ते रूक्षेऽबले गर्भवतीषु चापि |
(सु. क. अ. ३) |

Likewise, the effect of poison will become doubly powerful (incurable) in persons suffering from indigestion, those afflicted by diseases caused by increased pitta, and exposed to sun. It is also true in case of children, aged people, and those hungry and wounded / emaciated due to wounds, in those suffering from diabetes and skin diseases (leprosy), in those who have dryness of the body, malnourished (weak) and in pregnant women.

Other signs and symptoms of incurability of snake bite cases

शस्त्रक्षते यस्य न रक्तमेति राज्यो लताभिश्च न सम्भवन्ति ||२१||
शीताभिरद्भिश्च न रोमहर्षो विषाभिभूतं परिवर्जयेत्तम् |
जिह्मं मुखं यस्य च केशशातो नासावसादश्च सकण्ठभङ्गः ||२२||
कृष्णः सरक्तः श्वयथुश्च दंशे हन्वोः स्थिरत्वं च विवर्जनीयः |
वर्तिर्घना यस्य निरेति वक्त्राद्रक्तं स्रवेदूर्ध्वमधश्च यस्य ||२३||
दंष्ट्रानिपाताश्चतुरश्च यस्य तं चापि वैद्यः परिवर्जयेच्च |
उन्मत्तमत्यर्थमुपद्रुतं वा हीनस्वरं वाऽप्यथ वा विवर्णम् ||२४||
सारिष्टमत्यर्थमवेगिनं च ज्ञात्वा नरं कर्म न तत्र कुर्यात् |
(सु. क. अ. ३) |

If in a person who has been bitten by a snake – if bleeding does not occur in spite of a cut being made by a sharp instrument, if linear marks do not appear on the skin (at the site) even if beaten or tied with a creeper / rope, horripilations does not occur in spite of sprinkling with cold water (cannot bring the person back to consciousness by sprinkling cold water), he or she should be refused treatment (because they are incurable).

Irregularity / crookedness of the face, falling of hairs (or the person pulling off his hairs by himself), displacement / deformity of the nose, inability to hold the neck straight in position (hoarseness of voice), reddish black coloured swelling at the site of bite, and stiffness of the lower jaw (lockjaw) when seen in the patient who has been bitten by the snake should be rejected (because the presence of these symptoms indicates that the condition is incurable).

Similarly a person in whom thick wick-like saliva comes out of the mouth, bleeding occurs through both upper (nose, mouth etc) and lower (anal,

urethra etc) passages, and the physician attending such person not having expertise to remove poison (impression of four fangs are found at the site of bite) should also be refused treatment considering that it is incurable.
The person who after being bitten by snake has become insane (lost the mind balance), has many complications, feeble voice, and discolouration, who has developed signs of death and who does not have urges of the body (in whom the urges of defecation, urination etc are not manifested) should be rejected, the condition being incurable. (21-24)

Dushivisha

जीर्णं विषघ्नौषधिभिर्हतं वा दावाग्निवातातपशोषितं वा ||२५||
स्वभावतो वा गुणविप्रहीनं विषं हि दूषीविषतामुपैति |
(सु. क. अ. २) |

Dushivisha is a poison or poisonous substance which is very old, whose properties have been nullified as an effect of (after being mixed with) anti-poisonous drugs, which has been dried up by the forest fire, breeze and sunlight and by nature does not have powerful properties of poisons (having lesser properties in comparison to a strong poison). (25)

Properties of poor potency poisons

वीर्याल्पभावान्न निपातयेत्तत् कफान्वितं वर्षगणानुबन्धि ||२६||
तेनार्दितो भिन्नपुरीषवर्णो वैगन्ध्यवैरस्ययुतः पिपासी |
मूर्छां भ्रमं गद्गदवाग्वमिं च विचेष्टमानोऽरतिमाप्नुयाद्वा ||२७||
(सु. क. अ. २) |

Because of its poor potency and being associated with kapha (kapha dilutes the strong and intense properties of the poison), it does not kill the person (suddenly or even later). Such a poison remains inside the body for years without undergoing digestion. The person who is afflicted with such poison will have diarrhoea, discolouration, and bad smell from the body, bad smell from the mouth, thirst, fainting, giddiness, stammer, vomiting, unnatural body movements and restlessness. (26-27)

Symptoms of DushiVisha based on the place / organ in which it is located

आमाशयस्थे कफवातरोगी पक्वाशयस्थेऽनिलपित्तरोगी |
भवेत् समुद्ध्वस्तशिरोरुहाङ्गो विलूनपक्षस्तु यथा विहङ्गः ||२८||
(सु. क. अ. २) |

If Dushivisa is located in the stomach, diseases of kapha-vata origin get manifested. If DusVisha is located in the intestines, the person would become a patient of diseases of vata-pitta origin. Apart from this, due to the loss of hairs of the head and body, he appears like a bird whose wings have been cut off. (28)

Symptoms of dushivisha lodged in different tissues

स्थितं रसादिष्वथवा यथोक्तान् करोति धातुप्रभवान् विकारान् |
कोपं च शीतानिलदुर्दिनेषु यात्याशु पूर्वं शृणु तस्य रूपम् ||२९||
(सु. क. अ. २) |

If the dushiVisha is lodged in rasa and other tissues of the body, it produces the symptoms / diseases which are likely to develop in those tissues. The symptoms become severe and troublesome due to exposure to cold winds and on cloudy days. First make a note of its premonitory symptoms. (29)

Premonitory Symptoms of effect of DushiVishas

निद्रागुरुत्वं च विजृम्भणं च विश्लेषहर्षावथवाऽङ्गमर्दम् |
ततः करोत्यन्नमदाविपाकावरोचकं मण्डलकोठजन्म ||३०||
मांसक्षयं पादकरप्रशोथं मूर्छां तथा छर्दिमथातिसारम् |
दूषीविषं श्वासतृषाज्वरांश्च कुर्यात् प्रवृद्धिं जठरस्य चापि ||३१||
(सु. क. अ. २) |

Excessive sleep, feeling of heaviness of the body, yawning, looseness of the body parts, horripilations, and pains in the body parts (as if beaten), (later) feeling of intoxication after having meals, indigestion, loss of taste (tastelessness), manifestation of rashes and papules, depletion of muscles (emaciation), swelling of feet and hands, fainting, vomiting, loose motions (diarrhoea), dyspnoea (difficulty in breathing), thirst, fever and enlargement of abdomen – are the premonitory symptoms of effect of dushiVisha. (30-31)

Different diseases caused by DushiVisha

उन्मादमन्यज्जनयेत्तथाऽन्यदानाहमन्यत् क्षपयेच्च शुक्रम् |
गाद्गद्यमन्यज्जनयेच्च कुष्ठं तांस्तान् विकारांश्च बहुप्रकारान् ||३२||
(सु. क. अ. २) |

Some kinds of dushiVisha will produce insanity, some others would produce flatulence (enlargement of abdomen) and some other types would bring about loss of semen. Other types of dushivisa will cause stuttering / stammer and some others will cause skin disorders (leprosy) and many other kinds of diseases. (32)

Definition of Dushivisha

दूषितं देशकालान्नदिवास्वप्नैरभीक्ष्णशः |
यस्मात् सन्दूषयेद्धातून् तस्माद्दूषीविषं स्मृतम् ||३३||
साध्यमात्मवतः सद्यो याप्यं संवत्सरोत्थितम् |
दूषीविषमसाध्यं स्यात् क्षीणस्याहितसेविनः ||३४||
(सु. क. अ. २) |

Dushivisha is so called because it keeps vitiating the dhātus (tissues) often, being aggravated by the influence of deśa (habitat), kāla (season), anna (food) and divāsvapana (day sleep). Dusivisa of recent origin and present in those who have self-control (strong will) is curable. It becomes manageable after one year (can be cured but it keeps recurring when favourable conditions are available, hence needs monitoring throughout life). It is incurable in those who are emaciated (weak) and are habituated to getting indulged in unhealthy foods and life activities. (33-34)

Garavisha

Symptoms of persons affected by Garavisha

सौभाग्यार्थं स्त्रियः स्वेदं रजो नानाङ्गजान् मलान् |
शत्रुप्रयुक्तांश्च गरान् प्रयच्छन्त्यन्नमिश्रितान् ||३५||
तैः स्यात् पाण्डुः कृशोऽल्पाग्निर्गरश्चास्योपजायते |
मर्मप्रधमनाध्मानं हस्तयोः शोथलक्षणम् ||३६||
जठरं ग्रहणीदोषो यक्ष्मा गुल्मः क्षयो ज्वरः |
एवंविधस्य चान्यस्य व्याधेर्लिङ्गानि दर्शयेत् ||३७||

Women expecting wealth (or other benefits or to take someone under their control and influence) administer sweat, menstrual blood, excretions (waste products) produced by different body parts, or artificial poison provided by enemies mixed with food. Poisons administered in this form are called Garavisha (homicidal poison).

Effect of Garavisha (symptoms of impact of garavisha) – The person affected by garavisa becomes pale, emaciated, and would have poor digestion. These things will produce garavisha in the body of the person who has consumed them. The person will have pain in vital organs of the body, distension of the body, symptoms of swelling in their hands, abdominal disorders (abdomen enlargement), duodenal disorders, tuberculosis, abdominal tumour, emaciation (consumption), fever and symptoms of many such (allied) diseases. (35-37)

Lutavisha

यस्माल्लूनं तृणं प्राप्ता मुनेः प्रस्वेदबिन्दवः |
तस्माल्लूतास्तु भाष्यन्ते सङ्ख्यया ताश्च षोडश ||३८||
(सु. क. अ. ८) |

The droplets of sweat of the sage Vaşistha (who had become angry with Viswamitra at the abduction of Kamadhenu, the cow) which fell on the grass become converted into Lūtās (spiders). Lutas are of sixteen kinds. (38)

General Symptoms of Spider bite

दंशकोथः प्रवृत्तिः क्षतजस्य च |
ज्वरो दाहोऽतिसारश्च गदाः स्युश्च त्रिदोषजाः ||३९||
पिडका विविधाकारा मण्डलानि महान्ति च |
शोथा महान्तो मृदवो रक्ताः श्यावाश्चलास्तथा ||४०||
सामान्यं सर्वलूतानामेतद्दंशस्य लक्षणम् |
(सु. क. अ. ८) |४२|

When bitten by these spiders, putrefaction at the site of the bite occurs. Apart from this, there will be bleeding, fever, burning sensation, diarrhoea and other symptoms (diseases) caused by the increase of all the three doshas together. Papules of different kinds, big patches, profound soft swelling, red or black in colour and movable are formed. These are the general symptoms of spider bite. (39-40)

Symptoms of bite of Dushivisha type of spiders

दंशमध्ये तु यत् कृष्णं श्यावं वा जालकाचितम् ||४१||
ऊर्ध्वाकृति भृशं पाकं क्लेदशोथज्वरान्वितम् |
दूषीविषाभिर्लूताभिस्तद्दष्टमिति निर्दिशेत् ||४२||
(च. चि. अ. २३) |

Below mentioned are the features (symptoms) found in person bitten by dushivisha type of spiders (spiders having slow acting poisons) –
Blackish or blackish blue colour at the centre of the site of spider bite
Appearance of network (like structure) at the site of bite

Elevation of skin around the bite
Severe suppuration
Exudation
Swelling
Fever (41-42)

Symptoms of bite of sauvarnika etc spiders
शोथाः श्वेताः सिता रक्ताः पीता वा पिडका ज्वरः |
प्राणान्तिकाश्च जायन्ते श्वासहिक्काशिरोग्रहाः ||४३||
(च. चि. अ. २३) |
Bite of Sauvarnika etc eight types of spiders' cause swelling, along with papules which are white, red or yellow in colour, fever, dyspnoea (difficulty in breathing), hiccough and headache. The poisons of these types of spiders are said to be quick acting and fatal. (43)

Symptoms of Musika Dushivisha
आदंशाच्छोणितं पाण्डुमण्डलानि ज्वरोऽरुचिः |
लोमहर्षश्च दाहश्चाप्याखुदूषीविषार्दिते ||४४||
(च. चि. अ. २३) |
The symptoms of poisoning by musika (rat) visha include bleeding from the site of bite, appearance of white coloured patches, fever, loss of taste, horripilation and burning sensation. (44)

Symptoms of incurability of poisonous rat bite
मूर्छाङ्गशोथवैवर्ण्यक्लेदशब्दाश्रुतिज्वराः |
शिरोगुरुत्वं लालासृक्छर्दिश्चासाध्यमूषिकैः ||४५||
(च. चि. अ. २३) |
The symptoms of incurability when bitten by a poisonous rat include – fainting, swelling of body parts, discolouration, wetness / moistness of the body, deafness, fever, heaviness of the head, excessive salivation and blood vomiting. (45)

Symptoms of Krkalasa Damsa (bite by chameleon)
कार्ष्ण्यं श्यावत्वमथवा नानावर्णत्वमेव वा |
मोहोऽथ वर्चसो भेदो दष्टे स्यात् कृकलासकैः ||४६||
(च. चि. अ. २३) |
The symptoms caused by bite of chameleon include blackish or blackish

blue discolouration or appearance of different colours on the skin (site of bite), delusion and diarrhoea. (46)

Symptoms of Vrscika damsa - Scorpion sting

दहत्यग्निरिवादौ च भिनत्तीवोर्ध्वमाशु च |
वृश्चिकस्य विषं याति दंशे पश्चात्तु तिष्ठति ||४७||
दष्टोऽसाध्यश्च हृद्घ्राणरसनोपहतो नरः |
मांसैः पतद्भिरत्यर्थं वेदनार्तो जहात्यसून् ||४८||
(च. चि. अ. २३) |

The symptoms of scorpion sting include – Immediately after the sting by scorpion the person would experience a severe burning sensation as if burnt by fire and splitting pain at the site of sting. Following this the poison quickly ascends upwards and later once again becomes limited to (settled in) the site of sting.

If the scorpion sting has caused destruction of (diseases of) heart, loss of functions of nose and tongue, it should be considered as an incurable condition. Similarly, if the muscles (after undergoing putrefaction) around the site of scorpion sting falls off and if the person suffers from severe pain, the person will die soon. (47-48)

Symptoms of Kanabha Dasta – wasp sting

विसर्पः श्वयथुः शूलं ज्वरश्छर्दिरथापि च |
लक्षणं कणभैर्दष्टे दंशश्चैवावसीदति ||४९||
(च. चि. अ. २३) |

Erysipelas (or ulcer spreading from one place to the other), swelling, pain, fever and vomiting are the symptoms found in a person stung by a wasp. Apart from this, the surroundings (muscles etc) of the sting would fall off. (49)

Symptoms of Ucchitinga Damsa – bite by poisonous crab

हृष्टलोमोच्चिटिङ्गेन स्तब्धलिङ्गो भृशार्तिमान् |
दष्टः शीतोदकेनेव सिक्तान्यङ्गानि मन्यते ||५०||
(च. चि. अ. २३) |

Horripilations, stiffness (sustained erection) of penis, and severe pain are the symptoms found in a person bitten by ucchitinga (poisonous crab, variety of scorpion). (50)

Symptoms of bite by Poisonous frogs, fishes and leeches

एकदंष्ट्रार्दितः शूनः सरुजः पीतकः सतृट् |
छर्दिर्निद्रा च सविषैर्मण्डूकैर्दष्टलक्षणम् ||५१||
मत्स्यास्तु सविषाः कुर्युर्दाहं शोथं रुजं तथा |
कण्डूं शोथं ज्वरं मूर्छां सविषास्तु जलौकसः ||५२||
(च. चि. अ. २३) |

Bite by poisonous frogs – causes symptoms including swelling, pain and yellow discolouration at the site of bite, thirst, vomiting and excessive sleep.
Bite by poisonous fish – causes symptoms including burning sensation, swelling and pain.
Bite by poisonous leeches – causes symptoms including itching, swelling, and fever and fainting. (51-52)

Symptoms of bite by house lizard, centipede, mosquitoes, bees

विदाहं श्वयथुं तोदं स्वेदं च गृहगोधिका |५३| (च. चि. अ. २३) |
दंशे स्वेदं रुजं दाहं कुर्याच्छतपदीविषम् ||५३|| (च. चि. अ. २३) |
कण्डूमान् मशकैरीषच्छोथः स्मान्मन्दवेदनः |
असाध्यकीटसदृशमसाध्यं मशकक्षतम् ||५४|| (च. चि. अ. २३) |
सद्यःप्रस्राविणी श्यावा दाहमूर्छाज्वरान्विता |
पिडका मक्षिकादंशे तासां तु स्थगिकाऽसुहृत् ||५५||
(च. चि. अ. २३) |

Bite by house lizard - will cause severe burning sensation, swelling, pricking pain and perspiration.
Bite by the centipede - will cause excessive sweating, pain and burning sensation.
Bite by ordinary mosquitoes - will cause itching, slight swelling and mild pain. Bite of poisonous mosquitoes will be incurable just like the bit of poisonous insects.
Sting by bee – will produce immediate discharge (of blood), blackish discolouration, burning sensation, fainting, fever and papules. Among all the bees, the sting of sthagika variety of bee will be fatal. (53-55)

Symptoms of bite by animals of four or two legs

चतुष्पद्भिर्द्विपद्भिश्च नखदन्तविषं च यत् |
शूयते पच्यते वाऽपि स्रवति ज्वरयत्यपि ||५६||

Assault by the claws and teeth of animals of four or two legs will cause swelling, suppuration (putrefaction), discharges (exudation) and fever. (56)

Symptoms of effect of poison in tiger etc wild animals

श्वशृगालतरक्ष्वृक्षव्याघ्रादीनां यदाऽनिलः |
श्लेष्मप्रदुष्टो मुष्णाति सञ्ज्ञां सञ्ज्ञावहाश्रितः ||५७||
तदा प्रस्रस्तलाङ्गूलहनुस्कन्धोऽतिलालवान् [१] |
अव्यक्तबधिरान्धश्च सोऽन्योन्यमभिधावति ||५८||
प्रमूढोऽन्यतमस्त्वेषां खादन् विपरिधावति |
तेनोन्मत्तेन दष्टस्य दंष्ट्रिणा सविषेण तु ||५९||
सुप्तता जायते दंशे कृष्णं चातिस्रवत्यसृक् |
दिग्धविद्धस्य लिङ्गेन प्रायशश्चोपलक्षितः ||६०||
येन चापि भवेद्दष्टस्तस्य चेष्टां रुतं नरः |
बहुशः प्रतिकुर्वाणः क्रियाहीनो विपश्यति ||६१||
दंष्ट्रिणा येन दष्टश्च तद्रूपं यस्तु पश्यति |
अप्सु चादर्शबिम्बे वा तस्य तद्रिष्टमादिशेत् ||६२||
त्रस्यत्यकस्माद्योऽभीक्ष्णं दृष्ट्वा स्पृष्ट्वाऽपि वा जलम् |
जलत्रासं तु तं विद्याद्रिष्टं तदपि कीर्तितम् ||६३||

In animals like dogs, fox, hyena, bear, tiger etc, when Vata is vitiated by increased kapha attacks and destroys the nervous system, the consciousness (intelligence) of these animals get hampered and they become rabid. In such animals the tail, lower jaw and shoulders will drop down, saliva starts dribbling from their mouth in large quantities. The animals appear blind and deaf to a certain extent and run towards each other. Among these the one which has gone excessively mad will run amuck everywhere and run to bite the others. If bitten by such rabid animals there will be loss of sensation at the site of bite, discharge of black coloured blood in excess (or there will be blackish discolouration at the site and severe bleeding). There will be symptoms of wounds caused by poisonous weapons.

The person who has been bitten by a rabid animal such as a dog etc will repeatedly keep imitating all the actions of that animal (whichever animal has bitten) and produces sounds (cries, shouts) similar to that animal. He will not be able to do any of his activities (becomes unconscious) and will face death. If one sees the image / reflection of the animal which has bitten him instead of his reflection in the water or mirror it shall be considered as a fatal sign. If the person bitten by a rabid animal becomes afraid of seeing or touching water it is known as Jalatrasa – hydrophobia. This is also a fatal sign. (57-63)

Another fatal sign

अदष्टो वा जलत्रासी न कथञ्चन सिद्ध्यति |
प्रसुप्तो वोत्थितो वाऽपि स्वस्थस्त्रस्तो न सिद्ध्यति ||६४||
(सु. क. अ. ७) |

In spite of not being bitten by a rabid animal, if a person develops fear towards water, the condition should be considered as incurable. Similarly, if a healthy person develops fear towards water while sleeping or after waking up (in woken state) the condition shall be considered to be incurable. (64)

Nirvisha Purusha Laksana

प्रशान्तदोषं प्रकृतिस्थधातुमन्नाभिकामं सममूत्रविट्कम् |
प्रसन्नवर्णेन्द्रियचित्तचेष्टं वैद्योऽवगच्छेदविषं मनुष्यम् ||६५||
(सु. क. अ. ६) |

Symptoms of person relieved from poison

Aggravation of doshas coming down (all the increased dosas getting back to normal), all the tissues coming back to normal state (become pure), developing desire for food, proper and timely elimination of urine and faeces, restoration of (becoming normal and pleasant) normal colour and complexion, functioning of the senses and mind and activities and behaviour – should be considered by the physician as the symptoms of the person completely relieved of poison. (65)

इति श्रीमाधवकरविरचिते माधवनिदाने विषनिदानं समाप्तम् ||६९||

Thus ends the chapter on Visharoga Nidanam in Madhava Nidana text written by Acharya Madhavakara.

70

Madhava Nidana Chapter 70 Anukramanika (Contents Of Treatise)

Contents of Rugviniscaya treatise

ज्वरोऽतिसारो ग्रहणी चार्शोऽजीर्णं विसूचिका |
अलसश्च विलम्बी च क्रिमिरुक्पाण्डुकामलाः ||१||
हलीमकं रक्तपित्तं राजयक्ष्मा उरःक्षतम् |
कासो हिक्का सह श्वासैः स्वरभेदस्त्वरोचकः ||२||
छर्दिस्तृष्णा च मूर्छाद्या रोगाः पानात्ययादयः |
दाहोन्मादावपस्मारः कथितोऽथानिलामयः ||३||
वातरक्तमूरुस्तम्भ आमवातोऽथ शूलरुक् |
पक्तिजं शूलमानाह उदावर्तोऽथ गुल्मरुक् ||४||
हृद्रोगो मूत्रकृच्छ्रं च मूत्राघातस्तथाऽश्मरी |
प्रमेहो मधुमेहश्च पिडकाश्च प्रमेहजाः ||५||
मेदस्तथोदरं शोथो वृद्धिश्च गलगण्डकः |
गण्डमालाऽपची ग्रन्थिरर्बुदः श्लीपदं तथा ||६||
विद्रधिर्व्रणशोथश्च द्वौ व्रणौ भग्ननाडिके |
भगन्दरोपदंशौ च शूकदोषस्त्वगामयः ||७||
शीतपित्तमुदर्दश्च कोठश्चैवाम्लपित्तकम् |
विसर्पश्च सविस्फोटः सरोमान्त्यो मसूरिकाः ||८||

क्षुद्रास्यकर्णनासाक्षिशिरःस्त्रीबालकामयाः |
विषं चेत्ययमुद्दिष्टो रुग्विनिश्चयसङ्ग्रहः ||९||

Jwara, Atisāra, Grahani, Arśas, Ajirna, Visucikā, Alaska, Vilambikā, Krimiroga, Pāndu, Kāmalā, Halimaka, Raktapitta, Rājayaksmā, Urahksata, Kāsa, Hikkā, Swāsa, Swarabheda, Arocaka, Chardi, Trsnā, Mürchā, etc., Pānātyaya, etc., Dāha, Unmāda, Apasmāra, Vātavyādhis, Vātarakta, Urustambha, Amavāta, Sula, PaktijaSūla, Anāha, Udāvarta, Gulmaroga, Hrdroga, Mutrakrchra, Mutrāghāta, Asmari, Prameha, Madhumeha, Prameha pidakās, Medoroga, Udararoga, Sotha, Vrddhi, Galaganda, Gandamālā, Apacī, Granthi, Arbuda, Slīpada, Vidradhi, Vranaśotha, Two kinds of Vranas, Bhagna, Nadivrana, Bhagandara, Upadamsa, Sukadosa, Twakrogas (kustha), Sītapitta, Udarda, Kotha, Amlapitta, Visarpa, Visphota, Romāntika, Masūrika, Ksudrarogas, Asyarogas (mukharoga), Karnarogas, Nasikarogas, Aksirogas (netra rogas), Sirorogas, Strīrogas, Balarogas and Visa rogas are the contents of the treatise Rugviniscaya. (1-9)

Efforts of Madhava in compiling the contents of rugviniscaya

सुभाषितं यत्र यदस्ति किञ्चित्तत् सर्वमेकीकृतमत्र यत्नात् |
विनिश्चये सर्वरुजां नराणां श्रीमाधववेनेन्दुकरात्मजेन ||१०||

The best descriptions regarding rugviniscaya (methods for diagnosis and understanding diseases) in human beings found in different places (texts) have been compiled here with great effort, by Sri Madhava, son of Indukara, for understanding of all diseases. (10)

यत् कृतं सुकृतं किञ्चित् कृत्वैवं रुग्विनिश्चयम् |
मुञ्चन्तु जन्तवस्तेन नित्यमातङ्कसन्ततिम् ||११||

Whatever good I have done by creating (writing) this treatise 'Rugviniscaya' with good intention, may all the living beings keep getting rid of chain of diseases permanently with its (Rugviniscaya treatise) help.

इति श्रीमाधवकरविरचितं माधवनिदानं समाप्तम् ||७०||

Thus ends RogaVinischaya of Madhavakara.

Easy Ayurveda Publications: Books

All our book publications are available at
www.EasyAyurveda.com/Books

English Books:
Charaka Samhita Volume 1,2,3 and 4 - English Translation
Ashtanga Hrudayam Sutrasthanam - English Translation
Living Easy With Ayurveda
Easy Ayurveda Home Remedies
Tridosha Made Easy
Ayurveda Tarka

Hindi Books:
Ayurved Samadhan

Kannada Books:
Sugama Jivanakkagi Ayurveda
Ayurveda Santvana

Malayalam Books
Ayurveda Asvasam
Jeevitha Soukhyathinu Ayurvedam
Lalithamaya Ayurveda Veettu Vaidyangal

All our book publications are available at:
www.EasyAyurveda.com/Books

Easy Ayurveda Video Classes And Courses

Every week we conduct weekly online classes on various Ayurveda topics.
This is attended by 400+ students from different parts of the world.
The classes videos, audiobook and notes are provided to the students.

Learn more about it here

EasyAyurveda.com/video-classes

Online Video Courses

Reverse Type2 Diabetes Naturally
Treat Chronic Heart Diseases with Ayurveda
Marma Therapy Course
Learn ECG in 7 days
Ayurvedic Herbology
Prakriti - Dosha Body Type
Ayurvedic Cooking
Ayurvedic Remedies

Buy them at EasyAyurveda.com/Books

www.ingramcontent.com/pod-product-compliance
Ingram Content Group UK Ltd.
Pitfield, Milton Keynes, MK11 3LW, UK
UKHW040556210726
13854UKWH00007B/995